Immunology

RAJ KHANNA

Formerly Professor
Department of Biochemistry
University of Lucknow

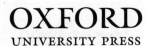

OXFORD

UNIVERSITY PRESS

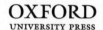

OXFORD
UNIVERSITY PRESS

YMCA Library Building, Jai Singh Road, New Delhi 110001

Oxford University Press is a department of the University of Oxford.
It furthers the University's objective of excellence in research, scholarship,
and education by publishing worldwide in

Oxford   New York
Auckland   Cape Town   Dar es Salaam   Hong Kong   Karachi
Kuala Lumpur   Madrid   Melbourne   Mexico City   Nairobi
New Delhi   Shanghai   Taipei   Toronto

With offices in
Argentina   Austria   Brazil   Chile   Czech Republic   France   Greece
Guatemala   Hungary   Italy   Japan   Poland   Portugal   Singapore
South Korea   Switzerland   Thailand   Turkey   Ukraine   Vietnam

Published in India
by Oxford University Press

ISBN-13: 978-0-19-806826-6
ISBN-10: 0-19-806826-3

Typeset in Baskerville
by Innovative Processors
Printed in India by Shri Krishna Printer, Noida, UP
and published by Oxford University Press
YMCA Library Building, Jai Singh Road, New Delhi 110001

This book is dedicated to the
fond memory of my dear father
Shri Harbans Lal

List of Icons

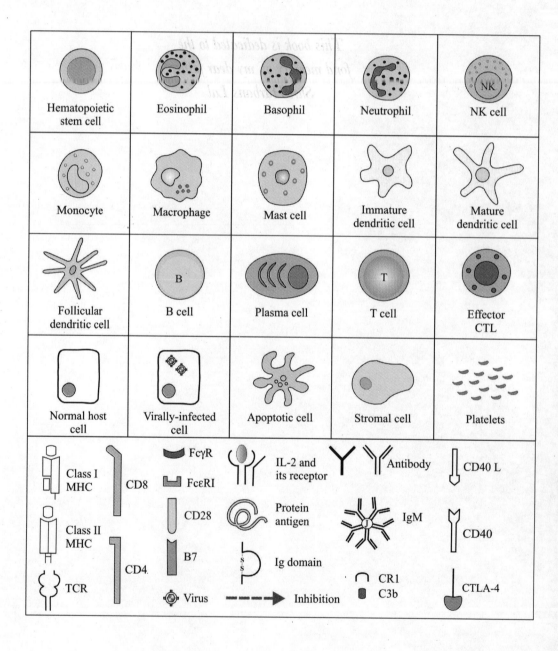

Foreword

The immune system is a complex network of cells which work continuously against attack from bacteria and other potentially life-threatening organisms that surround us in the environment. In effect, the immune system basically and literally protects/saves human lives from all possible threats from 'nonself'. This textbook of immunology has been written extremely well by Prof. Raj Khanna, who has been a dedicated faculty member and a popular teacher of biochemistry and immunology both for undergraduate and postgraduate students. Since the field of immunology is day by day becoming more and more specialized, there has been a need to have a textbook that covers all aspects of basic and applied knowledge that differentiates 'self' from 'nonself'. Based on the contents and topic areas covered, this book has done exactly that.

The approach and plan of chapters have been well thought of, wherein providing a brief introduction preceding the main text has set the background for each chapter. The inclusion of learning objectives at the start and summaries and review questions at the end provide uniqueness to this book. All along, the text is accompanied by numerous illustrations (many in colour) and this along with the simple and explanatory style of writing should appeal to students. According to me, the book has fulfilled its aim of providing readers with an easy and thorough understanding of the immune system and its functioning.

While going through the book, I observe that the first half of the book deals with basic immunology. The early chapters cover the following in a comprehensive manner:

+ Elements of the innate and adaptive immune system and its functioning
+ Toll-like receptors and their role in discriminating self from nonself and in initiation of adaptive immune responses
+ Structure of antibodies, how they recognize antigens, and how the vast antibody repertoire is generated
+ Organization of the MHC and the role of products that are encoded within it in T cell activation, and antigen processing and presentation

The above mentioned chapters have set the stage for an understanding of discussions in the later chapters on how the immune system responds to antigens:

+ Development of B and T lymphocytes and their differentiation to mature cells, their activation and central role in immune responses to protein antigens
+ Effector mechanisms of cell-mediated and humoral immunity including the complement system, which defend against different types of microbes

The last set of chapters deal with different areas of clinical importance and how the immune system at times fails to maintain good health. Some of the areas included are as follows:

+ Immune response to different types of infectious agents, diseases such as tuberculosis, malaria, SARS, and influenza

- Hypersensitivity diseases of which commonest is allergy
- Transplantation and graft rejection and its overall modulation
- Donor-specific tolerance currently under investigation
- Phenomenon of immunological tolerance and how it relates to autoimmune disease
- Immunodeficiency disorders, both congenital and secondary, with special emphasis on AIDS which is afflicting people worldwide
- Tumour immunology and cancer vaccines
- Manipulation of the immune system to fight disease by vaccination, immunotherapies based on cytokines and antibodies, and cell-based therapies

While adhering to the outline of most immunology courses and all the essentials in this subject area, the author has included certain descriptions which are currently under research investigations, namely mannose-binding lectin (MBL) activating complement and helping in clearance of apoptotic cells, pattern-recognition receptors of the innate immune system, cancer vaccines versus traditional vaccines, T regulatory cells, and donor-specific tolerance—a future perspective. Inclusion of these aspects shows the maturity and foresightedness of the author.

This textbook *Immunology* would be extremely useful and inspirational to students and researchers alike.

Lalit M. Srivastava
PhD, FAMS, FCBI, Dr B.C. Roy National Awardee
Professor, Senior Consultant, and Head
Department of Biochemistry, Sir Ganga Ram Hospital
Rajinder Nagar, New Delhi–110060

Formerly, Professor and Head
Department of Biochemistry
AIIMS, New Delhi

Preface

In the last few decades, immunology has developed very rapidly. It has contributed significantly to our understanding of the complexities of various infections and diseases. Advancement in research tools has facilitated better comprehension of the complex functioning of the immune system. Immunology has become a major branch of life sciences and is included in the curricula of undergraduate and postgraduate courses such as biotechnology, biochemistry, and microbiology.

Immunology is a study of the ways in which the immune system works to protect the body against infections. The subject also discusses the structural and biological features of various components that comprise the immune system. Although different organisms have different mechanisms of immunity, the basic functionality of the immune system remains more or less the same. Thus, a basic understanding of the important concepts of immunology is essential for a clearer view of the complex phenomena pertaining to the subject. This book would bring clarity to the basic concepts and will help to comprehend the subject in a better and easier way.

About the Book

This book is a textbook for undergraduate students of biotechnology, biochemistry, microbiology, and medical biochemistry. However, the scope of this book is not limited to that of an undergraduate coursebook and can be used as a reference book by postgraduate students as well.

This book provides a thorough treatment of all relevant topics in a student-friendly style, which will help the students grasp the concepts easily. Effort has been made to make the subject simple for students.

The book begins with an overview of the immune system accompanied by coloured illustrations. This will familiarize students with the immune system components and functioning and will make comprehension easier as they read through the text. The book then proceeds to an introduction of the immune system, covering all major aspects and giving an in-depth knowledge of various immune components and immunological processes.

A suitable number of figures and tables are given in each chapter to ensure a better understanding of the concepts involved. A list of the icons used in these figures has also been included right at the beginning of the book. The learning objectives at the beginning of every chapter define the scope of the chapter and the point-wise summary at the end will help the students in their last minute preparations for examinations. Most chapters include exhibits that provide additional information and some important and interesting facts. Multiple-choice questions are given at the end of each chapter, which will enable students to evaluate their understanding of the concepts grasped in the chapters.

Content and Organization

This book contains 18 chapters which provide a comprehensive treatment of the subject. There are two appendices at the end of the book.

Chapter 1 introduces the immune system. It gives an introduction to innate and adaptive immunity, humoral and cell-mediated immunity, components of the immune system, clonal selection of lymphocytes, and immune dysfunction and its consequences.

Chapter 2 deals with innate immunity in detail. It starts with the barriers and defences the body has against infection followed by the receptors involved in innate immunity. Inflammation and phagocytosis are also covered. The chapter ends with evasion of innate immunity by microbes.

Chapter 3 introduces the lymphoid system. Primary and secondary lymphoid organs are discussed. The chapter also includes lymphocytes and antigen-presenting cells, and ends with lymphocyte circulation.

Chapter 4 discusses antigens and antibodies. Immunoglobulin structure and its various types and sub-types are presented. The chapter also covers primary and secondary antibody responses, and polyclonal and monoclonal antibodies. It concludes with antigen–antibody interactions.

Chapter 5 discusses the major histocomaptibilty complex and its organization, the inheritance pattern of MHC genes, and class I and class II types of MHC molecules. Antigen processing and presentation pathways for protein antigens, and presentation of lipid antigens are included.

Chapter 6 focuses on antibody diversity including the germline organization of immunoglobulin genes, somatic hypermutation, class-switching, and the assembly and secretion of antibody molecules. The chapter also discusses B lymphocyte maturation and selection.

Chapter 7 discusses general concepts related to cytokines including their properties, functional classification, cytokine receptors and signal transduction, cytokine-associated pathophysiology, and therapeutic uses of cytokines and cytokine antagonists.

Chapter 8 is devoted to T lymphocytes. The topics discussed are T cell receptor complex, germline organization of TCR genes, generation of receptor diversity, and maturation and activation of T cells. Signal transduction in T cells and their differentiation are also included in this chapter.

Chapter 9 covers the effector mechanisms of cell-mediated immunity. Sequential events that occur in cell-mediated immunity are described. Also discussed are TH1 and TH2 cells and their balance and functionality. Effector functions of cytotoxic T lymphocytes are also covered.

Chapter 10 discusses B lymphocyte activation covering antigen receptor–co-receptor complex, thymus-dependent and thymus-independent antigens, signalling pathways, and regulation of B cell responses.

Chapter 11 deals with effector mechanisms of humoral immunity. It discusses antibody-mediated effector mechanisms and antibody function at mucosal and other sites. The chapter also discusses the complement system, microbial evasion of humoral immunity, and immunopathology.

Chapter 12 deals with the different types of immune responses mounted by the body against viruses, bacteria, fungi, and protozoa and worms. Immunopathology caused by infection and superantigens are also considered in this chapter.

Chapter 13 discusses vaccination and vaccine strategies. The topics included are the requirement and aims of a successful vaccine, types of vaccines, and adjuvants. Some newer approaches to antigen delivery are also discussed.

Chapter 14 focuses on hypersensitivity reactions. Different types of hypersensitivity reactions—Type I, Type II, Type III, and Type IV—and the immune components and mechanisms involved in the different types are discussed in detail.

Chapter 15 covers immunologic tolerance and autoimmunity. Topics presented are the mechanisms in induction of self-tolerance, autoimmunity, some common autoimmune diseases, treatment of autoimmune diseases, and some animal models.

Chapter 16 deals with immunodeficiency diseases, including primary and secondary immunodeficiency diseases, their treatment and animal models. The chapter also discusses the various aspects of HIV and AIDS in detail.

Chapter 17 discusses transplantation and graft rejection. Topics covered are types of grafts, transplantation antigens, graft rejection, and typing for RBC and MHC antigens. The chapter also discusses immunosuppressive drugs and different types of transplantation.

Chapter 18 focuses on tumour immunology, discussing immunogenicity of tumours, tumour antigens, immune responses to tumours, and how tumours evade these responses. The concluding part of the chapter covers approaches to cancer immunotherapy and cancer vaccines.

The book also contains two appendices. Appendix 1 comprises immunological techniques and their principles and applications. Appendix 2 presents a cumulative glossary covering the important terms used in the book.

Acknowledgements

Foremost, I owe special thanks and gratitude to my mother, my brother Ram, and all my family members for their loving and enduring support and encouragement during the writing of this book. I am deeply indebted to all of them.

I would like to express my sincere gratitude to my respected teachers, Late Prof. P.S. Krishnan (Founder Head of the Department of Biochemistry, University of Lucknow), and Prof. G.G. Sanwal (Former Head, Department of Biochemistry, University of Lucknow) for always having shown confidence in me and encouraging me. I also extend my thanks to all my colleagues at the Department of Biochemistry for their kind cooperation.

I would specially like to thank Dr L.M. Srivastava (Senior Consultant and Chairperson, Department of Biochemistry, Sir Ganga Ram Hospital, New Delhi) for providing valuable suggestions through his expertise in the subject. I would like to express my appreciation and gratitude to Dr Rajendra Prasad (Professsor, Jawaharlal Nehru University) for his constant encouragement. My sincere thanks are due to Dr Nibhriti Das (Professor, Department of Biochemistry, AIIMS) for her enthusiastic support and helpful suggestions, and to Dr D.N. Rao (Professor, Department of Biochemistry, AIIMS) for kindly providing photographs of patients with autoimmune disease.

I gratefully acknowledge my appreciation to the editorial team of Oxford University Press for patiently helping to bring the book to publication. My sincere thanks are due to them for their assistance and the cooperation that they have shown.

I would also like to thank Dr Kishore B. Challagundla, Department of Molecular Medical Genetics, Oregon Health & Science University , USA and Mr Gopal Joshi for helping with the literature survey, and Mr Mukul Tewari for technical assistance.

It is my students who have been my main motivation behind writing this book. I hope the book will be of value to all the students of immunology and will answer the questions that they generally have about the immune system. It would be rewarding for me if the book succeeds in creating amongst them an interest and fascination for this exciting field.

Raj Khanna

Contents

List of Abbreviations

Ab	antibody
ADCC	antibody-dependent cell-mediated cytotoxicity
ADEPT	antibody-directed enzyme prodrug therapy
AFP	α-fetoprotein
Ag	antigen
AICD	activation-induced cell death
AID	activation-induced cytidine deaminase
AIDS	acquired immunodeficiency syndrome
ANAs	anti-nuclear autoantibodies
APC	antigen-presenting cell
APP	acute-phase protein
AZT	3'-azido 3'-deoxythymidine
β_2m	β_2 (beta$_2$) microglobulin
BALT	bronchus-associated lymphoid tissue
BCR	B cell receptor
Btk	B cell-specific tyrosine kinase (or Bruton's tyrosine kinase)
C	complement
CALT	cutaneous-associated lymphoid tissue
CAM	cell adhesion molecule
CD	cluster of differentiation
CDR	complimentarity determining region
CEA	carcinoembryonic antigen
CLIP	class II-associated invariant chain peptide
CMI	cell-mediated immunity
CR1	complement receptor type1 (also CR2)
CRP	C-reactive protein
CTL/Tc	cytotoxic T lymphocyte/cytotoxic T cell
CTLA-4	cytotoxic T lymphocyte antigen-4
CTL-P	CTL-precursor
DC	dendritic cell
DTH	delayed-type hypersensitivity
EBV	Epstein–Barr virus
ECF-A	eosinophil chemotactic factor-A
ECP	eosinophil cationic protein
ELISA	enzyme-linked immunosorbent assay
Fab	fragment, antigen binding (monovalent)
F(ab')$_2$	fragment, antigen binding (divalent)
FACS	fluorescence-activated cell sorter
Fc	fragment, crystallizable
FCA	Freund's complete adjuvant
FcRn	neonatal Fc receptor
FcγR	Fc receptor for Fc fragment of IgG
FDC	follicular dendritic cell
FIA	Freund's incomplete adjuvant
FR	framework region
GALT	gut-associated lymphoid tissue
G-CSF	granulocyte-colony stimulating factor
GlyCAM-1	glycosylation-dependent cell adhesion molecule-1
GM-CSF	granulocyte monocyte-colony stimulating factor
GVHD	graft-versus-host disease
H-2	mouse major histocompatibility complex
HAART	highly active antiretroviral therapy
HAMA	human anti-mouse antibody
HBsAg	hepatitis B surface antigen
HEV	high endothelial venule
HIV	human immunodeficiency virus
HLA	human leukocyte antigen
HSC	haematopoietic stem cell
h-v-g	host-versus-graft
HVR	hypervariable region
ICAM-1	intercellular adhesion molecule-1
IDC	interdigitating dendritic cell
IEL	intraepithelial lymphocyte
IFN	interferon
Ig	immunoglobulin
IgG	immunoglobulin G (also IgM/IgA/IgE/IgD)
IL-1Ra	interleukin-1 receptor antagonist
IL-2	interleukin-2 (also IL-1, IL-4, etc.)
iNOS	inducible nitric oxide synthase
ISCOM	immunostimulating complex
ITAM	immunoreceptor tyrosine-based activation motif

ITIM	immunoreceptor tyrosine-based inhibition motif
IVIG	intravenous immune globulin
JAK	Janus kinase
Ka	association (affinity) constant (generally in Ag–Ab interactions)
kDa	kilo Daltons (unit of molecular mass)
LAK	lymphokine-activated killer cell
LFA-2	lymphocyte function antigen-2
LGL	large granular lymphocyte
LPS	lipopolysaccharide
LTB4	leukotriene B4
mAb	monoclonal antibody
MAC	membrane attack complex
MALT	mucosa-associated lymphoid tissue
MASP	MBL-associated serine protease
MBL	mannose-binding lectin
MBP	major basic protein (also myelin basic protein)
MCP	monocyte chemotactic protein
M-CSF	monocyte-colony stimulating factor
MHC	major histocompatibility complex
MIF	macrophage migration inhibition factor
MIP	macrophage inflammatory protein
MLR	mixed lymphocyte reaction
MPO	myeloperoxidase
MR	mannose receptor
NADP	nicotinamide adenine dinucleotide phosphate
NCF	neutrophil chemotactic factor
NF-AT	nuclear factor of activated T cells
NFκB	nuclear factor kappa B
NK	natural killer cell
NOD	non-obese diabetic mouse
(NZB × NZW) F_1 mouse	New Zealand black mouse × New Zealand white mouse F_1 hybrid
$(\cdot O_2^-)$	superoxide anion
PALS	periarteriolar lymphoid sheath
PAMP	pathogen-associated molecular pattern
PCD	programmed cell death
PCR	polymerase chain reaction
PDGF	platelet-derived growth factor
PGD_2	prostaglandin D_2
p-IgR	poly-Ig receptor

PLCγ	phospholipase Cγ
PMN	polymorphonuclear neutrophil
PPD	purified protein derivative
PRR	pattern-recognition receptor
PSGL-1	P-selectin glycoprotein ligand-1
RF	rheumatoid factor
RhD	Rhesus D
RIA	radioimmunoassay
ROI	reactive oxygen intermediate
RSS	recombination signal sequence
SARS	severe acute respiratory syndrome
SARS-CoV	SARS-associated corona virus
SCID	severe combined immunodeficiency
SDS–PAGE	sodium dodecyl sulfate–polyacrylamide gel electrophoresis
sIgA	secretory immunoglobulin A
SIV	simian immunodeficiency virus
SMAC	supramolecular activation cluster
STAT	signal transducer and activator of transcription
TAA	tumour-associated antigen
TAP	transporter associated with antigen processing
TCR	T cell receptor
TD	thymus-dependent (antigen)
TdT	terminal deoxyribonucleotidyl transferase
T_{DTH}	T cells of delayed-type hypersensitivity
TGF-β	transforming growth factor-β
T_H	T helper cell
TI	thymus-independent (antigen)
TIL	tumour-infiltrating lymphocyte
TLR	toll-like receptor
TNF	tumour necrosis factor
T_{reg}	T regulatory cell
TSA	tumour-specific antigen
VCAM-1	vascular cell adhesion molecule-1
V_H	variable part of Ig heavy chain
V_L	variable part of Ig light chain
VLA	very late antigen
WBC	white blood cell
X-L	X-linked
ZAP-70	zeta-associated protein of 70 kDa

An Overview of the Immune System

The functioning of the immune system is mysterious and complex. To facilitate understanding of the way the immune system recognizes and responds to antigens/microbes, various events that lead to activation of an immune response are summarized in the following sections (Figs 0.1 and 0.2). Although what is diagrammed and outlined in the following text is a broad guide, constant reading and referring to these while going through the chapters will help to clear questions and doubts that are bound to arise.

OVERVIEW 1—INNATE DEFENCE MECHANISMS

Epithelial barriers of the host represent the first line of defence against infection. If a pathogen breaches these barriers, an important question arises. How does the immune system sense that an infection has occurred? The innate immune system is made aware of an infection through *pattern-recognition receptors* (*PRRs*). These receptors of innate immunity recognize conserved microbial structures called *pathogen-associated molecular patterns* (*PAMPs*), which are only present in microbes and are lacking in our own cells. This is important as it helps to spare self-tissues from immune attack. Once the pathogen has been recognized, the innate immune system responds by bringing together various effector mechanisms which provide immediate defence. These include phagocytic cells (macrophages and neutrophils), complement proteins, acute-phase proteins, e.g., C-reactive proteins (CRP) and mannose-binding lectin (MBL), antibacterial peptides (defensins), besides other elements. The initial recognition event by PRRs is thus converted to an effector response. Some PRRs, e.g., mannose receptors, facilitate phagocytosis of the microbe, whereas others such as toll-like receptors (TLRs) are involved in signalling. Both events (recognition and effector response) release cytokines which promote development of an *inflammatory response,* an immediate defensive response to infection/injury in which blood cells and also proteins (e.g., acute-phase and complement proteins) leave blood vessels and enter tissues. Inflammatory mediators released (one source is the mast cell) have important roles in coordinating various events that trigger inflammation. Innate mechanisms can in many cases, on their own, rid the body of the foreign invader. But, if the pathogen persists, the presence of danger signals (PAMPs) is communicated to cells of adaptive immunity, namely T and B lymphocytes, and adaptive immune responses are activated. Signalling through TLRs is significant as it, along with cytokines of innate immunity, instructs development of the subsequent adaptive immune response.

OVERVIEW 2—ADAPTIVE IMMUNE RESPONSE

Immature dendritic cells (DCs), located at portals of pathogen/antigen entry, are efficient at capturing antigen after which they migrate to local lymph nodes—sites where adaptive immune responses are initiated (there are other sites also). Dendritic cells undergo maturational events on their journey,

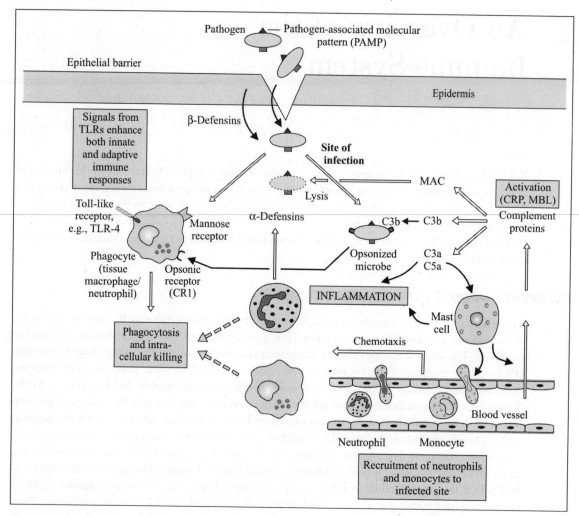

Fig. O.1   Innate immunity provides early defence against microbes. Some of the major elements of innate immunity including phagocytes, complement proteins, acute-phase proteins (CRP and MBL), and anti-microbial peptides (defensins) are shown here. C3a and C5a are complement breakdown products which induce degranulation in mast cells with release of inflammatory mediators. C3b, which is also a product of complement activation, coats microbes (opsonized microbes) and promotes phagocytosis.
Note: Natural killer (NK) cells, which recognize and kill cells harbouring viruses, and also some other elements of innate immunity are omitted.
MAC, membrane attack complex (a complex of complement proteins that induces microbial lysis); CRP, C-reactive protein; MBL, mannose-binding lectin (both CRP and MBL activate complement but pathways differ)

signals from toll-like receptors promoting the maturation process. Mature DCs which on their way to the lymph nodes have upregulated expression of costimulatory molecules and class II major histocompatibility complex (MHC) molecules are efficient antigen-presenting cells (APCs) devoid of phagocytic activity. They present antigenic peptide–MHC complexes to rare recirculating naïve T cells (cells not yet been exposed to antigens) which on encountering a specific peptide–MHC complex undergo clonal expansion and differentiation to effector T cells (T helper cells, Tн, and cytotoxic T lymphocytes, CTLs). The process is dependent on costimulatory signals provided by dendritic cells. Thus, an adaptive immune response is triggered. Effector T cells exit the lymph nodes via efferent

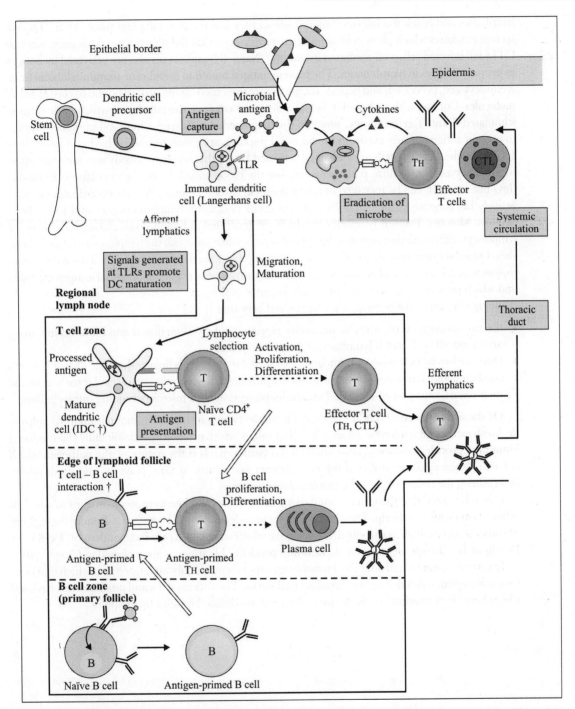

Fig. 0.2 Adaptive immunity—a specialized form of host defence. Shown here is the response to a microbial protein antigen which is dependent on T cell help. B cells are activated by the same antigen that has been recognized by T cells as a peptide—MHC complex on the DC surface.

Note: Germinal centre events (late events) which characterize humoral responses to protein antigens and which generate memory B cells are not depicted in the figure. Memory T cells are also not shown. IDC, interdigitating dendritic cell

† Mechanism of T helper cell-mediated activation of B cells is detailed in Chapter 10. Only signal 1 for T cell is shown here.

lymphatics and reach the infected/injured site as they can traverse inflamed tissue. Here, TH cells secrete cytokines which allow activation of macrophages to kill the phagocytosed microbe, whereas CTLs kill infected cells (cell-mediated immunity). Naïve B lymphocytes also are activated by antigen in primary follicles in lymph nodes. The protein antigen bound to membrane immunoglobulin (mIg) is endocytosed, processed, and peptide fragments are presented on the surface bound to class II MHC molecules. Contact with activated T helper cells at the edges of the follicles, to which both antigen-stimulated B and T cells migrate, provides the help needed to initiate a humoral immune response to protein antigens. Early events in the humoral response are characterized by IgM and low-affinity IgG antibodies. Plasma cells are end-stage activated B cells that secrete antibody into the circulation, where it serves to neutralize pathogens entering the bloodstream. From the circulation, antibodies (IgG but not IgM) can be recruited to infected sites in tissues. Plasma cells, however, do not circulate actively but migrate to the extrafollicular regions of peripheral lymphoid organs and to the bone marrow. Memory T and B lymphocytes which are generated in lymph nodes during the process of lymphocyte differentiation stay on in lymphoid organs, while some exit the lymph nodes for peripheral sites. On subsequent exposure to the same pathogen, they afford quick protection. This is the *memory response* which is more rapid and more intense than the response triggered on initial antigen exposure and which protects against re-infection with the same pathogen.

Being relevant to the context, it is emphasized here that

- the two broad arms of adaptive immunity represented by cell-mediated and humoral immunity are mediated by T and B lymphocytes, respectively; and
- there are two broad classes of pathogens (extracellular and intracellular) which the immune system combats in different ways—humoral immunity provides defence against extracellular pathogens and their toxins, whereas cell-mediated immunity protects against microbes residing intracellularly.

Of the two major subsets of T cells, the TH2 subset (which stimulates humoral immunity) helps to deal with extracellular microbes/toxins. The TH1 subset (which promotes predominantly cell-mediated immunity) provides defence against intracellular pathogens. It is the nature of the pathogen which determines the cytokine profile in the environment and which, in turn, plays an important role in determining the course of the adaptive immune response.

It is to be noted that the events summarized in Overview 2 relate to protein antigens to which B cells respond with T cell help. These are called thymus-dependent (TD) antigens. Besides these, there are other antigens, such as carbohydrate antigens, which stimulate B cells independent of T cell help. Details of B cell responses to these thymus-independent (TI) antigens are included in Chapter 10.

In summary, innate and adaptive immune responses form a highly integrated unit which functions to provide optimal defence against invading pathogens. The various steps and processes involved and which have been summarized in the preceding text are detailed in relevant chapters.

The Immune System
An Introduction

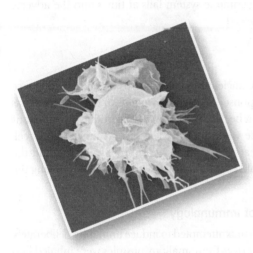

Immunity refers to the resistance of the body to infectious diseases. Various cells and molecules that have a role in protecting the body and in conferring resistance to infection, along with lymphoid organs/tissues, comprise the *immune system*. These elements work together to mount a response to the wide range of pathogens including viruses, bacteria, fungi, and parasites that are present in the environment, and also against foreign molecules such as toxins. This response is referred to as the *immune response*. Since pathogens are diverse, the immune system has evolved to cope with them in ways that provide optimal defence. Although protection against pathogens is the major function of the immune system, it protects against anything that poses a threat to survival, such as abnormal cells that multiply uncontrolled and lead to cancer. The immune system, therefore, is critical for survival but it may sometimes fail to function properly. Such failures of the immune system can have severe consequences on the host.

There are two types of immunity: innate immunity and adaptive immunity. Innate immunity is an ancient form of host defence present in both invertebrates and vertebrates. It provides the immediate first line of defence against infection. Adaptive immunity, however, evolved relatively late in evolutionary terms and is present only in vertebrates. The innate immune system presents various defensive barriers to pathogens and may on its own deal effectively with foreign invaders. But some pathogens succeed in evading innate defences. In such cases, the more specialized adaptive immune responses are called into play in which B and T lymphocytes play a pivotal role. These cells perform different functional roles and give rise to humoral and cell-mediated immunity, respectively. Both innate and adaptive immune systems are highly interdependent and interact with each other in various ways.

This opening chapter is a broad overview of the various defence systems of the body that protect against infectious diseases. The chapter also introduces some key concepts that will recur throughout the text. It highlights the major features of innate and adaptive immunity, and humoral and cell-mediated immunity. The various elements that comprise the immune system have also been introduced. These will be described in detail in later chapters. The origin of blood cells (haematopoiesis) and clonal selection of lymphocytes are discussed. The way the immune system fails at times and the adverse consequences that arise due to failure are briefly reviewed.

IMMUNOLOGY—A BRIEF HISTORY

The history of the science of immunology dates back to ancient Egyptian records which have reference to probably the earliest description of an immune response. An event analogous to inflammation has been used to describe the death of a pharaoh due to a bee sting. It is not very certain when humans first realized that they are better at fighting a disease when they get it a second time. The Greek historian, Thucydides, in 430 BC, described the great plague that swept through Athens and the way the survivors (including the historian himself) could care for the sick without fear of catching the disease on second contact.

Early Vaccination Attempts Marked as the Beginning of Immunology

It was in the fifteenth century that the Chinese and the Turks attempted to induce immunity deliberately to prevent smallpox caused by the variola virus. Dried crusts from smallpox pustules were inhaled into the nostrils or inserted into small cuts in the skin in order to prevent disease. This technique, called *variolation*, became quite common in the Middle East from where it was introduced to western countries

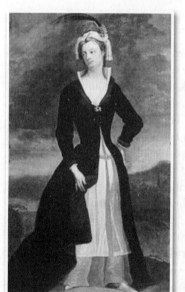

by Lady Mary Wortley Montagu (Fig. 1.1). Some early records indicate that the primary aim was to 'preserve' the beauty of the daughters of the royal families and no mention has been made about saving lives.

The origin of immunology as a science can be traced back to early vaccination studies and is usually linked to the English physician, Edward Jenner. He was puzzled by the observation that milkmaids who had contracted the mild disease, cowpox, caused by the vaccinia virus were later immune to smallpox , a severe disfiguring disease which leaves behind scars on the body (Fig. 1.2).

In the late eighteenth century, Jenner inoculated a young boy with pus from lesions of a dairy maid who had cowpox, and later deliberately exposed the boy to smallpox. This failed to cause the disease, which indicated that the initial inoculation with cowpox virus had a protective effect. The term *vaccination* (from the Latin word *vacca* meaning 'cow') was coined for the process described in the preceding text of inducing acquired

Fig. 1.1 Lady Mary Wortley Montagu. It was due to her efforts that variolation spread in the West. She herself had facial scars from the disease and had lost her brother due to smallpox.

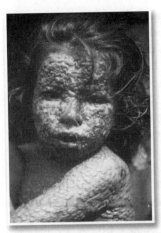

Fig. 1.2   A child with smallpox.

immunity. There was widespread acceptance of Jenner's method which, today, remains the most effective method for preventing infection. Smallpox was the first disease to be eradicated worldwide by a programme of vaccination, a significant achievement that was formally announced by World Health Organization (WHO) in 1980.

Induction of immunity to cholera by Louis Pasteur in 1879 was another major advance in immunology. Credit is due to him also for introducing the concept of *attenuation* (weakening of a pathogen), which led to the development of attenuated strains for use as vaccines. Louis Pasteur produced a vaccine for rabies, and it was in 1885 that he administered the first attenuated vaccine to a young boy who had been bitten several times by a rabid dog.

Early Studies on Mechanisms of Immunity

It was through Robert Koch in the late nineteenth century that it came to be known that infectious diseases are caused by pathogens (disease-causing organisms) of which four broad categories are recognized (Table 1.1).

Table 1.1   Major categories of human pathogens. Some examples of pathogens and the diseases caused by them are shown. Note that *C. albicans* infects individuals with immune deficiency.

Category	Pathogen	Disease
Viruses	Human immunodeficiency virus (HIV) Influenza virus Hepatitis B virus	Acquired immunodeficiency syndrome (AIDS) Influenza Hepatitis B
Bacteria	*Mycobacterium tuberculosis* *Clostridium tetani* *Bordetella pertussis*	Tuberculosis (TB) Tetanus Whooping cough
Fungi	*Candida albicans*	Candidiasis
Parasites ♦ Protozoa	*Plasmodium spp.* *Trypanosoma cruzi* *Leishmania spp.*	Malaria Trypanosomiasis Leishmaniasis
♦ Worms	*Schistosoma mansoni*	Schistosomiasis

It was in Koch's laboratory that von Behring and Kitasato, in the early 1890s, discovered tetanus and diphtheria toxin and made some interesting observations. They showed that transfer of serum from animals immune to tetanus and diphtheria to unimmunized animals conferred immunity. Thus, *passive immunization* was introduced. These experimental observations helped in understanding the mechanisms of immunity. The term *antibody* was later coined for the protective component that was present in serum.

In the late nineteenth century, studies by the Russian biologist Elie Metchnikoff (Fig. 1.3) led to the discovery of phagocytes, which are the principal components of innate immunity. He observed that these cells are immediately available to fight a wide range of pathogens and that they could ingest and digest them, unlike antibodies which are produced only after infection and are specific to the pathogen.

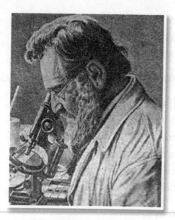

Fig. 1.3 Elie Metchnikoff (1845–1916). He is known for his work on phagocytes. He won the Nobel Prize (with Paul Ehrlich) for Physiology or Medicine in 1908 for his research on cellular immunity.

In 1902, Portier and Richet discovered anaphylaxis in their studies on sea anemone. Another significant achievement was the development of Bacillus Calmette-Guerin (BCG) vaccine in the 1920s for immunization against tuberculosis. A major triumph in the history of immunology came when Jerne, Talmadge, and Burnet proposed and developed the *clonal selection theory* of antibody production (1955–1959). At about the same time, the inactivated and attenuated polio vaccines, which are in widespread use today for preventing paralytic polio, were developed by Salk and Sabin, respectively.

The development of a method for the production of monoclonal antibodies by G. Kohler and C. Milstein, for which they were awarded the Nobel Prize for Physiology or Medicine in 1984, is worth mentioning. Development of this technology has benefited research in almost all areas of biomedical sciences. Monoclonal antibodies are widely being used clinically for diagnosis, imaging, and therapy, particularly cancer immunotherapy. There are a plethora of other uses also.

There have been several other milestones, some of which have been highlighted at relevant places in the book.

INNATE AND ADAPTIVE IMMUNITY

Immunity in vertebrates is of two types: *innate* and *adaptive*.

Innate (or Natural) Immunity

This provides early protection against invading microbes. Its major features include the following:

- It is *inborn* (constitutive) as it is always present, it is available at short notice, and no prior activation is needed.
- It shows broad specificity for structures shared by classes of microbes.
- It occurs in the same way on second or subsequent exposure (secondary response) to the microbe, that is, the primary response (first exposure) is *unchanging*.

Although innate mechanisms can effectively deal with many infectious microbes, some pathogens have very cleverly evolved ways to evade innate immunity (see Chapter 12). In such cases, adaptive immune responses are activated to cope with the foreign invader.

Adaptive (or Acquired) Immunity

This type of immunity develops in response to infection. It differs from innate immunity in the following ways:

- It is highly *specific* for a particular pathogen/molecule.
- It is *slow* to develop.
- A second or subsequent exposure to the same pathogen is *rapid* and *more intense* than the first exposure.

The term 'acquired immunity' relates to the fact that immunity is acquired during development by learning. This allows the immune system to respond more efficiently every time it is exposed to the same pathogen. The key features of innate and acquired immunity are summarized in Table 1.2.

Table 1.2   Some key features of innate and adaptive immunity—a comparison.

Feature	Innate immunity	Adaptive immunity
Specificity	Broadly specific	Fine specificity
Response time	Rapid response (hours)	Slow response (days)
Response on second exposure to pathogen	Same as primary response (no memory)	Much more rapid and intense than the primary response (memory)

It is relevant to emphasize here that the innate and adaptive immune systems are not independent. Various signals produced during the activation of innate immunity guide development of the adaptive immune response. The two together form a highly coordinated system that aims to provide optimal host defence against invading pathogens (see Chapter 3). It is to be kept in mind that defects in components of either of the two forms of immunity affect functioning of the immune system and host defence against infection.

FEATURES OF ADAPTIVE IMMUNE RESPONSES

Some salient features of adaptive immunity are elaborated in the following text:

Specificity

The immune system can detect small chemical differences in foreign molecules. For instance, it can distinguish between aminobenzene and its carboxy-derivative *o*-aminobenzoic acid, and between two proteins differing in just one amino acid residue. An individual who has suffered from measles (rubeola virus) will be immune to the measles virus and will not be protected against mumps if it has not been contracted before. Adaptive immune responses, therefore, are highly specific.

Memory

This refers to the ability of the immune system to remember previous contact with an organism. It allows an individual to mount a more rapid and more intense immune response when confronted with the same pathogen at some later time. This explains why some diseases like chickenpox occur only once in a lifetime. However, for some diseases caused by pathogens which vary their surface components, such as influenza virus, more than one attack can occur. The memory response forms the basis of vaccination which is used to immunize individuals against infectious diseases (see Chapter 13).

Diversity

Lymphocytes, the central cells of adaptive immunity, are capable of generating tremendous diversity in antigen receptors. We shall learn in later chapters that this involves unique mechanisms such as random rearrangements of a limited number of receptor gene segments (see Chapter 6). The tremendous diversity created in antigen receptors allows recognition of myriads of antigenic structures in the environment to which our body is exposed.

Self-discrimination

Another key feature of the immune response is its ability to recognize and respond to molecules that are foreign (nonself) and to ignore those molecules that are self. In this context, it is necessary to define the terms 'nonself' and 'self'. 'Nonself' refers to anything that is not part of the host which is self. It is nonself that is generally recognized as foreign by the immune system and is the target of an

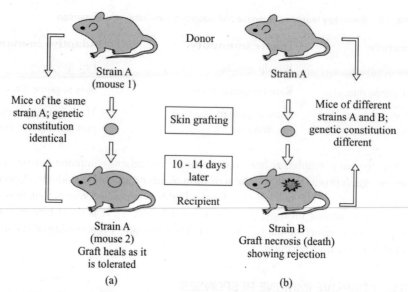

Fig. 1.4 Skin grafting in mice. As graft was of the self-type in (a), it is accepted. In (b), graft is of the nonself type so it is rejected (see Chapter 17).

immune response. This can be illustrated by a simple experiment based on skin grafting in mice (Fig. 1.4). Self-discrimination is an essential feature as it prevents damaging immune reactions against our own cells and tissues. But occasionally, the immune system fails and immune responses to self-antigens do occur leading to *autoimmunity*.

An important decision that the immune system has to make is whether it should mount a response or not. Some fundamental aspects related to the way the innate immune system distinguishes between 'self' and 'nonself' and the way it decides whether to respond or not will be taken up in Chapter 2.

There are two types of adaptive immune responses: *humoral* and *cell-mediated*. Their distinct roles in immune defence are described later in this chapter.

HAEMATOPOIESIS

Haematopoiesis is a term used for the process that generates all the different types of blood cells. During foetal development, haematopoiesis occurs in the yolk sac and later in the liver and the spleen. After birth, this function is gradually assumed by the bone marrow. By puberty, haematopoiesis occurs in the marrow of the flat bones, particularly the pelvis and the sternum, where it continues throughout life. *Haematopoietic stem cells (HSCs)* are undifferentiated cells in the bone marrow. These cells have the capacity for *self-renewal*, that is, they divide continuously giving rise to new stem cells. They are pluripotent stem cells which give rise to lymphoid and myeloid progenitors from which all other specialized cells in blood develop. The development of mature blood cells from HSCs is depicted in Fig. 1.5.

As HSCs are difficult to grow in vitro, it is still not fully understood the way they undergo differentiation. The particular lineage that differentiates from HSCs is determined by the HSC microenvironment. The bone marrow stroma supports haematopoiesis, both structurally and functionally. *Stromal cells* form a meshwork in the bone marrow and secrete cytokines called *haematopoietic cytokines*, which are essential for differentiation of precursor cells into the relevant cell types (see Chapter 7). Other critical cell types include fibroblasts, endothelial cells, smooth muscle cells, and immune cells. Contact of responding precursor cells with stromal cells and interaction with particular cytokines is

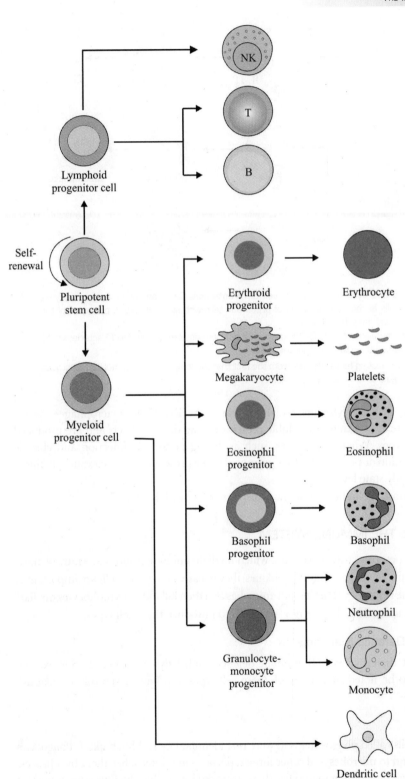

Fig. 1.5 Haematopoiesis. All cells in blood originate from a pluripotent haematopoietic stem cell. The figure depicts development of the different lineages. Cytokines play an important role in haematopoiesis.

Note: Although most dendritic cells belong to the myeloid lineage, some also originate from lymphoid precursor cells.

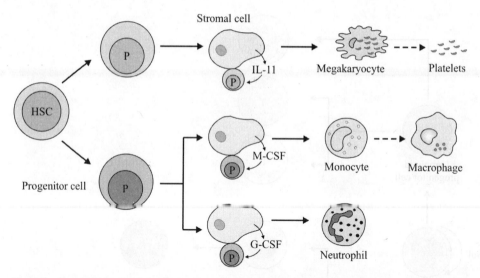

Fig. 1.6 Stromal cells and cytokines in stem cell differentiation. Development of megakaryocytes, monocytes, and neutrophils is shown. Interaction of precursor cells with stromal cells in presence of the relevant cytokine(s) is critical for differentiation.

M-CSF, monocyte-colony stimulating factor; G-CSF, granulocyte-colony stimulating factor; IL-11, interleukin-11 (many cytokines are referred to by the term 'interleukin').

Note: The term colony stimulating factor derives from the fact that these substances stimulate the growth of various leukocytes in vitro to form clumps or colonies.

essential (Fig. 1.6). Many of these cytokines are also produced by T cells and macrophages. As will be seen in the following text, cytokines are soluble proteins having diverse effects and are produced by many different cell types. When need arises, such as during periods of infection and chronic inflammation, differentiation of precursor cells is promoted in the presence of the relevant cytokine(s) in order to maintain steady state levels.

HSCs have an important use in bone marrow transplantation (see Chapter 17).

CELLULAR COMPONENTS OF THE IMMUNE SYSTEM

There are various cell types, primarily leukocytes, which mediate immune responses. Many of these cells participate through the soluble mediators (cytokines) they release. Phagocytic cells are important in mediating innate immune responses. They engulf microbes and then kill them. Lymphocytes mediate specific or adaptive immunity. The chapter now proceeds to introduce these cell types.

Cells Involved in Host Innate Defence Mechanisms

The essential features of the cells involved in innate defence are briefly considered in the text that follows (Fig. 1.7). It is to be noted that many of these cell types also have a key role in adaptive immunity.

Macrophages

These are specialized cells called phagocytes and were first identified by E. Metchnikoff. Phagocytes are eating cells which bind to microbes and other foreign particles and internalize them by a process called *phagocytosis*. The ingested foreign material is then destroyed intracellularly. This is an important

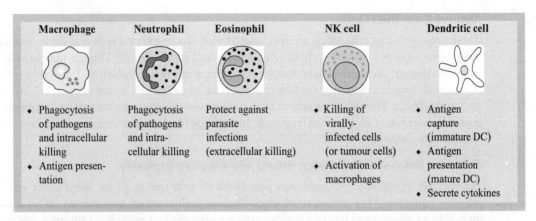

Fig. 1.7 Cell types involved in innate immunity and their function(s). Activation of eosinophils is dependent on both triggering of complement activation (alternative pathway, innate) by parasites and by antibody (adaptive, see Chapter 2).
DC, dendritic cell (bridges innate and adaptive immunity)

first line of defence against infection. Macrophages are the mature forms of *monocytes* which are small spherical cells with a single-lobed, often bean-shaped nucleus. Monocytes, which perform many of the functions attributed to macrophages, circulate for only a few hours before migrating from the bloodstream into tissues. Here, they differentiate into macrophages which remain in tissues and never re-enter the circulation. Macrophages and other phagocytic cells such as neutrophils (described in the following text) use nonspecific receptors that allow binding to a wide range of microbial structures. These receptors of innate immunity are introduced in brief later in the chapter and in greater detail in Chapter 2. Besides phagocytic activity, presenting antigens and delivering activating signals to T cells is another very important role of macrophages which is critical in adaptive immunity.

Granulocytes

Their name derives from the abundant granules present in the cytoplasm. They are short-lived cells having the ability to migrate into tissues after which they never return to the bloodstream. They represent about 65 per cent of all white blood cells (WBCs; mean number 7,500 μl^{-1}) and include *neutrophils, eosinophils,* and *basophils*. They are also called *polymorphonuclear leukocytes* due to their multilobed nucleus. The term, however, is often used synonymously with neutrophils (called PMNs) which are the most numerous among granulocytes. Neutrophils are the major phagocytic cells involved in killing bacteria. Eosinophils deal with multicellular parasites such as worms. As parasites are too large to be engulfed and destroyed intracellularly, eosinophils are involved in extracellular killing of their targets (see Chapter 11). They discharge their function by releasing the contents of their granules on receiving an appropriate stimulus, a process called *degranulation*. Basophils have a role in inflammatory reactions and more importantly, are implicated in allergic disease (see Chapter 14). Like basophils, eosinophils are also involved in allergic reactions.

Mast Cells

These cells are found fixed in tissues, particularly at epithelial surfaces, and do not circulate in the blood as do basophils. They resemble basophils both structurally and functionally. Mast cells are characterized by the presence of abundant granules containing inflammatory mediators, many of which are also present in basophil granules. They are involved in inflammation and are the major effector cells of allergic responses (see Chapter 14).

Natural Killer (NK) Cells

These are circulating cells which are specialized to kill virally-infected cells and some tumour cells. They have features common to both lymphocytes and myeloid cells. Though they belong to the lymphoid lineage, they lack antigen-specific receptors, a distinctive feature of T and B lymphocytes. Also, unlike lymphocytes, they contain characteristic granules and so are also called *large granular lymphocytes (LGLs)*. They kill their targets by releasing cytotoxic granule contents and enzymes which lead to breakdown of DNA of the target cell. In response to a foreign stimulus, they secrete cytokines that activate macrophages.

Dendritic Cells—A Link between Innate and Adaptive Immunity

Dendritic cells represent a heterogeneous population of cells that lie at the interface of innate and adaptive immunity. They are a type of specialized cells called *antigen-presenting cells (APCs)* which also include macrophages and B cells. Dendritic cells are very efficient as antigen capturing cells and have a major role to play in activation of T cells by antigen. Precursor dendritic cells after being released into the circulation from the bone marrow take up residence in tissues where they are constantly on the watch out for foreign invaders. We will learn more about these cells (and also other APCs) in Chapter 3. For the time being, remember that these cells, besides their role in innate immunity, are crucial for initiating adaptive immune responses in peripheral lymphoid organs leading to T cell activation.

The way the cells of innate immunity, described in the preceding text, sense that an infection has occurred is covered in Chapter 2. It suffices here to know that innate immunity cells recognize distinctive molecular structures present only on microbes called *pathogen-associated molecular patterns (PAMPs)* and which are absent on host cells. This happens with the help of receptors which have broad specificity and are called *pattern-recognition receptors (PRRs)*. Of these, the *toll-like receptors (TLRs)* are of particular interest. It is with the help of these receptors that innate cells are able to discriminate nonself from self-components. Some soluble elements, too, can recognize microbial structures.

Cells of Adaptive Immunity

Lymphocytes and the products they release are the central components of adaptive immune responses. These responses are more powerful and help to rid the body of those microbes that resist innate defence mechanisms. As a reminder, cells involved in innate defence also participate in adaptive immune responses.

Lymphocytes

As lymphocytes occupy a central position in immunity, their study is essential for learning about adaptive immune responses. They are the smallest of the leukocytes and are almost spherical in shape having only a small amount of cytoplasm separating nuclear and plasma membranes. They are long-lived cells capable of entering and leaving body tissues. These cells carry memory of previous encounter with antigen, unlike neutrophils and other cell types of innate immunity. These cells are of two types, namely *B* and *T lymphocytes*, also referred to commonly as B and T cells. Natural killer cells, also of the same lymphoid lineage, function in a major way in innate immunity and have been introduced in the preceding text.

In birds, B lymphocytes are produced in a gut-associated lymphoid organ called the *bursa of Fabricius*. Early studies on antibody production in birds revealed that removal of the bursa led to a failure to produce antibody. This is how antibody producing cells came to be known as B (bursa-derived) lymphocytes. The name turned out to be very appropriate as B cells, in humans, are derived from the *bone marrow*. T lymphocytes, too, just as B cells, have their origin in the bone marrow, but they mature after migrating to the *thymus* (T for thymus), a bilobed organ situated above the heart. This is unlike

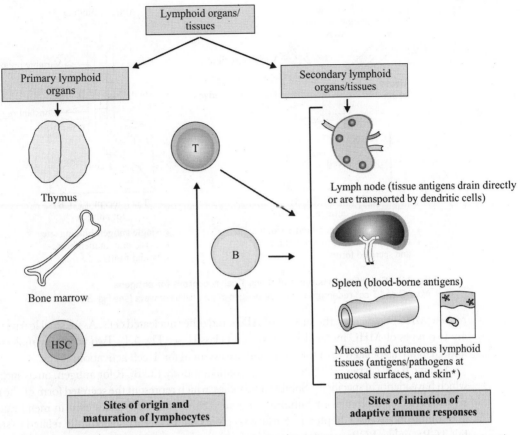

Fig. 1.8   Organs/tissues of the immune system. Both B and T cells originate in the bone marrow. Whereas maturation of B cells occurs in the bone marrow, these events for T cells occur in the thymus. Mature B and T cells then migrate to secondary lymphoid organs/tissues where immune responses are triggered.
* Immune responses are initiated in lymph nodes draining the area.

B cells which mature in the bone marrow itself. The bone marrow and thymus are, therefore, important sites and are called the *primary or central lymphoid organs* (Fig. 1.8). Once lymphocytes have completed their maturation at these sites, they migrate via the circulation to *secondary* or *peripheral lymphoid organs/tissues*, where adaptive immune responses are initiated (see Chapter 3). These include *lymph nodes, spleen,* and *mucosal* and *cutaneous* lymphoid tissue.

Lymphocyte Receptors and Recognition of Antigen

Before proceeding to B and T lymphocyte antigen receptors which determine specificity of the adaptive immune system, it would not be out of place to first define an *antigen* here. An antigen, as we shall see in Chapter 4, is a molecule that can interact with specific lymphocyte receptors or with secreted antibody (also called *immunoglobulin* usually written as *Ig*). Lymphocyte receptors include *B cell receptor (BCR)* which is a membrane-bound antibody on B cells, and *T cell receptor (TCR)* on T cells. Although antibody, both membrane-bound and secreted, can bind to a wide range of substances such as simple chemicals, sugars, small peptides, and large protein molecules in their native form, the TCR reacts largely with peptide fragments derived from partial degradation of proteins inside cells. These peptide fragments need to be presented to the T cell by peptide display molecules called *major histocompatibility*

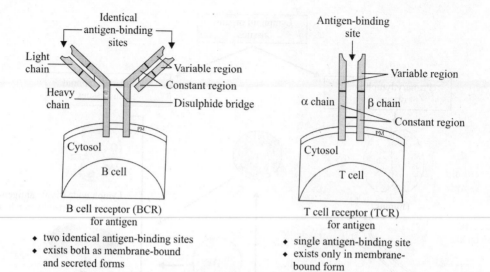

Fig. 1.9 **Simplified structures of B and T cell receptors for antigens.**
Note: B and T cell receptors recognize antigen in very different ways (see Fig. 3.11).

complex (MHC) molecules on the surface of APCs and other nucleated cells. As we shall learn later, there are two types of MHC molecules—class I and class II (see Fig. 5.4). Two accessory molecules CD4 and CD8 are associated with the TCR and are essential for T cell activation.

A single B cell carries ~10^5 molecules of bound antibody, the BCR for antigen, on its surface all of which have identical specificity. Soluble antibodies, which represent the secreted form of the receptor, serve as effector molecules of humoral immunity. Structural differences exist in membrane-bound and soluble forms (see Chapter 4). Surface receptors on T cells are structurally related to surface Ig, but TCRs, unlike BCRs, are not secreted.

Antigen receptors on lymphocytes are comprised of two parts (Fig. 1.9). There is a *constant (C) region* in which the amino acid sequence is the same in all receptors expressed on different cells. The other part is the *variable (V) region* in which the amino acid sequence is unique to each receptor. This variable part is the region that determines antigen specificity and contributes to antigen binding. Each mature lymphocyte entering the circulation from central lymphoid organs carries receptors of only a single specificity. But as specificity of each lymphocyte varies, an enormous range of different specificities is available.

Lymphocytes Require Two Signals for Activation

Normally, lymphocytes are in a resting state. They become functionally active only when they encounter an antigen. Initially, when an antigen enters the body, the number of lymphocytes available to fight the pathogen is very small. For an effective immune response to protect the host, a specific lymphocyte must proliferate and differentiate into *effector cells* which function to eliminate (or help to eliminate) the pathogen that triggered the immune response. Two signals are needed for lymphocytes to proliferate and differentiate into effector cells (Fig. 1.10). *Signal 1* is provided by binding of antigen to the lymphocyte receptor and is important for initiating an immune response. Another signal called the *costimulatory signal* or *signal 2* is also needed. It is so called because it is needed along with the antigen to activate lymphocytes. For B cells, the second signal is generally delivered by a T cell. Signal 2 to T cells is delivered by specialized APCs such as dendritic cells and macrophages. The *dual signal requirement* for activation of T and B cells is described in more detail in Chapters 8 and 10, respectively.

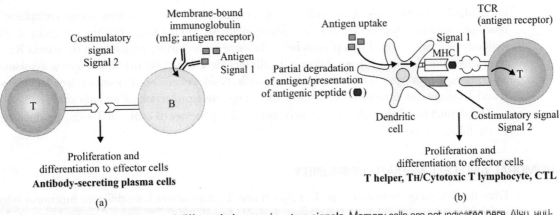

Fig. 1.10 **Lymphocyte expansion and differentiation requires two signals.** Memory cells are not indicated here. Also, antigen uptake by DC into endosome is not shown.

Lymphocytes are Activated by Antigen to Effector Cells and Memory Cells

On activation by an antigen, specific lymphocytes proliferate and differentiate into effector cells which function to eradicate infecting microbes (Fig. 1.11). Effector B cells are called *plasma cells* which

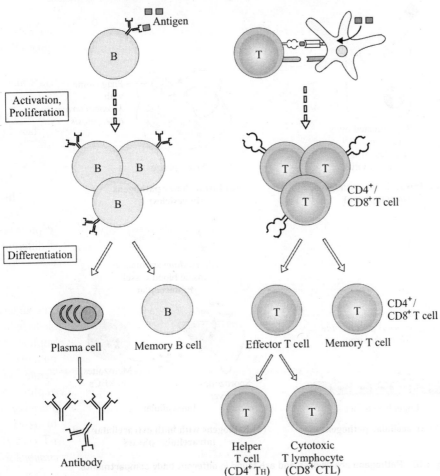

Fig. 1.11 **Adaptive immune responses.** B cells are activated by directly binding to antigen and secrete antibody molecules. T cells, however, recognize antigen displayed on cells and are activated to TH cells and CTLs. TH cells secrete cytokines and CTLs lyse virally-infected cells. Adaptive immunity also generates memory B and T cells which help to eliminate the same invader if encountered again.

are antibody-secreting cells. These cells are characterized by a very prominent rough endoplasmic reticulum, an adaptation to their role in antibody synthesis. Do not forget that the specificity of the antibody molecule secreted by a plasma cell is the same as the surface antibody on the parent B cell from which the plasma cell arose. Effector T cells include *T helper* (*TH*) *cells* which secrete cytokines, and *cytotoxic T lymphocytes* (*CTLs*) which kill target cells. Besides effector cells, some antigen-stimulated B and T cells persist as *memory cells*. These confer long-lasting protection on an individual.

The distinct functional roles of the two classes of lymphocytes (B cells and T cells) are discussed in the following text.

HUMORAL AND CELL-MEDIATED IMMUNITY

From the foregoing discussion, it is clear that B and T lymphocytes have different functional roles in adaptive immunity which is of two types: *humoral immunity* (by *B cells*) and *cell-mediated immunity* (by *T cells*). It is emphasized here that the type of host defence mechanism(s) activated depends on the nature of the pathogen. Broadly, there are two classes—*extracellular* and *intracellular* (Fig. 1.12).

Humoral immunity mediated by antibodies is the major defence mechanism against extracellular microbes and their toxins. On the other hand, immunity mediated by T lymphocytes or cell-mediated

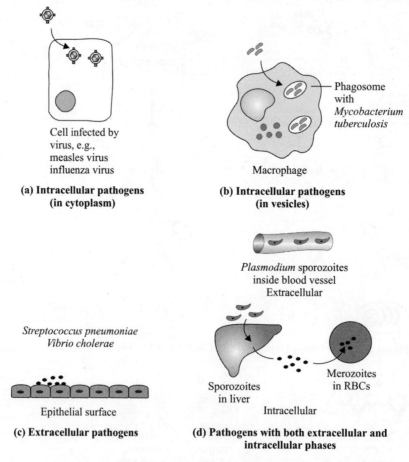

Cell infected by
virus, e.g.,
measles virus
influenza virus

**(a) Intracellular pathogens
(in cytoplasm)**

Phagosome
with
*Mycobacterium
tuberculosis*

Macrophage

**(b) Intracellular pathogens
(in vesicles)**

Plasmodium sporozoites
inside blood vessel
Extracellular

*Streptococcus pneumoniae
Vibrio cholerae*

Epithelial surface

(c) Extracellular pathogens

Sporozoites
in liver

Merozoites
in RBCs

Intracellular

**(d) Pathogens with both extracellular and
intracellular phases**

Fig. 1.12 Pathogens are diverse and are found in different body compartments.

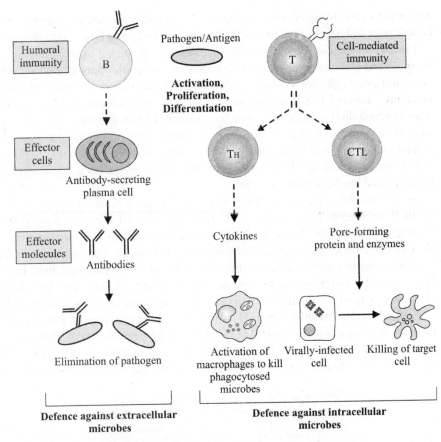

Fig. 1.13 Humoral and cell-mediated immunity.
Note: Cytokines secreted by TH cells also activate B cells and cytotoxic T cells (see Fig. 3.9).

immunity protects against intracellular microbes that survive inside phagocytes or which infect nonphagocytic cells. This is necessary as antibodies cannot penetrate the interior of cells harbouring intracellular pathogens. T helper cells have a pivotal role in immunity. By secreting cytokines, they deliver activating signals to macrophages to kill phagocytosed microbes. Cytotoxic T lymphocytes directly lyse target cells such as virally-infected cells (Fig. 1.13).

SOLUBLE COMPONENTS OF THE IMMUNE SYSTEM

Lysozyme, present in various secretions, such as tears and saliva, is protective in nature as it can lyse the cell walls of many bacteria. The *complement system*, also a component of humoral immunity, comprises several proteins found in plasma and also in other body fluids and tissues. It provides a quick protective mechanism against infectious microbes before adaptive immune responses come into play. There are three major pathways of complement activation which are triggered differently. An important product of complement activation is C3b which promotes phagocytosis by neutrophils and macrophages. Other important roles of the complement system include inflammation (the body's protective response to infection) and microbial lysis (see Fig. 2.3). We will see more about these proteins in Chapter 2 and then again in greater detail in Chapter 11. *Acute-phase proteins* (*APPs*) are synthesized mainly in liver hepatocytes during infection in response to cytokines released by macrophages. They activate complement and help in clearance of pathogens besides having other important roles (see Box 2.1).

Cytokines are potent soluble proteins/glycoproteins produced in small amounts in response to microbes and other external stimuli. It is through cytokines that leukocytes communicate with each other and other cells (see Chapter 7). Macrophages are the major source of cytokines in innate immunity, whereas T helper lymphocytes are the principal producers in adaptive immune responses. They exhibit a diverse range of actions on various cell types. *Interferons (IFNs) type I* and *II* represent a family of cytokines so named because they interfere with viral replication in cells. They act early to limit viral spread and make adjacent cells resistant to viral infection (Fig. 1.14). Type I IFNs are more potent, whereas type II IFN, produced by T lymphocytes, has a role in regulation of immune responses and has weak antiviral action.

Serum *antibodies* or immunoglobulins which mediate humoral immunity are the secreted forms of the BCR for antigen. They are glycoproteins and are secreted when B cells are activated by binding of antigen to membrane-bound Ig. A typical antibody molecule is composed of two identical *heavy (H) chains* and two identical *light (L) chains* which are held together by disulphide linkages (Fig. 1.15).

The two binding sites for antigen in the *Fab* regions exhibit the same specificity. In other words, they bind to two identical *epitopes* on the same or on different antigen molecules. An epitope is a small part of an antigen to which an antibody can bind. The binding is a non-covalent reversible interaction.

Antibody molecules differ in their H chains which are of five types: μ, γ, α, ε, and δ. On this basis, there are five major Ig classes: *IgM, IgG, IgA, IgE,* and *IgD* (see Chapter 4). Differences in heavy chain constant regions confer unique biological properties on the antibody class. The constant region of heavy chains of different antibody classes called the *Fc region* can bind to distinct receptors called *Fc*

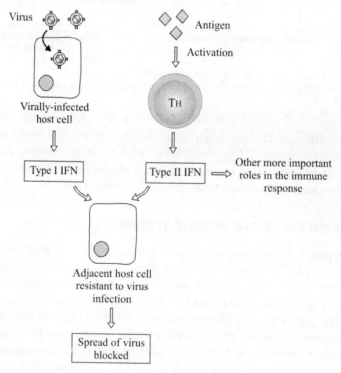

Fig. 1.14 Interferons (IFNs). IFNs act early to limit viral spread before the adaptive immune response develops.

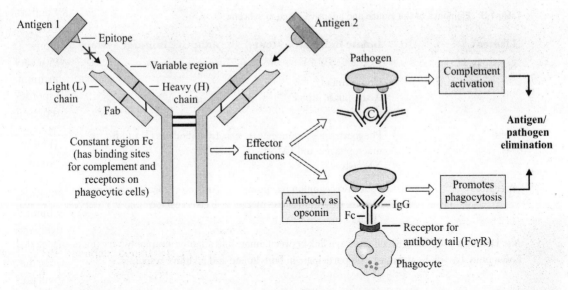

Fig. 1.15 Simplified structure of an antibody molecule showing functional parts. The Fab region binds antigen whereas the constant Fc region or the antibody tail mediates biological activity. Binding of antibody occurs to antigen 2 due to complimentarity in shape and not to antigen 1. Complement (C) product C3b-coated targets are also readily engulfed by phagocytes (not shown). Both antibody and C3b are called opsonins.

receptors or *FcRs* on phagocytic cells and killer cells such as NK cells. For instance, IgG binds to *FcγRs*, whereas IgE binds to *FcεRs* (see Chapter 11).

Although many microbes adhere well to the surface of phagocytes through nonspecific receptors and are readily phagocytosed, there are some microbes which are resistant. However, if coated with antibody and complement split product C3b which bind to Fc receptors and complement receptors, respectively, on the phagocyte membrane, they are readily ingested. Antibody and complement products which enhance phagocytosis are called *opsonins* and the process of coating of microbes with opsonins is referred to as *opsonization*, a term which in Greek means to make tastier (see Chapter 11).

The various elements of the innate and adaptive immune systems discussed in the preceding text are summarized in Table 1.3. The major elements of innate immunity are depicted in Fig. 1.16.

Interestingly, though innate defence mechanisms are found in both vertebrates and invertebrates and also in plants, adaptive immunity emerged with the vertebrates. Some features of evolution of the immune system in various species and development of adaptive immunity are briefly considered in Box 1.1.

CLONAL SELECTION OF LYMPHOCYTES

Each individual possesses an enormously large number of mature lymphocyte clones. A clone comprises identical cells which arise from a single progenitor cell. The specificity of antigen receptors expressed by a clone is different from receptor specificity of another clone. Hence, a wide range of lymphocyte specificities is available which is referred to as the *pre-immune repertoire*. The diverse receptor specificities are generated during maturation of lymphocytes in central lymphoid organs before their encounter with an antigen.

An antigen entering the body selects a specific lymphocyte with which it can react with high-affinity. This event called *clonal selection* is responsible for the specificity of the immune response. The

Table 1.3　Elements of the innate and adaptive immune system.

Element	Innate immune system	Adaptive immune system
Soluble factors	Lysozyme Complement Acute-phase proteins Cytokines	Antibody (B cells) and cytokines (T cells)
Cells	Phagocytes, e.g., monocytes/macrophages, and PMNs NK cells	Lymphocytes (T and B)
Receptors	Pattern-recognition receptors (PRRs), e.g., toll-like receptors (TLRs)	Antigen-recognition molecules (B cell and T cell receptors)

Note: Dendritic cells (DCs) which serve as a link between innate and adaptive immunity have not been included. Eosinophils, basophils, and mast cells participate in both innate and adaptive responses.

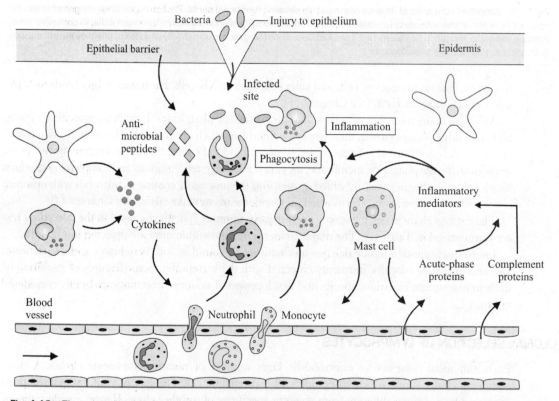

Fig. 1.16　Elements of the innate immune system. Key components of the innate immune system are shown here. Dendritic cells and macrophages activate an inflammatory response in tissues by secreting cytokines. Complement proteins are activated in tissues by microbes. They, along with other soluble proteins, also exit blood vessels with the plasma. NK cells are not shown.

Box 1.1 Evolution of the immune system

Comparative immunology which studies the immune system in different phylogenetic groups has made it possible to follow evolution of the immune system. The most ancient elements are those that are present in simple organisms, whereas those present only in higher animals are more recent in evolution. As even the simplest animal species have to deal with potential threats, elements of an immune system can be detected in almost all living organisms. Even Paramecium, a simple single-celled creature, defends itself in a way that is similar to phagocytosis in humans.

Innate immunity is an ancient form of defence found in all multicellular plants and animals studied. Invertebrates are equipped with only natural immune responses, and elements of adaptive immunity, such as lymphocytes and antibodies have not been detected. Antimicrobial peptides are the earliest defence molecules and are found in invertebrates. In addition, organisms of nonvertebrate phyla have other defence mechanisms which are based on phagocytosis and soluble mediators, similar to cytokines in higher species. Coagulation of haemolymph, initiated by activation of proteolytic cascades, helps to entrap foreign invaders.

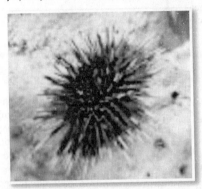

Fig. 1.17 Sea urchin, an echinoderm, has early forms of the complement system for defence.

The toll molecule in the fruit fly *Drosophilia* is a receptor for PAMPs and provides defence against fungal infection. PAMPs, introduced earlier in the chapter, are molecular patterns found only in microbes and not in host cells. On activation, the toll molecule initiates the ancient signalling toll pathway that is present in both invertebrates and vertebrates. It generates signals that activate innate immune responses and also the more specialized adaptive immune responses which are present only in vertebrates. Early forms of the complement system predate vertebrates and are found even in lower orders such as echinoderms, e.g., sea urchin (Fig. 1.17).

Specialized adaptive immune responses are more recent in evolutionary terms and emerged at about the same time as vertebrates. The early jawless vertebrates, such as lampreys, lacked organized lymphoid tissue and failed to mount an adaptive immune response. Neither T nor B lymphocytes have been detected in these jawless fishes. But the jawed cartilaginous fishes such as sharks, which are further up in the evolutionary scale, developed organized lymphoid tissue, T cell receptors, immunoglobulins, and MHC molecules. This led to the emergence of adaptive immunity.

clonal selection of B lymphocytes is depicted in Fig. 1.18. The selected lymphocyte on stimulation proliferates and differentiates into plasma cells (effector cells) that secrete large amounts of antibody, and memory cells. These have specificity identical to the parent lymphocyte that was selected. The concept behind clonal selection, called the *clonal selection theory*, was proposed and developed by Neils Jerne, David Talmadge, and F. MacFarlane Burnet in the 1950s and gained wide acceptance. *Clonal selection of lymphocytes forms the basis of adaptive immunity.*

Following encounter with pathogen/antigen, there is a change in the pre-immune repertoire. As lymphocytes with specific receptors have proliferated, their numbers are increased enormously compared to those lymphocytes that were not stimulated by antigen. This tremendous increase helps to mount an effective immune response that clears the pathogen from the body.

The memory cells that remain after the infection has been cleared are responsible for long-lasting immunity. These cells can be rapidly restimulated by antigen on second encounter at some later time. It is due to memory cell generation that the response generated on second contact with antigen, called the *secondary immune response*, is more rapid and more intense than the *primary immune response* stimulated on initial encounter (Fig. 1.19).

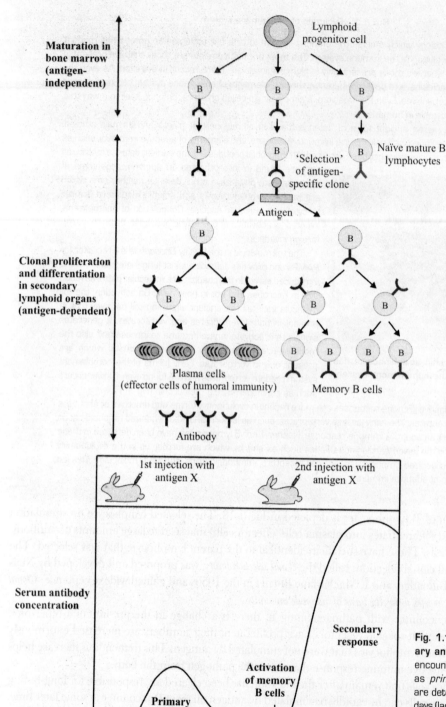

Maturation in bone marrow (antigen-independent)

Lymphoid progenitor cell

Naïve mature B lymphocytes

'Selection' of antigen-specific clone

Antigen

Clonal proliferation and differentiation in secondary lymphoid organs (antigen-dependent)

Plasma cells (effector cells of humoral immunity)

Memory B cells

Antibody

Fig. 1.18 Clonal selection of B lymphocytes. An antigen entering the body selects a particular clone having specific receptors for the antigen. The selected clone proliferates (clonal expansion) and differentiates to plasma cells and long-lived memory cells. The same principle, as depicted in the figure for B cells, applies to T lymphocytes.

1st injection with antigen X

2nd injection with antigen X

Serum antibody concentration

Secondary response

Activation of memory B cells

Primary response

Lag phase

1   2   3   4   1   2   3

Time (weeks)

Fig. 1.19 Primary and secondary antibody response. The first encounter with antigen X is known as *primary response*. Antibodies are detected in serum after several days (lag phase). A second encounter with the same antigen causes a *secondary response*. Note that the response is more rapid and intense on second exposure to antigen X due to stimulation of memory B cells.

IMMUNE DYSFUNCTION AND ITS CONSEQUENCES

The main focus of the discussion in the preceding text has been on the role of the immune system in protecting the host from invading pathogens. But sometimes the immune system fails to provide adequate protection, consequences of which can be very severe (Fig. 1.20). Some ways in which the immune system fails to function are discussed in the following section.

Hypersensitivity Reactions

Sometimes immune responses against harmless foreign substances such as pollen, dust, medications, and even a food molecule may in some individuals lead to severe pathological consequences and sometimes death. These responses are *hypersensitivity reactions* or *allergic reactions*. Hay fever and asthma are examples of such reactions. However, there are other categories of hypersensitivity also such as granulomatous hypersensitivity, consequences of which can be very severe (see Chapter 14). It is to be noted that mechanisms involved in hypersensitivity also afford protection against invading microbes.

Autoimmunity

The immune system normally avoids mounting a response against our body's own cells and tissues and initiates a response only against foreign antigens. But, at times, the ability to discriminate between self and nonself is lost and the immune system reacts against self-cells leading to autoimmunity. Some examples include Graves' disease, myasthenia gravis, and rheumatoid arthritis (see Chapter 15).

Immunodeficiency

This is a state that arises due to defects in one or more components of the immune system, either innate or specific. Immunodeficient individuals are at greater risk of infection than normal people, the nature of infection depending on the deficient component. Such a state may arise due to a genetic defect in which case the immunodeficiency manifests just after birth. This is called *primary immunodeficiency*. Severe combined immunodeficiency (SCID), a disorder with defects in both B and T cells, is a good example. An immunodeficient state may also arise later in life, called *secondary immunodeficiency*, due to loss in function of immune components by use of cytotoxic drugs, malnutrition, biologic agents, etc.

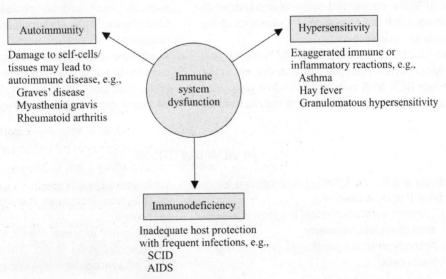

Fig. 1.20 Immune system can fail in various ways.

Acquired immunodeficiency syndrome (AIDS) is a secondary disorder in which infection by human immunodeficiency virus (HIV) leads to depletion of Tн cells and crippling of the immune system.

SUMMARY

♦ Immune responses protect against infectious agents, harmful molecules, such as toxins, and also cancer. They may be innate or adaptive (acquired). Invertebrates mount only innate immune responses.

♦ Innate immunity represents the first line of defence against infection. It is inborn, broadly specific, and unchanging.

♦ Specificity, immunologic memory, diversity, and self/nonself discrimination are key features of adaptive immunity.

♦ Innate and adaptive immunity do not function independently. Signals produced during activation of innate immune responses direct development of subsequent adaptive immunity.

♦ All cell types in blood arise from haematopoietic stem cells (HSCs). Differentiation and development of various cell types depend on interaction of progenitor cells with stromal cells, and cytokines.

♦ Immune system comprises specialized immune cells and soluble molecules. Cells involved in innate immunity include macrophages, granulocytes, NK cells, and mast cells. Neutrophils and macrophages are the major phagocytic cells.

♦ PAMPs are conserved molecular patterns in microbes that are recognized by receptors of the innate immune system.

♦ Central cells of adaptive immunity include B and T lymphocytes. Receptors of adaptive immunity, namely BCR on B cells and TCR on T cells, bind specifically to an antigen. This is the reason why adaptive immune responses are highly specific.

♦ Adaptive immune responses are of two types —cell-mediated and humoral. Broadly, there are two groups of pathogens. Intracellular pathogens stimulate cell-mediated immunity (CMI) in which T lymphocytes help in eradicating the microbe. Extracellular microbes stimulate humoral immunity in which antibodies help in pathogen clearance.

♦ Noncellular components of the immune system include lysozyme, complement proteins, acute-phase proteins, antibody, and cytokines. Complement proteins opsonize or directly lyse target cells and promote inflammation. Synthesis of acute-phase proteins is increased in infections. Antibodies (and also complement proteins) mediate humoral immunity. Cytokines allow communication between cells and tissues.

♦ Clonal selection involves recognition of an antigen by specific clones of B and T lymphocytes. These specific clones expand and differentiate to effector cells and memory cells. An immune response by effector cells helps to eliminate antigens, whereas memory cells provide long-term protection.

♦ Immune responses to harmless foreign substances, such as pollen, can sometimes cause injury to host tissues. These are hypersensitivity or allergic reactions.

♦ An immune response mounted against self-tissues can lead to autoimmune disease.

♦ Immunodeficient individuals suffer from various infections depending on the deficient component.

REVIEW QUESTIONS

1. Indicate whether the following statements are true or false. If false, explain why.
   (a) The term 'variolation' refers to a form of attenuation of virulent organisms.
   (b) Antibody protects against pathogens that reside inside cells.
   (c) Interferons kill viruses.
   (d) Infection increases the rate of haematopoiesis.
   (e) NK cells express highly specific antigen receptors as do B and T lymphocytes.
   (f) T cells recognize native unmodified antigen.

2. Self-assessment questions
   (a) What are the major ways in which natural immune responses differ from acquired immune responses? How can innate immune mechanisms involving phagocytes and complement be enhanced?
   (b) The immune system at times fails to function properly. Giving examples, explain the consequences of immune dysfunction.
   (c) Explain the terms 'clonal selection' and 'clonal expansion' with reference to B lymphocytes. How do these events affect an immune response?
   (d) What are haematopoietic stem cells? List some of their characteristics. What are their two major pathways of differentiation?
   (e) Name two antigen-binding molecules of the immune system. What is the nature of the signals needed by lymphocytes to proliferate and differentiate to effector cells?

3. For each question, choose the *best* answer.

   (a) Which is not a feature of the acquired immune response?
       (i) Ability to remember previous encounter with antigen
       (ii) Broad specificity for microbes
       (iii) Ability to distinguish self from nonself
       (iv) Diversity in recognition molecules
   (b) Immunological memory is a property of
       (i) Neutrophils
       (ii) Lymphocytes
       (iii) Macrophages
       (iv) NK cells
   (c) Humoral immunity involves
       (i) Processed antigen
       (ii) Antibody and complement
       (iii) An attack on intracellular microbes
       (iv) Cytotoxic T cells
   (d) An immunoglobulin is an
       (i) Antibody
       (ii) Enzyme
       (iii) Immunogen
       (iv) Epitope

Innate Immune Response to Infections

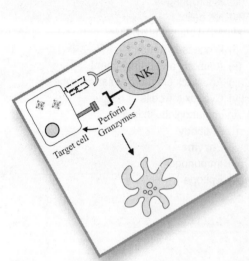

LEARNING OBJECTIVES

Having studied this chapter, you should be able to understand the following:

♦ The external barriers that provide the first line of defence against infection and the role of complement proteins, acute-phase proteins, and cytokines
♦ The features of granulocytes, macrophages, and NK cells and the way they mediate early defence
♦ Recognition of microbial components by receptors of innate immunity
♦ The role of innate immunity receptors in elimination of pathogens and generation of signals that guide both innate and adaptive immune responses
♦ Protective mechanisms such as inflammation and phago-cytosis triggered in response to microbial infection and the antimicrobial systems in phagocytes

Innate defence mechanisms are the natural mechanisms that are always present in healthy individuals. They are quick to respond as no prior activation is needed. In recent years, there has been increasing interest in innate defence systems and the way they afford protection against infection and tissue injury.

There are two broad categories of pathogens: extracellular and intracellular. These stimulate different types of innate immune responses which are best at eliminating the microbe. Phagocytes, the complement system, and acute-phase proteins (APPs) provide optimal defence against extracellular microbes such as bacteria and fungi. Defence against intracellular microbes, such as viruses, is largely mediated by natural killer (NK) cells, whereas macrophages protect against some intracellular bacteria and fungi. Cytokines released by immune cells, particularly macrophages, have a crucial role to play.

To mount an attack the innate immune system must recognize the microbe as foreign. This depends on the use of *pattern-recognition receptors (PRRs)* which are recognition molecules of the innate immune system and which recognize broad classes of microbes. Recognition is followed by the response or the effector phase which helps in elimination of the pathogen from the body. The adaptive immune system, on the other hand, depends on highly specific antigen receptors on B and T lymphocytes to recognize foreign material. Whereas innate immune mechanisms recognize microbial antigens, adaptive responses are directed against non-microbial antigens too. In addition, cells of innate immunity do not clonally expand as do lymphocytes in adaptive immunity. The clonal selection and expansion of lymphocytes has been described in Chapter 1 and is the basis of adaptive immune responses.

Although innate immunity can operate independently of the adaptive immune system, it is linked to it in many ways. Besides providing rapid and effective initial defence against infection, innate immunity generates signals that direct subsequent adaptive immune responses. Conversely, effector molecules of adaptive immunity such as antibodies enhance innate defences. Cooperation between the two arms of the immune system is important as it provides optimal defence against invading pathogens (see Chapter 3).

This chapter introduces various host innate defence mechanisms which consist of epithelial barriers, and soluble factors including complement proteins, APPs, and cytokines. Cellular defences such as phagocytes (which include neutrophils and macrophages) and NK cells are covered. Other aspects focused on include the PRRs and their role in both elimination of pathogens and generation of signals that direct innate and adaptive immunity. Events that occur in an inflammatory response, phagocytosis of microbes, and antimicrobial systems in phagocytes are discussed. The way microbes evade innate immunity is briefly described in the concluding part of this chapter.

EXTERNAL BARRIERS TO INFECTION

External barriers represent the first line of defence against infectious microbes (Fig. 2.1). Body surfaces are protected by *epithelia* which include skin, and linings of the gastrointestinal, respiratory, and

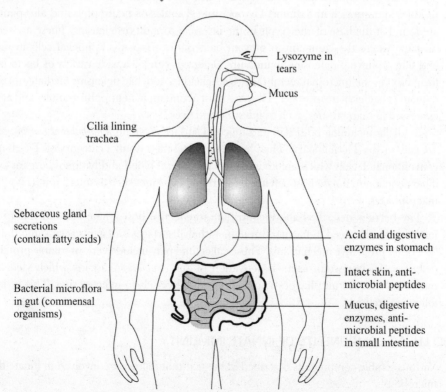

Fig. 2.1 **External barriers provide early defence against infection.**

genitourinary tracts (mucosal epithelia). These provide an effective barrier, and infection occurs only when a pathogen penetrates these barriers or colonizes them. An intact skin prevents most pathogens from entering the body. But when the integrity of the skin is breached as in burn victims (due to skin loss), and in wounds, infection poses a major problem.

Mucus, a viscous fluid secreted by membranes which line inner body surfaces, is an important protective barrier. It prevents bacteria from adhering to epithelial cells. Besides, due to its adhesive properties, it entraps microbes which can then be expelled by coughing, sneezing, and ciliary movement.

Presence of fatty acids in sweat and sebaceous secretions lowers the pH. This has an inhibitory effect on many bacteria. *Acid pH* of the stomach and also *digestive enzymes* constitute a major barrier. Washing action of tears and saliva, and also peristaltic movements in the gut, help to remove pathogens from the body.

A different kind of mechanism is the competition on epithelial surfaces between *normal bacterial flora (commensals)* and pathogenic microbes for essential nutrients and attachment sites. Normal flora is beneficial as it prevents growth of many pathogens. Therapy with antibiotics causes overgrowth of pathogens as non-pathogenic flora is killed.

Epithelial surfaces are not merely physical barriers as they also produce potent microbicidal substances.

Lysozyme, a bactericidal enzyme present in tears, nasal secretions, and saliva cleaves the peptidoglycan walls of many bacteria. *Antimicrobial proteins* which represent an important part of innate immune defence include *defensins* and *cathelicidins*. Defensins are cationic peptides which have 29–40 amino acid residues and are rich in arginine. Cytoplasmic granules of neutrophils and also paneth cells which are found at the base of the crypts in the intestine contain α-defensins. These are secreted into the intestine where they function to prevent bacterial overgrowth. Epithelial cells in respiratory tract and skin produce β-defensins abundantly. Defensins can kill a wide variety of bacteria through pore formation in the microbial membrane. Cathelicidins, too, like defensins mediate microbial killing by damaging bacterial membranes. They are most abundant in neutrophil granules and are constitutively expressed in many tissues, such as intestine and liver.

Epithelia including both skin and mucosal surfaces contain *intraepithelial lymphocytes (IELs)* which are cells of the T cell lineage. They, however, represent a distinct category of T cells and differ from conventional T cells which are abundant in peripheral blood and lymphoid organs (see Chapter 3). They function in innate host defence by secreting cytokines such as interferon (IFN)-γ and activating macrophages.

The barriers described above contribute to effective host innate immunity, but if an infectious microbe does succeed in passing through epithelial surfaces and gains access into the body, it has to face other protective mechanisms. Those called into play include various soluble proteins and cellular defences. An important event is activation of the *complement* cascade which yields inflammatory mediators that recruit phagocytic cells from blood vessels to infected sites. This is described in the following section.

NON-CELLULAR COMPONENTS OF INNATE IMMUNITY

Various soluble components described in the text that follows are involved in innate defence against microbes.

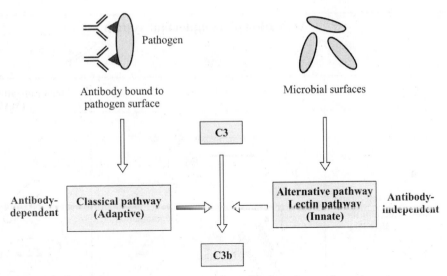

Fig. 2.2 Complement activation. The alternative and lectin pathways of complement activation provide nonspecific innate immunity, whereas the classical pathway is linked to the adaptive immune system.

Complement Proteins

These comprise a group of serum proteins/glycoproteins synthesized mostly by liver cells. They circulate in blood in an inactive form and respond rapidly to microbes. Their activation is a cascade reaction, similar to the blood coagulation system, with each component sequentially acting on others (see Chapter 11). The complement system, like antibody, is an important component of humoral immunity. There are three distinct pathways leading to complement activation: *classical pathway*, *alternative pathway*, and the *lectin pathway*. The central event in activation of the complement system is the conversion of the most abundant complement protein C3 to C3b (Fig. 2.2).

The complement system can be activated by the following factors:

Binding of Antibodies to the Pathogen Surface

This activates the classical pathway (adaptive). It is to be remembered that the classical pathway of complement cannot recognize pathogens directly, and it is only with the help of an antibody that complement proteins are guided to the microbe.

Microbial Surfaces

Acute-phase proteins such as *C-reactive protein (CRP)* and *mannose-binding lectin (MBL)*, described in the text that follows, bind to microbial surfaces and activate the alternative and lectin pathways, respectively, independent of the antibody (innate).

Complement proteins perform many important functions in innate defence, some of which are depicted in Fig. 2.3. These include the following functions:

Clearance of pathogens C3b a product of complement activation deposits on the pathogen surface and marks it as foreign for phagocytic cells. As phagocytes have receptors for C3b, they recognize the pathogen and engulf it. It is reminded here that molecules such as complement and also antibody which enhance phagocytosis are called opsonins and the coating of microbes with opsonins is termed opsonization.

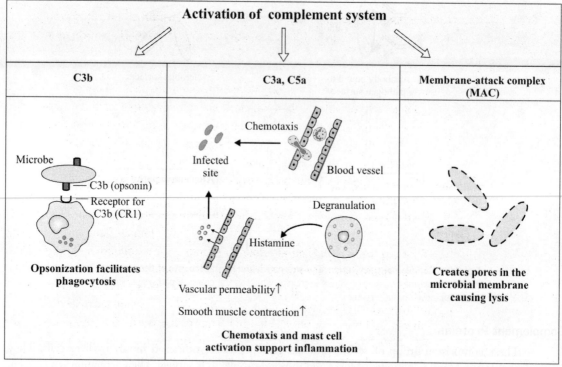

Fig. 2.3 **Role of complement proteins.** Activation of complement system yields products that have important roles in opsonization (C3b), inflammation (C3a, C5a), and microbial lysis (MAC). C3a and C5a are complement breakdown products.

Activation of inflammation Inflammation is a protective response to tissue injury/infection in which various defensive cells and molecules accumulate at infected sites being drawn from blood vessels. C3a and C5a have a major role in attracting phagocytes from blood vessels to the infected area (chemotaxis). They induce degranulation of mast cells at affected sites. The histamine released increases capillary permeability and smooth muscle contraction promoting inflammatory reactions. The events in inflammation are described in a later part of this chapter.

Cell lysis All pathways of complement activation finally lead to formation of a macromolecular structure called the *membrane attack complex (MAC)*. This forms a channel in the lipid bilayer of the target cell. Disruption of the hydrophobic barrier leads to disturbed ionic gradients and, consequently, cell death.

Additionally, the complement system (adaptive) has a major role in the clearance of immune complexes (ICs). It is relevant to mention here that the system is tightly controlled by many regulatory proteins. This is necessary as uncontrolled complement activation can cause undue damage to nearby host cells and tissues. Complement proteins and their roles are described in greater detail in Chapter 11.

Acute-phase Proteins

These proteins are produced by hepatocytes in response to infection and help in bacterial clearance. Their production increases during the *acute inflammatory response*, a defensive mechanism that takes place in infected tissues (the term 'acute' indicates that the response is of short duration). Its aim is to rid the body of the foreign invader. The response which is localized at the infected site may also affect distant regions in which case it is *systemic* and is termed the *systemic acute-phase response* (Fig. 2.4).

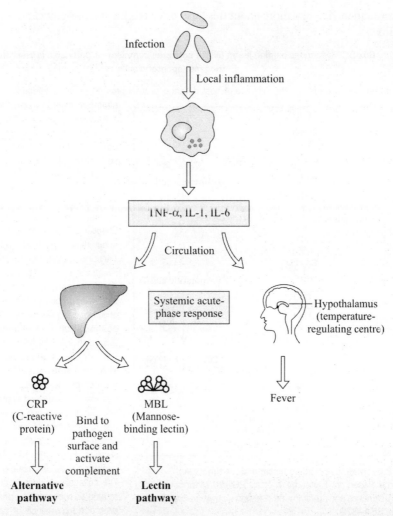

Fever

Fig. 2.4 **Systemic acute-phase response.** This accompanies local inflammation and is marked by production of acute-phase proteins (CRP and MBL) and induction of fever.

Whereas the local response is characterized by entry of neutrophils and monocytes/macrophages into infected sites, the systemic response is marked by synthesis of *acute-phase proteins*. Cytokines that induce their synthesis include tumour necrosis factor (TNF)-α, interleukin (IL)-1, and IL-6 released by activated macrophages at injured sites into the circulation. These cytokines, besides inducing synthesis of APPs, also induce fever by acting on the hypothalamus. Some APPs include CRP and MBL. C-reactive protein binds to phosphorylcholine on bacterial surfaces and activates complement via the alternative pathway. It belongs to the *pentraxin* family, members of which are pentameric proteins in which five identical polypeptides are held together by non-covalent forces. Its level may increase 1,000-fold during an immune response. Mannose-binding lectin is a member of the *collectin* family of proteins. It has multiple subunits, each having a collagenous tail and a globular head. It binds to mannose residues and initiates the lectin pathway of complement activation. Besides, it has a key role in the clearance of cells that have undergone *apoptosis* (Box 2.1). This is a form of cell death (*programmed cell death* or *PCD*) in which apoptotic cells are cleared by phagocytosis without inducing inflammation. There is more about this form of cell death and its significance in the immune system in Box 3.1.

Box 2.1 Mannose-binding lectin (MBL) activates complement and helps in clearance of pathogens/apoptotic cells

The innate immune system, the first line of host defence, protects not only against infectious microbes and apoptotic cells but also from damaged self-tissues. It recognizes targets through pattern-recognition receptors which may be soluble molecules or receptors on the surface of cells of innate immunity. Some receptors are also located intracellularly. MBL is a soluble pattern-recognition molecule and is structurally homologous to the complement protein C1q (see Chapter 11). It is composed of trimeric subunits having a lectin globular domain. Through this, it recognizes mannose residues in carbohydrates in the cell walls of many microorganisms, and also in apoptotic cells that arise during physiological processes. This facilitates opsonization and phagocytosis (Fig. 2.5). Deficiency of MBL is a risk factor for infectious diseases. Binding of MBL to bacterial surfaces activates the complement system via the lectin pathway. Host cells stay protected from MBL binding and complement activation due to presence of sialic acid residues. These block access of MBL to terminal sugars. However, MBL can bind to apoptotic cells as these lose sialic acid. The collagenous domain of MBL is free to bind to receptors on phagocytic cells promoting clearance of apoptotic cells and also pathogens by phagocytosis.

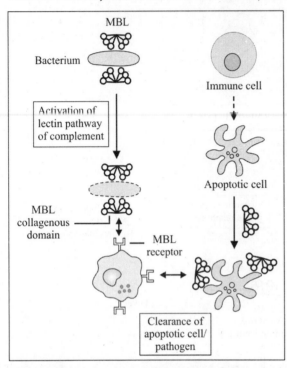

Fig. 2.5 Mannose-binding lectin and its functions.
Source: Based on: Tsutsumi, A. et al. (2005), 'Mannose binding lectin: Genetics and autoimmune disease', *Autoimmunity Reviews*, 4, pp. 364–372.

Interferons

Interferons represent a family of cytokines which include type I (IFN-α/IFN-β) and type II (IFN-γ) interferons. Type I IFNs, released by virally-infected cells, dendritic cells, and also macrophages, provide defence against many viruses by making nearby cells resistant to viral infection (see Fig. 12.3). This limits viral spread. Besides, they activate NK cells to kill virally-infected cells. Interferon-γ is produced by T lymphocytes and also NK cells. Although all three cytokines induce an antiviral state in cells, type I IFNs have strong antiviral action whereas IFN-γ has a more important role in regulation of immune responses (see Box 7.2). Other major cytokines of innate immunity are depicted in Fig. 2.8.

CELLULAR DEFENCES AGAINST INFECTION

The major effector cells of the innate immune system and their specialized roles in host defence are described in the following text. Though eosinophils and basophils contribute somewhat to innate defence, they have more important roles in adaptive immune responses.

Neutrophils

They represent 50–70 per cent of circulating white blood cells (WBCs) and are highly motile polymorphonuclear phagocytes. Neutrophil granules fail to stain well with basic or acidic dyes and, hence, they can be distinguished from basophils and eosinophils. They migrate from blood vessels into tissues particularly to inflammatory sites where they ingest foreign material. Neutrophils are short-lived cells and die soon after digesting and destroying the foreign matter. Figure 2.6 depicts a neutrophil ingesting anthrax bacteria.

Microbicidal substances and hydrolytic enzymes in neutrophils are contained in granules which are of two types:

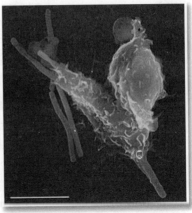

Fig. 2.6   Scanning electron micrograph (SEM) of a single neutrophil engulfing anthrax bacteria.

- Primary azurophil granules (a type of lysosome) which develop early and contain acid hydrolases, myeloperoxidase (MPO), and non-oxidative antimicrobial agents such as defensins, lysozyme, and bactericidal permeability increasing (BPI) protein.
- Secondary specific granules, which are smaller and more abundant, contain lactoferrin, most of the lysozyme, and proteolytic enzymes such as collagenase and elastase which can destroy different types of bacteria.

Both types of granules fuse with the phagosome and release their contents which help to digest the ingested matter. Phagocytosis and intracellular killing in neutrophils is described in a later section.

Neutrophils, unlike macrophages, do not produce TNF-α and have no antigen-presenting ability. They express FcγRs which recognize immunoglobulin G (IgG). The role of these receptors in promoting phagocytosis was introduced earlier in Chapter 1 and is described in greater detail in Chapter 11. When the target is too large to be phagocytosed, killing is extracellular unlike the intracellular killing in phagocytosis. This is called *antibody-dependent cell-mediated cytotoxicity (ADCC;* see Chapter 11). Besides, neutrophils express receptors for C3b, a product of complement activation that serves as opsonin, and also *PRRs* (such as toll-like receptors, TLRs) that recognize molecular patterns on microbes.

Neutrophils are the major cells involved in the inflammatory response to infection. They are the first cells to arrive at sites of inflammation followed by monocytes. We will learn more about the involvement of neutrophils in inflammation in the second half of this chapter.

Macrophages

Monocytes in blood and macrophages in tissues constitute the mononuclear phagocytic system. Macrophages are found at various sites in the body. They are either fixed in tissues, such as *Kupffer cells* in the liver or they may be wandering and highly motile, such as alveolar and peritoneal macrophages. They are also found fixed along the walls of blood and lymph vessels where they help to clear foreign material. Macrophage-like cells found in various tissues differ in both appearance and function and are known by specialized names (Table 2.1).

Lysosomal granules are very prominent in macrophages. They contain acid hydrolases and other digestive enzymes which destroy engulfed foreign material such as dead cells, immune complexes, antigen, or a pathogen. The steps in phagocytosis by both neutrophils and macrophages and mechanism of destruction of intracellular pathogens are essentially similar. Macrophages too, like neutrophils, express PRRs and receptors for opsonins. These have an important role in promoting phagocytosis and in signalling (see the text that follows).

Table 2.1 **Macrophage-like cells in various tissues.** Macrophages take up residence in tissues as fixed macrophages. They are known by specialized names according to their tissue location.

Macrophage-like cells	Location in body
Kupffer cells	Liver
Mesangial cells	Kidney
Microglial cells	Brain
Osteoclasts	Bone
Alveolar macrophages	Lung
Splenic macrophages	Spleen (white pulp)
Synovial macrophages	Synovial joint
Histiocytes	Connective tissue

Macrophages release TNF-α, IL-1, and IL-6 under the influence of bacterial products such as *lipopolysaccharide (LPS)* of Gram-negative bacteria. Although TNF-α plays a major role in containing local infection, it causes harm in excess. *Septic shock* is a severe clinical condition caused by systemic Gram-negative bacterial infections and is due to excess TNF-α production by macrophages. The condition is marked by a drop in BP (shock) and intravascular coagulation (see Chapter 7).

Eosinophils

Eosinophils represent about 2–5 per cent of blood leukocytes in a healthy individual. They have a bilobed nucleus and many cytoplasmic granules which stain with acidic dyes such as eosin. The major role of eosinophils is in defence against large parasites such as helminths, which, due to their large size cannot be phagocytosed. Many helminths trigger the alternative pathway of complement activation, and C3b deposited on their surface allows them to adhere to eosinophils via C3b receptors expressed on the eosinophil surface. This triggers degranulation which involves fusion of intracellular granules with the plasma membrane and release of cytotoxic granule contents such as *major basic protein (MBP)* which is toxic for helminths. The number of circulating and tissue eosinophils increases (eosinophilia) in parasite infections and allergy. They accumulate at sites of parasite infection, and also allergic reactions such as in lungs in persisting asthma—a type I hypersensitivity reaction (see Chapter 14). This process is promoted by cytokines released by T helper cells. Like neutrophils, eosinophils also express Fc receptors for both IgG (FcγR) and IgE (FcεR). Binding of eosinophils to antibody-coated targets also triggers degranulation. Although phagocytosis is not the primary function of eosinophils, they are capable of some phagocytosis and intracellular microbial killing.

Mast Cells/Basophils

Basophils are non-phagocytic cells which constitute less than 1 per cent of total WBCs. Their cytoplasm is densely granulated and stains with basic dyes such as methylene blue. They originate in the bone marrow in the same way as mast cells. Although basophils mature also in the bone marrow, maturation of mast cells occurs in tissues to which they migrate from the blood stream. Mast cells are generally found close to epithelia, blood vessels, and nerves, and also in gastrointestinal tract near smooth muscle cells and mucus-producing glands. Both mast cells and basophils have abundant granules containing histamine and other mediators in their cytoplasm. Mast cells can be triggered to release mediators during inflammatory reactions on binding of complement split products C3a and C5a to their surface receptors. Degranulation is also stimulated when antigen (allergen) cross-links specific IgE molecules bound to Fc receptors (FcεR) on the mast cell surface. The release of pharmacological mediators causes unpleasant symptoms of allergy (Chapter 14). Both mast cells and basophils release IL-4.

Natural Killer Cells

Natural killer cells belong to the lymphoid lineage and represent up to 15 per cent of blood lymphocytes (mean number = 2,600 μl^{-1}). Their name derives from the fact that NK cells can spontaneously kill their targets, which include virally-infected cells and tumour cells, without the need to undergo prior antigen-specific activation. In this respect they differ from cytotoxic T cells which require activating signals before they acquire the machinery to kill. Another important difference to be remembered is that while NK cells recognize class I MHC-negative targets, binding to peptide-associated class I MHC molecules is very essential for activation of cytotoxic T cells. It is only when MHC molecules are downregulated, as may occur in virally-infected cells and tumour cells, that susceptibility to killing by NK cells increases.

Although NK cells do not bear antigen-specific receptors as do B and T lymphocytes, they are able to distinguish their targets from normal host cells (Fig. 2.7).

There are two types of receptors expressed on NK cells:

Activating Receptors

They are lectins (carbohydrate-binding proteins) that interact with glycoproteins on the surface of cells infected by virus. This delivers an activating signal which by itself can trigger killing of the target cell to which an NK cell binds.

Inhibitory Receptors

Their ligands are class I MHC molecules. Receptor-ligand interaction delivers inhibitory signals which block cytotoxic activity of the NK cell. Virally-infected cells or tumour cells which have downregulated

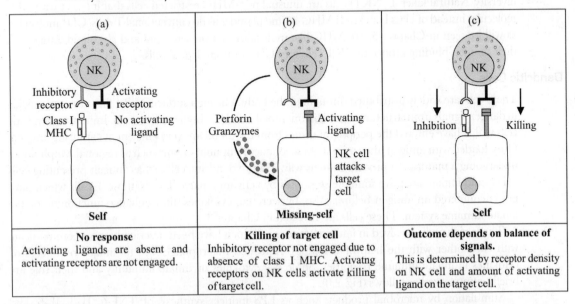

(a)	(b)	(c)
No response	**Killing of target cell**	**Outcome depends on balance of signals.**
Activating ligands are absent and activating receptors are not engaged.	Inhibitory receptor not engaged due to absence of class I MHC. Activatng receptors on NK cells activate killing of target cell.	This is determined by receptor density on NK cell and amount of activating ligand on the target cell.

Fig. 2.7 Missing-self hypothesis and NK cell killing. Absence of class I MHC molecules ('missing-self') on target cells (as in tumour cells and virally-infected cells) triggers killing by NK cells (b). Engagement of inhibitory receptors on NK cells by class I MHC dampens signals transduced through activating receptors (c).
Source: Based on Lanier, L.L. (2005), 'NK cell recognition', *Annual Review of Immunology*, 23, pp. 225–274.

class I MHC molecules ('missing-self') fail to deliver inhibitory signals leading to death of these cells by the lectin-carbohydrate interaction.

When both receptors are engaged, outcome depends on the balance of signals. Generally, the inhibitory influence predominates and NK cells are not activated to kill. Thus, healthy host cells stay protected.

Natural killer cells mediate killing through a *perforin/granzyme* pathway and another pathway mediated through *Fas* in which proteases called *caspases* are activated resulting in apoptotic death of the target cell. These mechanisms are comparable to mechanisms used by cytotoxic T cells to kill their targets and are described in Chapter 9.

Antibody-dependent cell-mediated cytotoxicity is an alternative mechanism used by NK cells to kill target cells, and provides an important link with adaptive immunity. As NK cells express FcγRs (FcγRIII) which interact with Fc tails of IgG, they can mediate ADCC (see Fig. 11.6).

Natural killer cells are a potent source of IFN-γ. Their activity is enhanced by

- type I IFNs produced by virus-infected cells,
- IL-12 secreted by activated macrophages and dendritic cells, and
- IL-2.

Natural killer cells activated in vitro with IL-2 are called *lymphokine-activated killer (LAK) cells*. They are being extensively studied for use in cancer immunotherapy (see Chapter 18).

NKT Cells

These cells are so called as they express markers common to both T lymphocytes and NK cells. They are part of innate defence mechanisms and are considered to be involved in protective responses against bacterial infections. Their precise role remains to be understood. In common with T lymphocytes, they express αβ T cell receptor (TCR) complexes on their surface, but the TCR α chains have limited diversity. Natural killer T (NKT) cells are unusual non-MHC restricted cells that interact with CD1 molecules instead of class I or class II MHC-bound peptides as do conventional T cells. CD1 molecules, as will be seen in Chapter 5, are MHC-like molecules that present lipid and glycolipid antigens in their antigen-binding groove to NKT cells and CD1-restricted γδ T cells.

Dendritic Cells

These cells are widely distributed throughout the body. Through surface TLRs, they respond quickly to danger signals from structures found on microbial cells but absent on host cells. Immature dendritic cells which have entered the peripheral tissues from the blood are very efficient at capturing antigen. Once loaded with antigen, they migrate to secondary lymphoid organs such as regional lymph nodes undergoing a maturation process on their way. Mature dendritic cells act as antigen-presenting cells (APC) and initiate adaptive immune responses by activating naïve T cells (those T cells which have not encountered an antigen before). Also, by secreting cytokines, they enhance functioning of the innate immune system. These cells are revisited in Chapter 3.

The various cells involved in innate defence and which have been described earlier communicate with each other with the help of cytokines. Activated macrophages are the major producers of cytokines in innate immune responses. Some key cytokines of innate immunity and their role are briefly summarized as follows (Fig. 2.8).

Stimulation by microbial products such as LPS induces synthesis of TNF-α, IL-1, IL-6, and *chemokines* (chemoattractant cytokines) such as IL-8 by activated macrophages. These perform several roles in host defence. In inflammation, they are the major cytokines that recruit polymorphonuclear neutrophils (PMNs) and monocytes to infected sites. But when produced in excess, they can have

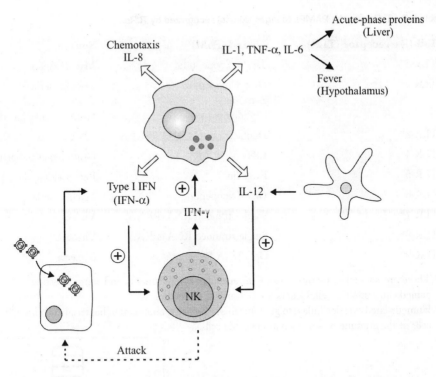

Fig. 2.8 Major cytokines of innate immunity. IFN-γ is involved in both innate and adaptive immunity.

disastrous effects. IL-12, also produced by macrophages in response to LPS, activates NK cells to release IFN-γ which, in turn, stimulates macrophages. Note that IFN-γ is also produced by T lymphocytes and is involved in both innate and adaptive immune responses. As described earlier, macrophages, dendritic cells, and also virally-infected cells produce type I IFNs which restrain spread of virus to adjacent uninfected cells (see Fig. 1.14) and activate NK cells to kill virally-infected cells.

PATTERN-RECOGNITION RECEPTORS OF THE INNATE IMMUNE SYSTEM

The innate immune system can detect the presence of microbes with the help of PRRs which are expressed in macrophages, dendritic cells, neutrophils, and many other cell types. Pattern-recognition receptors recognize conserved molecular structures in microbes called *pathogen-associated molecular patterns (PAMPs)* which are absent in mammalian cells. These receptors are encoded in the germline and have limited diversity, unlike the highly diverse antigen receptors on T and B lymphocytes. One such family of PRRs is represented by the *TLRs* of which more than 10 have been identified in mammals. The toll receptor was first identified in the fruit fly *Drosophilia melanogaster* in which it plays an important role in embryogenesis. Besides, it performs signalling functions in the adult fruit fly in response to infection. Several proteins homologous to toll were later identified in mammals. These evolutionary conserved receptors can recognize and be stimulated by different molecular patterns (PAMPs) found only in microbes, such as LPS and peptidoglycan (Table 2.2).

Different TLRs recognize different molecular patterns on microbes which allow detection of a wide range of pathogens by the immune system. They have very rightly been called 'sentinels of innate immunity' (Fig. 2.9).

Table 2.2   TLRs and the PAMPs (danger signals) recognized by TLRs.

Toll-like receptor (TLR)	Ligand (PAMP)	Source
TLR-1	Triacyl lipopeptide	Mycobacteria
TLR-2	Diacyl lipopeptide Zymosan Peptidoglycan	Mycobacteria Fungi Gram-positive bacteria
TLR-3*	Double-stranded RNA (dsRNA)	RNA viruses
TLR-4	LPS	Gram-negative bacteria
TLR-5	Flagellin	Bacterial flagella
TLR-6	Diacyl lipopeptide	Mycobacteria
TLR-7*	Single-stranded RNA (ssRNA)	Viruses
TLR-8*	Single-stranded RNA (ssRNA)	Viruses
TLR-9*	CpG DNA **	Bacteria

* These are located in membranes of intracellular compartments and sense infectious microbes that have gained entry into the cell. Others are cell surface molecules.

** Unmethylated cytosine linked to guanine; this sequence is abundant in bacterial and viral DNA and activates cells of the immune system such as dendritic cells.

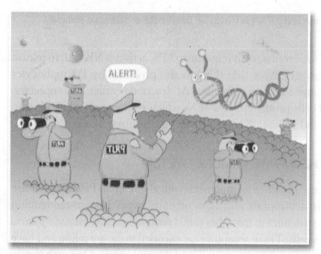

Fig. 2.9   Toll-like receptors: the sentinels of the innate immune system. Toll-like receptors (TLRs) play a critical role in activating early innate immunity which is necessary before adaptive immune responses are activated.
Source: Accessed from http://www.invivogen.com/ressource.php?ID=12 on 4 August 2010.

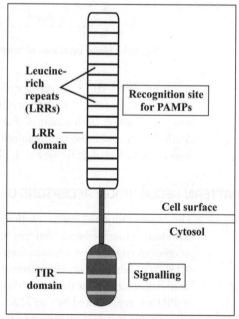

Fig. 2.10   Structure of a typical toll-like receptor (TLR). Different TLRs differ in their extracellular domain.

The structure of a typical TLR is shown in Fig. 2.10. The extracellular region has *leucine-rich repeats (LRRs)*, whereas the cytoplasmic domain is homologous to that of the IL-1 receptor and is called Toll/IL-1 receptor (TIR) domain. It is essential for cell signalling. Different TLRs differ structurally due to differences in number and arrangement of LRRs.

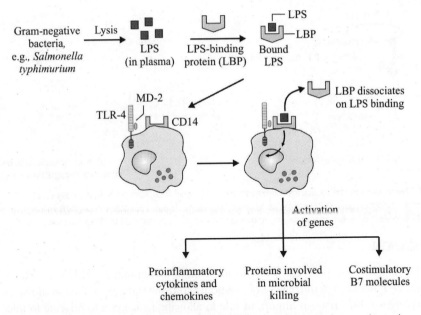

Fig. 2.11 LPS is a potent stimulator of macrophages. Stimulation of macrophages by LPS generates signals that stimulate both innate and adaptive immunity.

The effect of bacterial LPS in macrophages is mediated through a membrane protein CD14 which delivers LPS to TLR-4 (Fig. 2.11). MD-2 is an accessory protein associated with the extracellular domain of TLR-4 and is essential for LPS-induced signalling. Interaction of TLR-4 with LPS delivers signals to the cell nucleus resulting in activation of the transcription factor NFκB. This turns on genes encoding proteins that provide defence against invading pathogens including genes that encode proinflammatory cytokines and chemokines. Genes encoding costimulatory B7 molecules are also activated, which promote adaptive immune responses.

Besides TLRs, there are other receptors in the category of PRRs that recognize PAMPs. *Mannose receptors (MRs)* are lectins that recognize mannose in glycoproteins and glycolipids in microbial cell walls. Another PRR type with an important role is the *scavenger receptor (SR)* which helps in clearance of cell debris and apoptotic cells. Inability to clear apoptotic cells triggers inflammation and autoimmune reactions. Whereas TLRs are involved in signalling, MRs and SRs directly stimulate phagocytosis without the need for opsonins. They are unlike the *opsonic receptors* which can only recognize pathogens that have been coated with opsonins, namely, antibody and complement. Opsonic receptors include FcγR and CR1 which are receptors for IgG and C3b, respectively. Pattern-recognition receptors and opsonic receptors are represented in Fig. 2.12.

Recent evidence has shown the existence of an intracellular cytosolic mode of bacterial detection. This includes the *Nod family of receptor proteins* which detects different bacterial components and toxins. Two members of this family of proteins Nod1 and Nod2 recognize bacterial peptidoglycan. Whereas TLRs are membrane-bound and represent a mode of defence at the plasma membrane, Nod proteins sense danger signals in the cytosol.

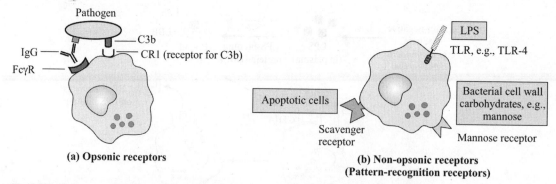

Fig. 2.12   Receptors of the innate immune system. (a) Opsonic receptors: Phagocytic cells express receptors for opsonins that promote phagocytosis. (b) Pattern-recognition receptors: These receptors recognize PAMPs on microbes. TLR-4 is involved in signalling whereas mannose and scavenger receptors directly lead to phagocytosis.

INFLAMMATION

The chapter now proceeds to events involved in inflammation. This is a protective response of the innate immune system triggered in response to tissue damage/infection in the body. As *cell adhesion molecules (CAMs)* play an important role in allowing leukocytes to migrate to infected sites, they are briefly introduced before describing the sequence of events that lead to an inflammatory response.

Cell Adhesion Molecules

Cell adhesion molecules are cell surface glycoproteins which facilitate adhesive interactions with other cells, in the circulation, in lymphoid tissues, or in the extracellular matrix (ECM). They have a role in

- differential migration of leukocytes from bloodstream into different tissues where the foreign body is present or to lymphoid tissues (*trafficking/homing*); this involves specific adhesive interactions between endothelial cells and leukocytes in which *homing receptors* play an important role (see Chapters 3 and 9); and
- cell-to-cell communication and activation of immune responses, e.g., during APC and Tн cell interactions leading to T cell activation.

Cell adhesion molecules are grouped into four major families (Fig. 2.13). These include

- integrins,
- mucin-like CAMs,
- selectins, and
- immunoglobulin superfamily CAMs.

Some representative members in each family are shown in Table 2.3. Adhesion molecules are expressed differently on various cell types. Some are constitutively expressed, whereas others are induced, such as during acute inflammation in response to cytokines released on cell activation.

Table 2.3   Cell adhesion molecule (CAM) families with representative members.

Integrins	Mucin-like CAMs	Selectins	Immunoglobulin superfamily CAMs
LFA-1 (β_2)	PSGL-1	L - Selectin	ICAM-1, -2, -3
VLA-4 (β_1)	GlyCAM-1	P - Selectin	LFA-2 (CD2)
VLA-6 (β_1)		E - Selectin	VCAM-1

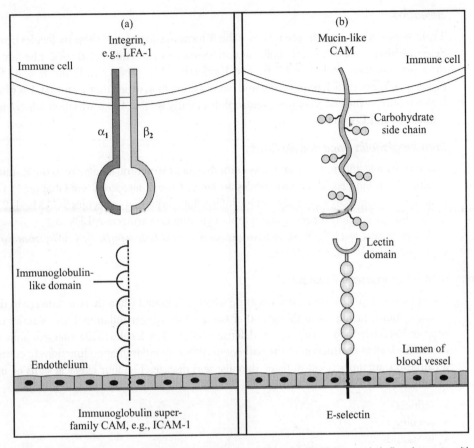

Fig. 2.13 Some selected cell adhesion molecules (CAMs). (a) ICAM-1 on endothelium interacts with LFA-1 ($\alpha_1\beta_2$ integrin) on neutrophils (and also lymphocytes and monocytes). (b) Lectin domain of E-selectin on the endothelium interacts with mucin-like CAMs on neutrophils.

Integrins

These are heterodimers composed of α and β subunits which are non-covalently associated with each other. Based on structure of the β subunits, there are five families which include β_1–β_5 integrins. The β_2 integrins which bind to molecules of the Ig superfamily play a major role in leukocyte–endothelial cell interactions. A noteworthy feature of integrins is that they exist in active and inactive states. Conformational changes occur on activation which increase affinity of integrins for their ligands. In *leukocyte adhesion deficiency (LAD)-type 1*, an inherited disease, leukocytes are unable to migrate to infected sites due to impaired integrin expression. Bacterial infections are common in such patients (see Chapter 16).

Mucin-like CAMs

They are extensively glycosylated proteins having an extended structure. The carbohydrate side chains provide binding sites for selectins, for example, GlyCAM-1 on endothelial cells binds to L-selectin on leukocytes, whereas PSGL-1 on neutrophils interacts with E- and P-selectin expressed on inflamed endothelium.

Selectins

Their name derives from the resemblance the *N*-terminal domains of these molecules bear with lectins. Selectins bind to carbohydrate molecules on leukocytes and endothelial cells. The family comprises three glycoproteins, including L-, P-, and E-selectins. The prefixes L, P, and E stand for leukocyte, platelet, and endothelial, respectively, and denote the cells in which they were first described. P-selectin is also found on the endothelium. Neutrophils in early stages of extravasation adhere to endothelial cells via P- and E-selectins.

Immunoglobulin Superfamily CAMs

Like many molecules in the immune system, they bear structural similarity to the distinctive domain structure found in Igs. All such molecules are part of the *Ig superfamily* (see Chapter 4). Cell adhesion molecules belonging to this family include intercellular adhesion molecules (ICAMs)-1, 2 and 3 which are binding targets for integrins, and lymphocyte function antigen-2 (LFA-2) .

It is to be noted that integrin family molecules generally bind to Ig superfamily CAMs, whereas members of the selectin family bind to mucin-like CAMs.

Events in an Inflammatory Response

Inflammation is a local protective response which is initiated when there is damage to tissues caused by a cut, burn, or infection, though other causes, too, trigger inflammation. A series of events are activated which help to recruit various defensive cells and molecules to the infected/injured site. These eventually lead to destruction of the pathogen. Although inflammation functions to control infection, it can also sometimes result in tissue damage and disease. The four classical signs of inflammation include

- redness,
- swelling,
- heat, and
- pain.

The various events in an inflammatory response are outlined as follows:

Release of Inflammatory Mediators

These are substances released from damaged host cells, mast cells, leukocytes, and other auxilliary cells. They also include complement breakdown products and bacterial products. Many mediators exert overlapping effects (Table 2.4).

Inflammatory mediators can diffuse away from the site of release due to their small size establishing a concentration gradient with the highest concentration at the site of production. This concentration gradient is important for drawing neutrophils from the blood to the infected site.

Vascular Changes

Endothelial cells respond to inflammatory mediators in various ways:

- They increase expression of adhesion molecules on their luminal surface.
- They assume a more rounded appearance which creates gaps between adjacent cells.
- They secrete cytokines which influence the inflammatory response.

Histamine is a key mediator released from mast cells. It causes vasodilation (increase in diameter of blood vessels) and increases capillary permeability at the injured site allowing more blood to flow into

Table 2.4 Major mediators of the acute inflammatory response.

Inflammatory mediator	Action
Histamine	Vasodilation Increased vascular permeability Upregulation of adhesion molecules on endothelium
C5a*	Increased vascular permeability
C3a*	Upregulation of adhesion molecules on endothelium and neutrophils Neutrophil chemotaxis
IL-8	Upregulation of adhesion molecules on neutrophils Neutrophil chemotaxis
Leukotriene B4 (LTB4)	Increased vascular permeability Upregulation of adhesion molecules on neutrophils Neutrophil chemotaxis
f Met. Leu. Phe. **	Increased vascular permeability Upregulation of adhesion molecules on neutrophils Neutrophil chemotaxis
PGD$_2$	Vasodilation Neutrophil chemotaxis Increased vascular permeability
IL-1 TNF-α	Upregulation of adhesion molecules on endothelium and neutrophils

* Complement breakdown products produced on complement activation.
** A sequence of three amino acids : formyl methionine, leucine, and phenylalanine (fMLP), and is a bacterial product.
Note: PGD$_2$ (a prostaglandin) and LTB4 (a leukotriene) are lipids derived from arachidonic acid in many cell types such as mast cells.

the area. This results in heating and reddening in the affected tissue. Plasma brings with it complement, antibodies, and other protective molecules to the target site. The pain that accompanies inflammation is due to pressure on sensory nerve endings by the swollen tissues, damage to nerve endings by bacterial toxins, and *bradykinin*. This is a vasoactive mediator released by the *kinin system,* an enzyme system in the plasma which has a role in the inflammatory response. Corticosteroids which are well known anti-inflammatory agents are often administered in inflammation to reduce pain.

Recruitment of Phagocytic Cells

Many mediators are chemoattractants. They recruit phagocytic cells, predominantly neutrophils, to the infected site where they phagocytose microbes and destroy them intracellularly. Other cells, too, namely monocytes/macrophages, small numbers of eosinophils and basophils, and lymphocytes (at a later stage), accumulate at sites of infection. The migration of neutrophils and other leukocytes to infected sites is dependent on adhesion molecules which have been briefly described earlier.

Sequential Events in Neutrophil Migration

The different stages involved in movement of neutrophils to infected sites from blood vessels are depicted in Fig. 2.14 and are outlined as follows:

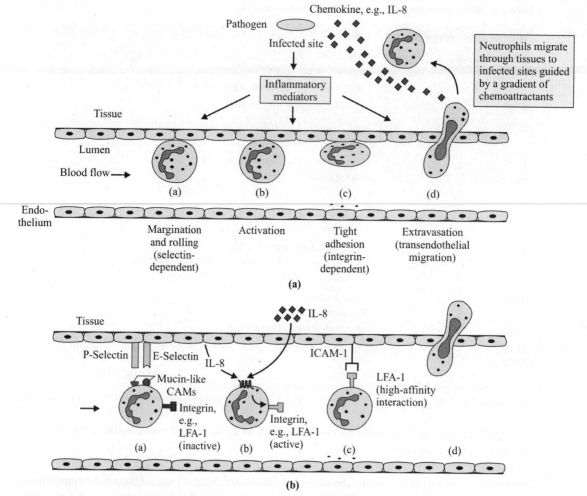

Fig. 2.14 Leukocyte migration from blood vessels to inflammatory sites. (a) Neutrophils move through tissues to infected sites by chemotaxis. (b) Interaction of leukocytes with endothelial cells mediated by CAMs is essential before they migrate out from the blood vessels.

Rolling

This depends on interactions between selectins expressed on inflamed endothelium with carbohydrate moieties on mucin-like CAMs on the neutrophil surface. Repeated formation and dissociation of these weak interactions cause neutrophils to roll on the endothelium.

Activation and Tight Adhesion

Binding of the chemokine IL-8 released by activated endothelium (and also macrophages) to receptors on neutrophils delivers activating signals. This induces conformational changes in the integrin LFA-1 due to which its affinity for ICAM-1 increases. This allows it to bind tightly to the endothelium.

Extravasation

Neutrophils which have stopped rolling due to firm binding to endothelial cells squeeze through gaps between endothelial cells and move into tissues. This escape into tissues of cells and fluid from the blood is referred to as *extravasation*, and the process of neutrophil (and also monocyte) exit from the blood vessel is called *diapedesis*.

Movement of Neutrophils to Sites of Inflammation

After squeezing through blood vessels, neutrophils move up a chemotactic gradient to the inflamed site where the pathogen is present. This process called *chemotaxis* is guided by IL-8 and low concentrations of inflammatory mediators such as C5a, fMLP, and LTB4. C5a is generated at the site of inflammation by complement activation, whereas LTB4 is produced by activated macrophages and mast cells. The bacterial product fMLP is an indicator of bacterial metabolism and represents a danger signal which is chemotactic for phagocytes. These mediators bind to specific receptors on neutrophils and contribute to directed migration and activation of these cells. Phagocytes are also attracted by molecules generated by the blood clotting system. Neutrophils on reaching the target site are activated by high concentration of mediators present at these sites where they eventually phagocytose the foreign matter.

Fever, a common and prominent feature of many infections, generally accompanies the inflammatory response and is due to excess secretion of IL-1 and also TNF-α and IL-6 from mononuclear phagocytes (see Fig. 2.4). These substances act on the thermoregulatory centre of the hypothalamus with resultant increase in body temperature. Fever-inducing substances (pyrogens) which are produced in the body are known as *endogenous pyrogens*, whereas bacterial components such as LPS are called *exogenous pyrogens*. Fever promotes body's defences in various ways such as by stimulating proliferation of antigen-activated lymphocytes and increasing bactericidal activity of phagocytic cells.

Healing Phase

After phagocytosing a large number of microbes and destruction of the invader, neutrophils die by apoptosis. Apoptotic cells are cleared by infiltrating macrophages, an essential step before the inflammatory site can be restored back to its original normal state. *Transforming growth factor (TGF)*-β is a major factor that plays a role in wound healing by stimulating division and proliferation of *fibroblasts*, cells with a distinctive elongated appearance which synthesize ECM proteins such as collagen. Enzyme systems in the plasma, such as the fibrinolytic (plasmin) system, have a major role in remodelling and regeneration of tissues. Plasmin dissolves fibrin and promotes formation of new blood vessels, a process called *angiogenesis*. Proliferation of fibroblasts and angiogenesis are two major events in the repair process and restoration of the pre-infective state.

PHAGOCYTOSIS AND INTRACELLULAR KILLING OF MICROBES

The phases involved in phagocytosis common to neutrophils and macrophages (Fig. 2.15) and intracellular killing mechanisms that lead to destruction of the pathogen (Fig. 2.16) are outlined as follows:

Phagocytosis

Phagocytosis is an important protective mechanism of the innate immune system. The way phagocytes internalize microbes is described here.

Adherence

Although many microbes adhere well to the surface of phagocytes and are readily phagocytosed, there are some microbes which are resistant. However, if coated with antibody and complement split product C3b, which bind to receptors on the phagocyte membrane, they are readily ingested.

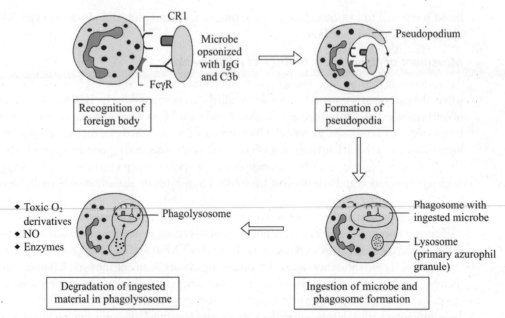

Fig. 2.15 Phagocytosis and microbial killing. For clarity, only one primary granule (enlarged) is shown.

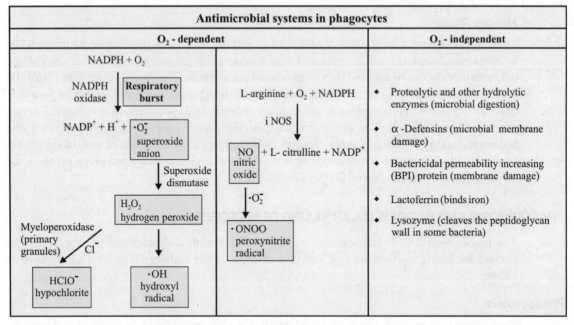

Fig. 2.16 Antimicrobial systems in phagocytic cells. Both O_2-dependent and O_2-independent mechanisms are involved in microbial killing (see main text for details). Each type of phagocyte differs slightly in the mix of killing mechanisms. Antimicrobial molecular species are shown in boxes.

Ingestion

After attachment of the microbe to the phagocyte surface, projections of the plasma membrane called pseudopodia extend around the microbe. These fuse and then pinch off from the plasma membrane into the cytoplasm forming a sac called a *phagocytic vesicle* or a *phagosome*. In phagocytes, lysosome fusion with the phagosome membrane forms a larger structure called the *phagolysosome* into which contents are released. Formation of the phagosome is important as it confines the microbe in a separate compartment where it can be subjected to killing by various toxic antimicrobial substances without causing damage to cytoplasmic contents.

Killing and Digestion

Killing of the ingested pathogen involves some major enzymes including

- *NADPH oxidase*, an enzyme present in the phagosome membrane, generates reactive oxygen intermediates (ROIs) which kill extracellular pathogens that have been phagocytosed,
- *Inducible nitric oxide synthase (iNOS)* present in the cytosol generates *nitric oxide (NO)* which defends against microbes present in the cytosol and in phagolysosome, and
- *Myeloperoxidase* present in primary granules converts Cl^- ions and H_2O_2 into hypochlorite ($HClO^-$), a potent antimicrobial agent.

Oxygen (O_2)-dependent and O_2-independent routes employed by phagocytes in microbial killing are discussed below.

Oxygen-dependent Mechanisms

When neutrophils and other phagocytic cells engulf bacteria, there is rapid increase in O_2 consumption and glucose oxidation. This increase in metabolism called the '*respiratory burst*' generates NADPH which is a substrate for the phagosomal enzyme NADPH oxidase. It catalyzes formation of superoxide anion ($\cdot O_2^-$) which generates other microbicidal products. The various reactive oxygen derivatives that are generated kill the bacteria in the phagolysosome. In *X-linked chronic granulomatous disease (CGD)*, there is diminished production of superoxide anion and other active derivatives of oxygen (see Chapter 16). Owing to this, bacterial killing is defective and patients suffer from frequent infections.

The production of superoxide anion by neutrophils indicates normal functioning and can be revealed by reduction of *nitroblue tetrazolium (NBT)*. The dye is yellow in the oxidized state, and on uptake by normal neutrophils, it is reduced to a blue-coloured product (formazan) in the phagolysosome (NBT test).

Nitric oxide generated in a reaction, catalyzed by inducible nitric oxide synthase, and also the peroxynitrite radical, contributes to antimicrobial activity of phagocytic cells. The enzyme (iNOS) is induced in phagocytes by various stimuli such as LPS which activates TLRs on macrophages, and exposure to certain cytokines.

Oxygen-independent Mechanisms

These include various enzymes, predominantly *acid hydrolases* present in lysosomal granules. The high pH in the lysosomes keeps these enzymes in an inactive state. Pumping of protons generated in the reaction catalyzed by NADPH oxidase (see above) into the phagosome by membrane enzymes reduces the pH to about 4.0. The low pH activates hydrolytic enzymes to kill and digest the microbe *Lysozyme* and also α-*defensins*, the cationic proteins in neutrophil granules, act within the phagolysosome. As described earlier, defensins have the ability to insert into microbial membranes and form pores killing ingested bacteria and fungi. Due to differences in membrane lipid composition, host cells stay protected. *Lactoferrin* present in secondary granules is bacteriostatic as it binds strongly to iron and makes it unavailable to bacteria.

After hydrolytic enzymes digest the killed microbe, degraded products are released to the exterior. Lysosomal digestion, besides being important for microbial killing, provides a pathway for antigen presentation in macrophages (but not in neutrophils). Proteolytic enzymes generate peptides which are displayed on the cell surface in association with MHC proteins providing signals for T cell activation.

In summary, O_2-dependent defences include reactive oxygen intermediates and reactive nitrogen intermediates. Oxygen-independent mechanisms increase the defences that phagocytes offer against microbes.

EVASION OF INNATE IMMUNITY BY MICROBES AND CHRONIC INFLAMMATION

Sometimes, the acute inflammatory response fails to clear the infectious agent, either due to a defective immune system or due to resistant microbes which are not easily degraded. A cell-mediated defence mechanism called *delayed-type hypersensitivity (DTH)* is activated against resistant intracellular pathogens (see Chapters 9 and 14). This is a chronic inflammatory reaction in which instead of neutrophils, $CD4^+$ T cells and mononuclear phagocytes increase in number at the inflamed site and play an important role.

Many bacteria are resistant to phagocytosis, and not all organisms engulfed trigger microbial killing mechanisms. For instance, capsular polysaccharides of *Pneumococcus* prevent phagocytosis. Some microbes have cell walls which are resistant to the contents of the lysosome, whereas others are resistant to attack by complement proteins. Catalase-producing organisms such as *Staphylococcus aureus* stay protected from ROIs produced in the phagosome. *Mycobacterium tuberculosis* prevents fusion of lysosomes and phagosomes and is able to proliferate inside macrophages within the phagosomes. There are other ways too, discussed in Chapter 12, by which some microbes cunningly resist innate defence mechanisms.

Owing to persisting pathogens/antigens, there is formation of a *granuloma* in which a lump resembling a tumour is seen to form (see Fig. 9.6). This is a hallmark of chronic inflammation and a manifestation of type IV hypersensitivity reactions. Granuloma formation which serves to isolate the resistant agent from the rest of the body occurs in tuberculosis and leprosy caused by mycobacteria. Eosinophil accumulation in parasite infections, such as by *Schistosoma mansoni*, and in the bronchial wall following asthmatic attacks are other instances of a chronic inflammatory reaction.

SUMMARY

- Various barriers provide the first line of defence against infection. These include external barriers such as epithelia and antimicrobial peptides, soluble proteins including complement proteins and acute-phase proteins, and cellular components such as phagocytes and NK cells.
- Complement proteins are activated sequentially by certain microbes (and by antibodies) to generate products that opsonize microbes for phagocytosis, stimulate inflammation, and lyse microbes.
- Acute-phase proteins are induced in hepatocytes in response to infection and include CRP and MBL. Both help in bacterial clearance by activating complement.
- Interferons are cytokines which interfere in viral infection and activate NK cells.

- Phagocytic cells include neutrophils and macrophages. They engulf foreign material and digest it intracellularly. Natural killer cells mediate early defence against viral infection by killing virally-infected cells.
- Dendritic cells represent an important link between innate and adaptive immunity.
- Cytokines of innate immunity include IL-1, IL-6, and TNF-α (stimulate inflammation), IL-12 (activates NK cells), IFN-γ (activates macrophages), and IFN-α/β (block viral infection).
- Innate immune system can detect broad classes of pathogens through a limited number of germline-encoded receptors called pattern-recognition receptors (PRRs). Toll-like receptors recognize various PAMPs and activate macrophages.

- Innate immune responses are important as they provide 'second signals' for activation of adaptive immune responses.
- Inflammation is a protective physiological response that brings leukocytes and plasma components (complement proteins, acute-phase proteins, and antibody) to infected/injured sites in tissues. Increase in vascular permeability facilitates movement of cells and fluid out of blood vessels.
- Arrival of leukocytes to inflammatory sites depends on chemokines and cell adhesion molecules (CAMs) expressed on endothelium.

- Phagocytosis of microbes at infected sites by neutrophils and macrophages involves ingestion, killing, and digestion of foreign material. Intracellular killing involves both O_2-dependent and O_2-independent mechanisms.
- Wound healing and regeneration of tissue restores the tissue to its normal state.
- Some microbes have evolved ways by which they can evade innate defence mechanisms. Persisting microbes stimulate chronic inflammatory reactions.

REVIEW QUESTIONS

1. Indicate whether the following statements are true or false. If false, explain why.
   (a) Acute inflammation is a non-specific event that occurs in response to any type of cellular injury.
   (b) NK cells bear receptors with specificity for class II MHC molecules.
   (c) NO is a product of activation of phagocyte NADPH oxidase.
   (d) Dendritic cells are involved in extracellular killing of target cells.
   (e) Generation of memory is not a feature of innate immunity.
   (f) LPS is a pattern-recognition receptor.

2. Self-assessment questions
   (a) A patient undergoing routine medical examination showed marked eosinophilia. What does this suggest?
   (b) What are the various mechanisms used by phagocytes to kill pathogens? How can functional activity of phagocytes be assessed?
   (c) NK cells do not bear antigen-specific receptors as do lymphocytes, yet they can recognize their targets. Explain how these cells distinguish normal host cells from target cells.
   (d) What are the basic steps involved in extravasation of polymorphonuclear neutrophils (PMNs) to infected sites?

   (e) How are toll-like receptors (TLRs) linked to both innate and adaptive immunity? Explain using TLR-4 as an example.

3. For each question, choose the *best* answer.
   (a) Killing by NK cells involves
      (i) interferons
      (ii) complement and perforins
      (iii) defensins
      (iv) perforins and proteases
   (b) Mast cells
      (i) express high-affinity receptors for IgE
      (ii) circulate in the blood stream
      (iii) can phagocytose microbes
      (iv) release IFN-γ
   (c) Which of the following is not used by macrophages to kill intracellular pathogens?
      (i) Proteolytic enzymes
      (ii) Nitric oxide
      (iii) Perforins
      (iv) H_2O_2
   (d) Of the following, what is not true for neutrophils?
      (i) Produce TNF-α
      (ii) Have C3b receptors
      (iii) Have NADPH oxidase
      (iv) Are phagocytic

The Lymphoid System and Cells of Adaptive Immunity

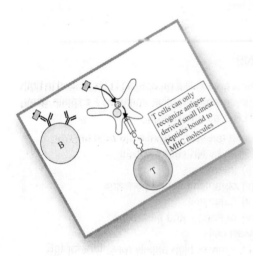

T cells can only recognize antigen-derived small linear peptides bound to MHC molecules

LEARNING OBJECTIVES

Having studied this chapter, you should be able to understand the following:

♦ The organization of the lymphoid system
♦ The different roles of primary and secondary lymphoid organs and tissues
♦ Major features and role of B cells and T cells and their types
♦ The way B and T cells differ in recognition of antigens and the role of MHC proteins
♦ The types and role of antigen-presenting cells
♦ The cooperation between the innate and adaptive immune systems to provide optimal defence
♦ Lymphocyte re-circulation, the factors that direct it, and its significance in initiation of immune responses

It is necessary to understand the organization of the lymphoid system to learn about the way immune responses are generated in vivo. The system comprises various organs and tissues, the major components being lymphocytes which are central to adaptive immunity. The lymphoid system is organized into either encapsulated organs or collections of diffuse lymphoid tissue. They are categorized into *central* (*primary*) and *peripheral* (*secondary*) lymphoid organs/tissues. Central lymphoid organs are sites where lymphocytes are produced from precursor cells. These are also the sites of lymphocyte maturation which, as we shall see, are different for B and T lymphocytes. Once mature, lymphocytes move to secondary or peripheral lymphoid organs/tissues. Their organization is highly regulated to allow immune responses to be initiated at these sites. Lymphatic vessels are also structures of the lymphoid system. They are located throughout the body and serve to connect various organs. These vessels drain fluid called lymph from various sites in the body and transport it to structures called the lymph nodes which are located along the lymphatic channels. The unique ability of lymphocytes to re-circulate throughout the body via blood and lymphatics has a major role in the development of adaptive immune responses.

This chapter focuses on the organization of lymphoid organs and their role in generation of immune responses. The salient features of lymphocytes and their types along with their functional roles are presented. The physiological importance of major histocompatibility complex (MHC) molecules and how peptide-MHC complexes are recognized by T cells is highlighted. The different types of antigen-presenting cells which are essential for T lymphocyte activation are described. The concluding sections of the chapter consider some of the ways innate and adaptive immune systems collaborate and also lymphocyte re-circulation and preferential homing on to lymphoid organs.

LYMPHOID ORGANS/TISSUES

The organs/tissues of the immune system are depicted in Fig. 3.1 (see also Fig. 1.8). Their organization and other features that are critical for maturation of lymphocytes and development of adaptive immunity are discussed in the following section.

Central (Primary) Lymphoid Organs

These include the *bone marrow* (in mammals) and *thymus*. They are called primary lymphoid organs as B and T lymphocytes, respectively, undergo maturation at these sites before they migrate to secondary

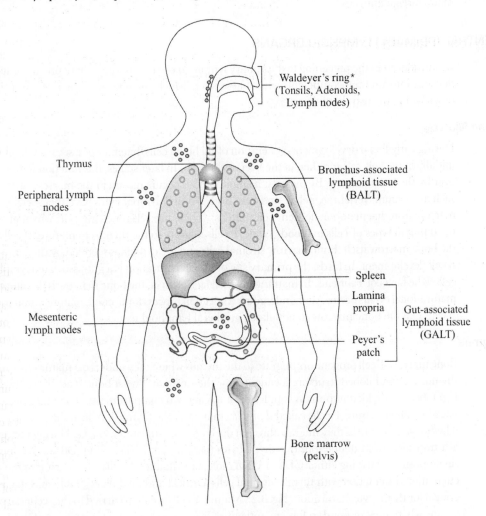

Fig. 3.1   Major lymphoid organs and tissues. *Ring of lymphoid tissues.

lymphoid organs as naïve mature lymphocytes. We shall learn later that it is at these primary sites that developing B and T cells acquire diverse antigen-specific receptors and immunocompetence (capability to mount an immune response).

Peripheral (Secondary) Lymphoid Organs/Tissues

These include *lymph nodes, spleen,* and *mucosa-associated lymphoid tissue (MALT)*. The first two are well-organized encapsulated organs, whereas MALT is unencapsulated. These are sites where naïve lymphocytes undergo proliferation and differentiation into effector cells in response to antigens. The location of lymph nodes along lymphatic vessels allows them to trap antigens from lymph or dendritic cells (DC). On the other hand, the spleen, which filters blood, traps blood-borne antigens. Mucosa-associated lymphoid tissue interacts with antigens/microbes that enter the body via gastrointestinal, respiratory, and genitourinary tracts. The intestinal mucosal system is known as *gut-associated lymphoid tissue (GALT)*, whereas *bronchus-associated lymphoid tissue (BALT)* is located in the lungs, particularly along the bronchi. The skin constitutes the *cutareous-associated lymphoid tissue (CALT)* which deals with many foreign antigens.

CENTRAL (PRIMARY) LYMPHOID ORGANS

As introduced in the preceding text, primary lymphoid organs are sites where precursor lymphocytes develop into immunocompetent cells. These sites, which include bone marrow and thymus, are described in the text that follows:

Bone Marrow

During early foetal development, generation of all blood cells (haematopoiesis, see Chapter 1) occurs initially in the yolk sac and then in the liver and spleen. In later stages, this function is gradually taken over by the bone marrow. By puberty, haematopoiesis occurs mostly in the marrow of the flat bones such as sternum, vertebrae, pelvis, and ribs. Both B and T lymphocytes have their origin in the bone marrow from haematopoietic stem cells (HSCs). These are self-renewing cells which give rise to all the different types of cells in blood. While T cells migrate to the thymus to mature, B cells mature in the bone marrow itself. Bone marrow stromal cells and the cytokines secreted by them are critical for B cell development. In birds, the primary site of B cell maturation is a gut-associated lymphoid organ called the bursa of Fabricius. In mammals, which lack a bursa, the bone marrow is the site where B cell maturational events occur. After undergoing a selection process for nonself, mature immunocompetent B cells exit the bone marrow to populate peripheral lymphoid tissues.

Thymus

Bone marrow T cell progenitors migrate to the thymus where they undergo a maturation process. The thymus is a flat bilobed structure located below the sternum (breast bone) and above the heart. The two lobes are divided into many lobules each having two compartments. The outer *cortex* is densely packed with immature T cells called *thymocytes* that enter the thymic lobule at the subcapsular region. Thymocytes mature as they migrate through the cortex into the inner *medulla*. During migration, there is a transition from double-positive thymocytes (bearing both CD4 and CD8 surface molecules) to single-positive (carrying either CD4 or CD8 molecules) mature T cells which exit into the peripheral circulation. Interaction with thymic stromal cells (cortical and medullary), DCs, and macrophages is critical for thymocyte maturation (Fig. 3.2). Mature T cells are then carried to the secondary lymphoid organs where they respond to foreign antigens.

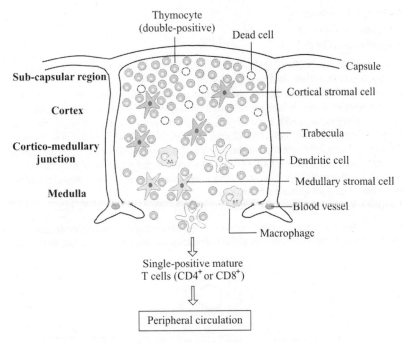

Fig. 3.2   Cellular organization of a thymic lobule. Thymocytes entering the thymic lobule mature as they migrate through the cortex and the medulla. Mature T cells then exit into the peripheral circulation.

Antigenic diversity of T cell receptors (TCRs) is generated during the process of T cell maturation in the thymus. Additionally, T cell precursors undergo an education process involving positive and negative selection (see Chapter 8) in which thymic stromal cells play a key role. It is only then that mature T cells are allowed to leave for secondary lymphoid organs. Interestingly, about 95–99 per cent of all thymocytes undergo programmed cell death (PCD), a pathway of cell death by apoptosis, in the thymus without ever maturing. Lymphocytes that undergo PCD include those that have either failed to make functional receptors, or those that have receptors with reactivity to self-components. The death pathway involves activation of endogenous enzymes that lead to deoxyribonucleic acid (DNA) fragmentation and eventually cell death. This process differs from cell death by necrosis which is induced due to cell damage by external causes such as poisoning or infection. The details of the process of apoptosis and more on its physiological importance are included in Box 3.1. The changes that occur during cell death by the two pathways are depicted in Fig. 3.3.

Box 3.1   Programmed cell death: a pathway of cell death by apoptosis

There are two major ways cells die—by necrosis or by apoptosis (Fig. 3.3). The word 'apoptosis' in ancient Greek describes the falling of leaves from trees, or petals from flowers. Deletion of the tail in developing human embryos is an example of cell death by apoptosis. It is a common process that gets rid of unwanted cells in the body and occurs throughout life. Its hallmark is disassembly of the cell in a highly ordered manner. Apoptosis can be triggered by γ-irradiation, treatment with glucocorticoids, withdrawal of critical growth factors, and activation of certain receptors. Expression of various genes that regulate apoptosis delivers signals (death signals) as a result of which the cell programmes itself to undergo death by apoptosis. On the other hand, protein products of other genes inhibit the process. Cells undergoing apoptosis detach from adjacent cells and show various morphological and biochemical changes which include

◆ cell shrinkage,

- blebbing at the membrane,
- chromatin condensation,
- fragmentation of DNA.

The cytoplasm and nucleus fragment into membrane-bound bodies containing intact organelles. These are called *apoptotic bodies*. As these are rapidly phagocytosed after being shed from cells undergoing apoptosis, cellular contents do not spill over into tissues. Inflammatory responses are, thus, avoided. It should be remembered here that scavenger receptors on phagocytic cells have an important role to play in the clearance of apoptotic cells. MBL too enhances clearance due to its ability to bind simultaneously to apoptotic cells and receptors on phagocytes (see Chapter 2). Apoptosis involves a family of protease enzymes called *caspases* which exist in the cytoplasm of most cells as inactive enzymes (see Chapter 15). Necrosis is another form of cell death which follows tissue injury and some infections. Uptake of necrotic cells is facilitated by Fc receptors and complement receptors. Unlike apoptosis, necrotic cells swell and burst releasing cellular contents that trigger inflammatory reactions.

Apoptosis is a normal physiologic process and has an important role in the following:

- *Immunological tolerance* During T cell development in the thymus, the thymocytes that fail the process of positive selection (or due to negative selection) undergo massive death by apoptosis and are phagocytosed

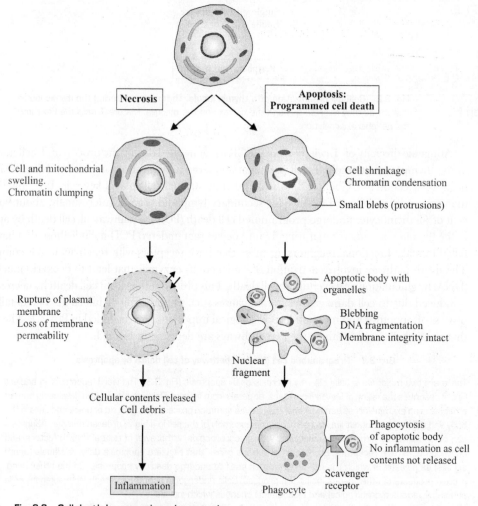

Fig. 3.3 Cell death by necrosis and apoptosis.

by thymic macrophages. The majority of B cells too, like thymocytes, undergo death by apoptosis during developmental processes in the bone marrow.

♦ *Immune homeostasis* Apoptosis is also important for maintenance of homeostasis in the immune system. Clonal expansion of T and B cells on activation by an antigen is followed by death of many activated cells after antigen clearance. Only memory cells are left behind. This helps to maintain a constant number of cells in the immune system. If activated cells were not eliminated, lymph nodes would burst due to continued proliferation on antigen encounter.

Thymectomy (surgical removal of the thymus) in neonates results in severe immunodeficiency. T cell numbers are drastically reduced and cell-mediated immunity (CMI) is impaired due to which neonates fail to survive. This shows the importance of the thymus in immunity. *DiGeorge syndrome* is a rare immune defect in which infants are born without a functional thymus (see Chapter 16). The size of the thymus and activity are maximum at birth and in early childhood. It gradually atrophies (shrinks) after puberty through adulthood, though remnants remain.

PERIPHERAL (SECONDARY) LYMPHOID ORGANS/TISSUES

These are sites where mature immunocompetent lymphocytes encounter antigens leading to initiation of adaptive immune responses. In mammals, organs/tissues which function as secondary sites include lymph nodes, spleen, mucosa-associated lymphoid tissue (MALT), and cutaneous-associated lymphoid tissue (CALT). These are described in the text that follows.

Lymph Nodes

These are small solid structures usually less than 1 cm in diameter, and are located in clusters in various regions throughout the body. They are found along the lymphatic system such as in neck, armpit, and chest, and are sites where T and B cells respond to antigens. Morphologically, lymph nodes can be divided into three regions (Fig. 3.4) as follows:

Cortex

This contains many *primary (unstimulated) lymphoid follicles* composed mostly of naïve B cells. On B cell stimulation by a protein antigen, primary follicles enlarge to form *secondary follicles* with *germinal centres*

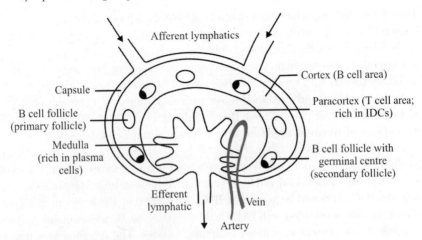

Fig. 3.4   Lymph node structure.

which are densely populated with B cells in a state of mitosis. In these secondary follicles, activated B cells proliferate profusely. It is in germinal centres that B cells undergo *affinity maturation*, a process that generates B cells bearing high-affinity receptors for an antigen (see Chapter 10). *Follicular dendritic cells (FDCs)*, unique cells found in lymphoid follicles and having long dendritic processes, have an important role to play in this process. Follicular dendritic cells express neither class II MHC molecules nor costimulatory molecules and, hence, cannot present antigenic peptides to T cells. These cells, however, express Fc receptors (FcRs) and complement receptors. Through these receptors, they trap antigen–antibody complexes and display them on their surface for long periods of time. Germinal centres are also sites where *memory cells* are formed.

Paracortex

This region, which lies between the cortex and the medulla, is the T cell area of the lymph node. It is rich in T lymphocytes with many interspersed *interdigitating dendritic cells (IDCs)*. IDCs are mature dendritic cells into which immature dendritic cells transform during their migration from the tissues to the lymph nodes. They are rich in class II MHC molecules and, hence, are efficient antigen-presenting cells (APCs). They display antigenic peptides, derived from antigens taken up in peripheral tissues, to naïve T cells resulting in their activation and differentiation into effector cells and memory cells. Effector cells migrate to sites of infection where they function to eliminate invading microbes.

Medulla

This constitutes the innermost layer of the lymph node and is rich in plasma cells. These plasma cells are transported to the medulla from the cortex via lymphatic vessels. The antibodies that they secrete enter the circulation where they eliminate microbes and neutralize toxins.

Naïve lymphocytes enter lymph nodes from tissues via afferent lymphatics, and from bloodstream through *high endothelial venules (HEVs)*. These are specialized venules through which lymphocytes extravasating from the bloodstream enter the paracortical region. Endothelial cells lining HEVs express adhesion molecules which bind selectively to receptors on re-circulating naïve lymphocytes allowing them to home to these sites. We will learn more about re-circulation of lymphocytes in the later part of this chapter.

Spleen

The spleen is the largest lymphatic organ located on the left side of the abdomen below the diaphragm. It resembles a lymph node in basic structure and function. A distinguishing feature is that the spleen, unlike lymph nodes, circulates blood only and not lymph as it lacks afferent and efferent lymphatics. It is organized into two main types of tissues: the *red pulp* and the *white pulp* (Fig. 3.5). The red pulp is densely packed with resident macrophages. The spleen very efficiently traps foreign substances carried in the blood and also blood-borne microorganisms. As it contains abundant phagocytes, it is an important site for phagocytosis. Besides ingesting and destroying microbes in the blood, it helps in clearance of worn-out red blood cells and also immune complexes.

Both the T- and B-dependent regions of the spleen, which are segregated as in lymph nodes, are localized in the white pulp which is found around small arterioles. Hence, it is here that the immune function of the spleen resides. The region called the *periarteriolar lymphoid sheath (PALS)* is rich in T cells and IDCs. It should be noted that IDCs are located in T cell regions of all peripheral lymphoid organs. In close association with PALS is the *marginal zone*. Besides containing macrophages, it is rich in naïve B cells present in primary lymphoid follicles. The splenic artery transports blood-borne antigens to the marginal zone from where they are carried to PALS after uptake by dendritic cells.

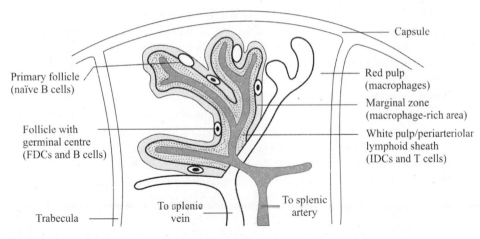

Fig. 3.5   A spleen lobule.

It is in PALS that dendritic cells activate T$_H$ cells which then activate B cells. During the course of a humoral immune response to a protein antigen, primary follicles develop into secondary follicles each having a germinal centre (as in lymph nodes). Here, proliferating B cells and plasma cells are present in large numbers. Specialized FDCs present in this region function in selection of B cells bearing high-affinity receptors for antigens. Plasma cells in the spleen actively synthesize antibodies that are released into the circulation.

Mucosa-associated Lymphoid Tissue

Many pathogens gain entry into the body through surfaces containing mucosal epithelial cells. So, unsurprisingly, a large part of the lymphoid tissue (about 50%) is associated with these surfaces which are collectively called *MALT*. Mucosa-associated lymphoid tissue, unlike other secondary lymphoid organs, is unencapsulated and includes tonsils and bronchial tissue, and *Peyer's patches* (in the small intestine), besides others. The intestinal mucosal system is known as *GALT* (Fig. 3.6). It performs the vital role of providing defence against microbes that enter via the intestinal tract. *Bronchus-associated lymphoid tissue* is structurally similar to Peyer's patches and is located in the lungs along bronchi.

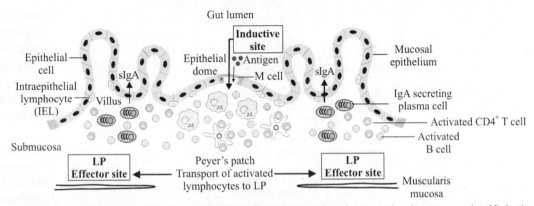

Fig. 3.6   Gut-associated lymphoid tissue (GALT). Peyer's patches are sites where naïve lymphocytes are primed (inductive sites). M cells are specialized to endocytose antigen from the lumen and pass it into the subepithelial tissue. Lymphocytes activated by antigen migrate to the lamina propria (LP) which is the effector site. Here, plasma cells secrete IgA (sIgA) into the gut lumen.

The organized lymphoid tissue of GALT is represented by Peyer's patches which form distinct nodules, unlike in the *lamina propria* in the connective tissue that underlies epithelia at mucosal sites. Peyer's patches are composed primarily of B cells organized in follicles, just as in lymph nodes, and which often have germinal centres. Small numbers of T cells and APCs are also present here. Peyer's patches function to trap antigens from the gastrointestinal tract and are sites where B and T cells interact with an antigen to initiate immune responses (*inductive sites*).

Uptake of foreign antigens/pathogens from the intestinal lumen is mediated by specialized *M cells*, so called because they have many microfolds on their luminal surface (Fig. 3.7). These cells are found scattered in the epithelial layer. Intraepithelial lymphocytes (IELs), unusual cells which have been introduced earlier in Chapter 2, are also found interspersed in the epithelial layer. Antigens after uptake by M cells are transported through the cell and released into a deep invagination on the internal side where the organized lymphoid tissue is located. Similar antigen uptake by M cells occurs in mucosal tissue of the respiratory and genitourinary tracts. Antigen-presenting cells (macrophages and DCs) found in Peyer's patches process the foreign matter after uptake and present it to T cells resulting in their activation. B cells, too, are activated in underlying lymphoid follicles in Peyer's patches. Activated lymphocytes then home on to the lamina propria.

Diffused clusters of cells present in the lamina propria include activated TH cells and large numbers of activated B cells and plasma cells. Here, TH cells which have migrated from Peyer's patches stimulate B cells to produce antibodies (*effector site*). It should be remembered that secretory immunoglobulin A (sIgA) is the major antibody isotype that provides defence at mucosal surfaces. It is transported across intestinal epithelial cells by a process called *transcytosis* (see Fig. 11.9).

Immune responses similar to those described in the preceding text also occur at other mucosal sites. Re-circulation permits lymphocytes stimulated in GALT to migrate to lamina propria in the respiratory mucosa, a major portal of entry of pathogens. This serves to defend against the same microbe which initiated the activation process.

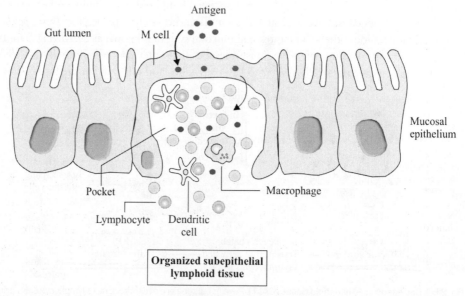

Fig. 3.7 M cells and their role in gut mucosal immunity. M cells function to endocytose antigen from the gut lumen and release it to the underlying lymphoid tissue.

Cutaneous-associated Lymphoid Tissue (CALT)

Many pathogens/antigens gain entry through the skin if the surface barrier is breached. Intraepithelial T lymphocytes, which are also present in mucosal epithelia, are found located in the skin epidermis whereas other immune cells are found in relatively low numbers. Keratinocytes, present in this region, contribute to the structural integrity of the epidermis and produce a wide range of cytokines. DCs and macrophages reside in the dermis. *Langerhans cells*, which are immature DCs, are efficient at trapping foreign material and transporting it to the regional lymph nodes. They undergo a maturation process on their way to the lymph nodes where they present antigen to re-circulating naïve T lymphocytes. Triggering of inflammatory reactions in the skin rapidly recruits leukocytes from the blood vessels to the site of inflammation. Type I (immediate) and Type IV hypersensitivity (contact dermatitis) reactions are initiated in the skin (see Chapter 14).

The chapter now proceeds to a discussion of T and B lymphocytes which are central to initiation of adaptive immune responses and which are responsible for its specificity and memory.

CELLS OF ADAPTIVE IMMUNITY—LYMPHOCYTES

As has been discussed earlier in the chapter, lymphocytes are produced in central lymphoid organs, but function in peripheral lymphoid organs/tissues where they respond to a specific antigen. A unique feature of lymphocytes is their ability to migrate into tissues and then return to the blood stream via lymphatic vessels. They are the only cells that produce high-affinity receptors for an antigen. Their receptors are clonally distributed, that is, there are many different clones of lymphocytes having distinct antigen specificities. All members of a clone express receptors of identical specificity.

Naïve lymphocytes leaving the central lymphoid organs have a large nucleus and a very small amount of cytoplasm. Like all other immune cells, lymphocytes express many cell surface molecules which are essential for their functioning. Cell surface molecules may be involved in recognition of antigen, cell–cell interaction and adhesion, and transduction of signals that lead to cell activation. A cell surface molecule which is defined by a cluster of monoclonal antibodies reacting with it is designated by a *CD (cluster of differentiation)* number. As new molecules are identified and characterized, they are labelled with a new CD number such as CD1, CD2, and so on. The list of CD molecules continues to grow and currently over 340 CD numbers have been assigned. It is relevant to mention here that some surface molecules on immune cells are unique to a particular cell type and are called *surface markers*. By using fluorescent monoclonal antibodies specific for a unique marker, cells in a mixed population can be identified (see Fig. 3.14).

There are three subpopulations of lymphocytes including the following:

- T lymphocytes
- B lymphocytes
- Null cells

Null cells are large granular lymphocytes and include natural killer (NK) cells which were introduced earlier in Chapter 2. They are a distinct lymphocyte subpopulation sharing features with both myeloid and lymphoid cells and form part of innate defence mechanisms. It is noteworthy that they lack the highly diverse antigen receptors that are expressed on the lymphocyte surface.

The chapter now turns to a description of the distinct structural characteristics of T and B lymphocytes, different T lymphocyte types and their functional roles, and the distinct ways T and B cells recognize antigen. In this context, the role of MHC molecules is elaborated.

T Lymphocytes

Early experiments showed that removal of the thymus (*thymectomy*) in mice soon after birth led to a drastic reduction in the number of T lymphocytes due to which susceptibility to infection ...creased. Antibody production, too, was to a large extent reduced. Some conclusions drawn were as follows:

- Thymus is essential for T cell development in early life.
- T lymphocytes play a critical role in defence against infection.
- T cells contribute to antibody production by B cells.

The experimental observations mentioned in the preceding text revealed the critical role of T cells in host defence.

Each mature T cell that leaves the thymus expresses a unique antigen-specific receptor called *TCR* on its membrane. Most T cells (αβ T cells) in the body express the αβ *TCR* that is composed of α and β chains, whereas a minority of T cells (γδ T cells) carry the γδ *TCR* with γ and δ chains (see Chapter 8). Some features of γδ TCR bearing T lymphocytes are described later in this chapter. The TCR is associated with several polypeptides collectively referred to as CD3; these are essential for T cell activation. CD3, which is invariant (identical on all T cells) and is expressed on T cells alone, is used as a marker to identify T cells. The αβ TCR is also associated with either CD4 or CD8, both are transmembrane molecules that have a role in transduction of signals in T cells. Later in Chapter 8, we will learn that immature T cells developing in the thymus express both CD4 and CD8 (double-positive cells), whereas mature T cells that exit the thymus are either CD4⁺ or CD8⁺ (single-positive cells). It would also be helpful here to refer back to Fig. 3.2 which depicts the transition from double-positive T cells to single-positive cells in a thymic lobule. Various molecules expressed on the T cell surface which are important for T cell functioning are shown in Fig. 3.8.

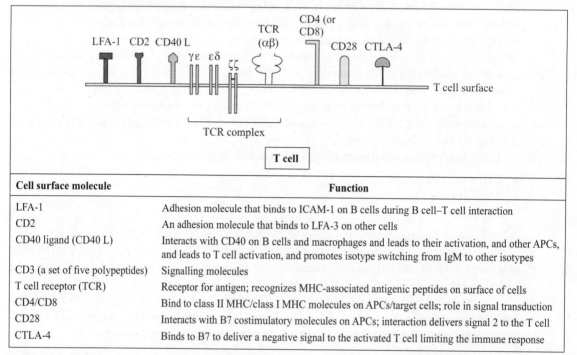

Cell surface molecule	Function
LFA-1	Adhesion molecule that binds to ICAM-1 on B cells during B cell–T cell interaction
CD2	An adhesion molecule that binds to LFA-3 on other cells
CD40 ligand (CD40 L)	Interacts with CD40 on B cells and macrophages and leads to their activation, and other APCs, and leads to T cell activation, and promotes isotype switching from IgM to other isotypes
CD3 (a set of five polypeptides)	Signalling molecules
T cell receptor (TCR)	Receptor for antigen; recognizes MHC-associated antigenic peptides on surface of cells
CD4/CD8	Bind to class II MHC/class I MHC molecules on APCs/target cells; role in signal transduction
CD28	Interacts with B7 costimulatory molecules on APCs; interaction delivers signal 2 to the T cell
CTLA-4	Binds to B7 to deliver a negative signal to the activated T cell limiting the immune response

Fig. 3.8 **T cell surface molecules and their functional roles.** Only four of the five polypeptides of CD3 are shown.

T Lymphocyte Types and Their Functional Roles

Recall from the introductory chapter that there are two types of adaptive immune responses. B lymphocytes produce antibodies that mediate *humoral immunity*, an important defence mechanism against extracellular pathogens and their toxins. T lymphocytes mediate *CMI* which protects against microbes that reside within phagocytic cells or infect non-phagocytic cells. Refer to Fig. 3.9 which depicts the different ways lymphocytes participate in elimination of antigen/pathogen. It is to be noted that CMI responses are of different types mediated by distinct classes of T cells. The major T lymphocyte types, including γδ TCR-bearing T lymphocytes, are shown in Fig. 3.10 . These and other minor T cell subpopulations are described in the following text.

T helper (TH) cells

These cells, in addition to TCR and CD3, express CD4 molecules and are designated CD4⁺ *TH cells*. They are critical to the development of an immune response and stimulate

- ◆ antibody production by B cells,
- ◆ killer activity of Tc cells, and
- ◆ phagocytic activity of macrophages.

There are two subsets of TH cells—*TH1* and *TH2*—which differ in the cytokines they secrete and, hence, in their functional roles. Further details about these cells and the types of immune responses they mediate are described in Chapters 8 and 9.

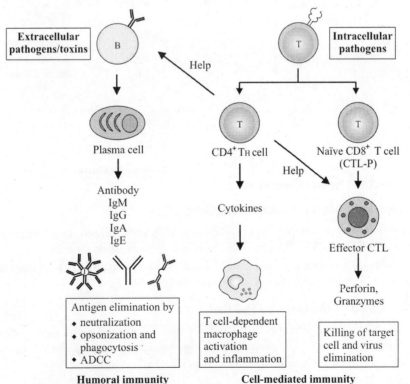

Fig. 3.9   Components of adaptive immunity. T lymphocytes provide help to B cells and CD8⁺ T cells. Besides, they activate macrophages to kill intracellular pathogens, and stimulate a local inflammatory response. Three ways of elimination of antigens/pathogens are depicted.

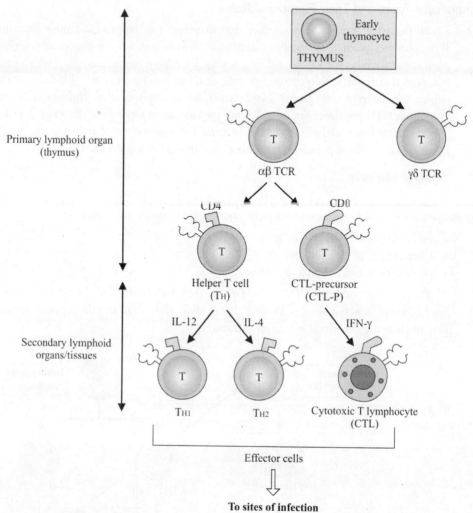

Fig. 3.10   Types of T lymphocyte.

Cytotoxic T Cells/Lymphocytes (Tc Cells/CTLs)

These cells express CD8 molecules in addition to TCR and CD3 and are designated *CD8⁺ Tc cells/CTLs*. They are effector cells which eliminate infected cells, particularly those infected by virus, tumour cells, and cells of a foreign graft. Naïve CD8⁺ T cells (CTL-precursors, CTL-P) need activating signals to acquire cytotoxicity and transform into effector cells.

CD4⁺ CD25⁺ T Regulatory (Treg) Cell

This T cell subpopulation regulates activity of other T cells and suppresses immune responses, unlike CD4-bearing TH cells. *Treg cells play a major role in maintenance of peripheral tolerance to self-antigens.* Refer to Chapter 15 for more information on Treg cells.

NKT Cell

This represents a minor αβ TCR - bearing T cell subpopulation considered to be involved in innate immune responses (see Chapters 2 and 5). It bears surface markers also expressed on NK cells.

γδ *TCR-bearing Lymphocytes*

Unlike αβ T cells which are abundant in peripheral circulation, γδ T cells are present in the circulation in only small numbers. These cells express antigen receptors of limited diversity and most lack the co-receptors CD4 and CD8. There are distinct subsets of γδ T cells which differ in anatomic distribution and functional role from T cells bearing αβ TCR. One subclass of γδ T cells accumulates in skin and mucosal epithelia such as in gastrointestinal tract. These cells, known as IELs, are part of innate immune mechanisms and were introduced in Chapter 2. Another unique feature of γδ T cells that sets them apart from αβ T cells is that they do not recognize MHC-peptide complexes. Hence, they are not dependent on antigen presentation by APCs and may recognize antigens directly. Some of these cells recognize microbial lipids and glycolipids associated with non-polymorphic class I MHC-like molecules called *CD1 molecules* (see Chapter 5).

Recognition of Peptide-MHC Complexes by T Cells

It is once again emphasized that T cells, unlike B cells cannot see native antigen, e.g., proteins in whole bacteria/virus, or protein. Rather, they recognize only short peptides derived from microbial antigens. These are presented on APCs, infected cells, tumour cells, or grafts bound to peptide-display molecules called major histocompatibility complex molecules (Fig. 3.11). These are membrane glycoproteins encoded by the *MHC*—a cluster of genes on chromosome 6 (see Chapter 5). There are two different classes of MHC molecules—class I and class II. They have a peptide-binding cleft in their extracellular domain. Peptide fragments generated from degradation of exogenous foreign proteins inside the cell

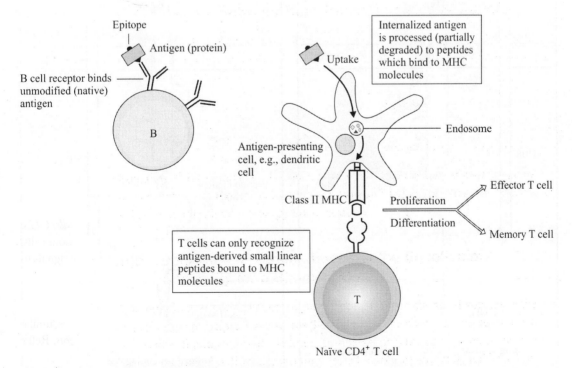

Fig. 3.11   Antigen recognition by B and T lymphocytes.
Note: Peptides derived from exogenous antigens generally bind to class II MHC molecules, whereas peptides derived from endogenous antigens, such as virally-derived proteins, bind to class I MHC molecules. The costimulatory second signal is not shown.

or from intracellular pathogens, a process called *antigen processing*, bind to newly synthesized MHC molecules and are transported to the cell surface. These peptide-MHC complexes are presented to T cells which recognize them with the help of the TCR. It should be noted that peptides derived from degradation of self-proteins are also presented on the surface complexed to MHC molecules. But these complexes are not recognized by T cells (see Chapter 5). When a naïve T cell encounters a specific peptide-MHC combination, the T cell proliferates and differentiates into effector T cells and memory T cells. *CD4$^+$ TH cells are activated by antigenic peptides bound to class II MHC molecules on the surface of antigen-presenting cells, whereas CD8$^+$ Tc cells recognize specific peptide bound to class I MHC molecules on APCs or target cells* (Fig. 3.12).

CD4 and CD8 molecules are important in many ways. They bind to class II and class I MHC molecules, respectively, on APCs or other cells, increasing the strength of the interaction between TCR and MHC-peptide complex. Interestingly, CD4 is used as a receptor by human immunodeficiency virus (HIV) to gain entry into CD4$^+$ TH cells (see Chapter 16). Normally, approximately 65 per cent of T cells in blood are CD4$^+$ TH cells and 35 per cent are CD8$^+$ Tc cells. But in some diseases, such as acquired immunodeficiency syndrome (AIDS), the CD4:CD8 ratio is reversed due to decline in CD4$^+$ TH cells and is an indicator of AIDS progression.

In summary, the two classes of MHC molecules (class I and class II) present antigens to the two different classes of T cells, namely, TH and Tc cells. Recognition of specific peptide-MHC complexes

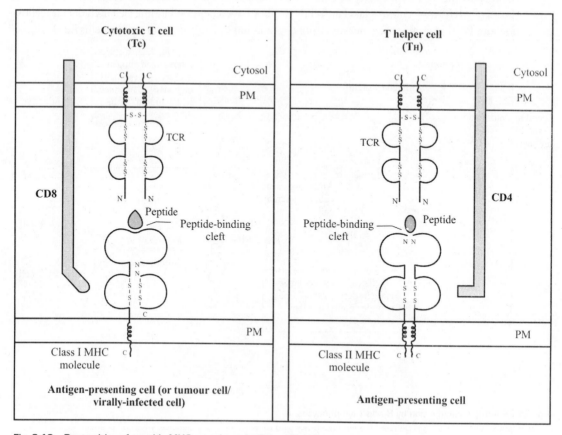

Fig. 3.12 Recognition of peptide-MHC complexes by Tc and TH cells.

along with other interactions activates T cells to undergo rapid cell division, a process called *clonal expansion*.

B Lymphocytes

Mature B cells which exit the bone marrow express membrane-bound antibody. This is monomeric IgM unlike the secreted form which is a pentamer (see Chapter 4). IgD, too, is expressed on the surface of a mature B cell and serves as a receptor for an antigen. The membrane-bound antibody along with *Ig-α/Ig-β* (signal-transducing molecules) forms the B cell receptor for an antigen. The B cell receptor (BCR) is associated with several other molecules which together form the *BCR complex*. Some important molecules expressed on the surface of a mature B cell are shown in Fig. 3.13.

B and T cells, which are morphologically very similar, can be distinguished on the basis of the antigen receptors they express or other surface markers. For instance, B cells can be identified using the fluorescent anti-IgM antibody (Fig. 3.14), whereas CD3, a pan T cell marker, can be identified

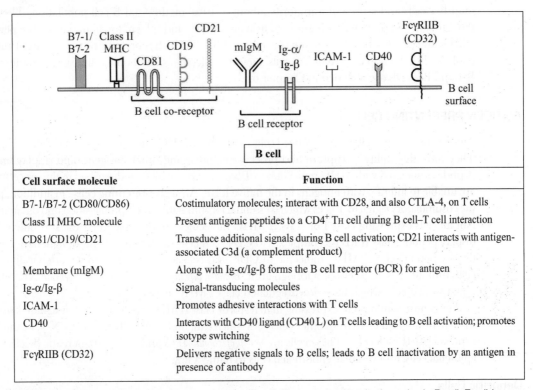

Cell surface molecule	Function
B7-1/B7-2 (CD80/CD86)	Costimulatory molecules; interact with CD28, and also CTLA-4, on T cells
Class II MHC molecule	Present antigenic peptides to a CD4$^+$ Tʜ cell during B cell–T cell interaction
CD81/CD19/CD21	Transduce additional signals during B cell activation; CD21 interacts with antigen-associated C3d (a complement product)
Membrane (mIgM)	Along with Ig-α/Ig-β forms the B cell receptor (BCR) for antigen
Ig-α/Ig-β	Signal-transducing molecules
ICAM-1	Promotes adhesive interactions with T cells
CD40	Interacts with CD40 ligand (CD40 L) on T cells leading to B cell activation; promotes isotype switching
FcγRIIB (CD32)	Delivers negative signals to B cells; leads to B cell inactivation by an antigen in presence of antibody

Fig. 3.13 Major surface molecules on a mature B cell. These molecules play key roles in B cell–T cell interactions.

Fig. 3.14 B cell identification. B cells can be detected by labelling with a fluorescent anti-IgM conjugate and viewing under UV light. The bound Ig on B cells is monomeric IgM.

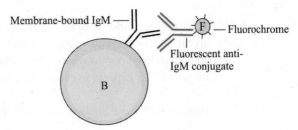

using anti-CD3. It is not to be forgotten at any stage that the receptor for antigen on B cells unlike TCRs can directly interact with an antigen. There are other points of distinction too. While T cells generally recognize only protein antigens, B cells can recognize a wide range of microbial structures including carbohydrates, lipids, and also proteins. It is to be noted that the unusual $\gamma\delta$ T cells recognize lipid antigens. The role of B cells as APCs is discussed in the following section.

On antigenic stimulation, B cells proliferate and differentiate into effector cells called plasma cells. These are end-stage cells that are actively engaged in antibody secretion (see Fig. 3.9). Although the majority of plasma cells are short-lived, some migrate to the bone marrow where they survive for long periods and continue to produce antibodies. Some progeny of antigen-activated B lymphocytes differentiate into memory cells which, on later exposure to the same antigen, rapidly mount an intense immune response (see Figs 1.18 and 1.19). Memory cells circulate in the blood from where they can be recruited to sites of infection, and are also found in lymph nodes and mucosal tissues.

B lymphocytes are of two types: *B-1* and *B-2 cells*. B-1 cells arise earlier in foetal development than B-2 cells and represent a minority (about 5–10%) of the total B cell population. These cells, though scarce in peripheral organs such as lymph nodes and spleen, are abundant in the peritoneal and pleural cavities. B-2 cells are the conventional B cells which represent the major part of the B cell pool. As they develop later than B-1 cells, they are called B-2 cells. Some other significant features of B-1 and B-2 cells are included in Chapter 6.

ANTIGEN-PRESENTING CELLS

Antigen-presenting cells are specialized cells which include DCs, macrophages, and B cells (Fig. 3.15). They have the ability to capture and process microbial and other antigens, and display antigenic peptides associated with MHC molecules to T lymphocytes which, as described in the preceding text, are unable to interact with antigens in the native form. Antigen-presenting cells , in addition, provide the costimulatory signal to T cells which is essential for stimulating their proliferation and differentiation. Not all cells expressing class I or class II MHC molecules are designated APCs. It is only cells that display peptide-class II MHC complexes to CD4$^+$ TH cells that are given this designation. Cells that display peptide-class I MHC molecule to CD8$^+$ TC cells are *target cells* and include virally-infected cells, tumour cells, and cells of a foreign graft. *Broadly, any nucleated cell can be a target cell.* NK cells , too, target similar cells which have downregulated class I MHC molecules.

Antigen-presenting cells expressing high levels of class II MHC molecules are designated *professional APCs* to distinguish them from other cell types which can, under the influence of IFN-γ, be induced to express class II molecules. These cells are *non-professional APCs* and include pancreatic β cells, thyroid epithelial cells, and vascular endothelial cells to name a few.

Dendritic Cells

These cells are unique among all APCs in many critical ways which are highlighted in the following points:

- Unlike macrophages and B cells, their primary function is antigen presentation.
- Their surveillance and migratory properties enable them to carry antigens captured at the periphery to secondary lymphoid organs where they stimulate naïve T cells.
- They (mature DCs) express exceptionally high levels of class II MHC and costimulatory molecules.
- They accumulate in T cell areas of lymphoid organs.

APC/FDC	Class II MHC	Costimulatory activity (B7 molecules)	Presentation to and activation/selection
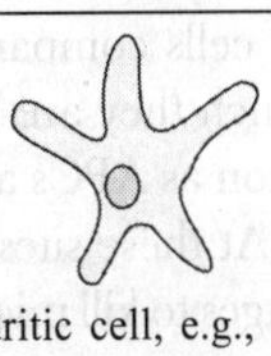 Dendritic cell, e.g., inter-digitating dendritic cell (IDC)	Constitutive expression	Constitutive expression	Naïve T cells (primarily)
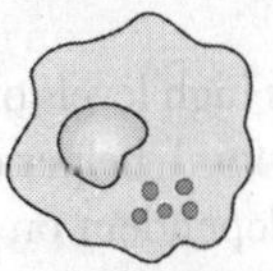 Macrophage	Inducible (by IFN γ)	Inducible (by bacterial products, e.g., LPS, and IFN-γ secreted by TH1 cells)	Effector and memory T cells (not very potent at activating naïve T cells)
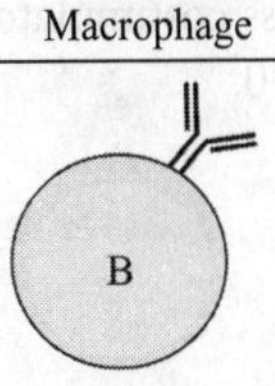 B cell	Constitutive expression	Inducible (on activation)	Only antigen activated B cells stimulate TH cells (primed). Resting B cells activate T effector cells and memory cells*
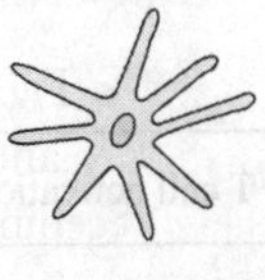 Follicular dendritic cell (FDC)	–	–	Activation and selection of B cells with high-affinity receptors for antigen (affinity maturation)

Fig. 3.15 Antigen-presenting cells. DCs, macrophages, and B cells are professional APCs. FDCs too are depicted here but are not in this category. They differ functionally as they express neither class II MHC molecules nor costimulatory molecules (see Chapter 10).

* Effector T cells and memory T cells do not require the second costimulatory signal for activation.

- Their extensive folds and extensions enable them to come into close contact with many T cells simultaneously.
- Their ability for cross-presentation is a distinguishing feature (see Chapter 5).

Immature DCs express low levels of class II MHC molecules. They express PRRs such as TLRs which enables them to sense the presence of danger signals such as PAMPs on microbes. This increases their phagocytic activity, and they engulf the infectious agent after which they migrate to secondary lymphoid organs maturing on the way. Mature DCs show decreased phagocytic activity, but they develop other capabilities such as presentation of antigenic peptides to T cells resulting in their activation. They express high density of class II MHC molecules, and also costimulatory B7 molecules which provide second signals for T cell activation (see Figs 8.6 and 8.7). These mature DCs are known as IDCs. Migration of DCs to secondary lymphoid tissues is guided by expression of specific chemokine receptors.

Macrophages

Resting macrophages express class I MHC molecules in high density. When they receive activation signals from inflammatory cytokines/bacterial products, they upregulate expression of both class

II MHC and costimulatory B7 molecules. However, even in activated macrophages expression of these molecules is lower compared to dendritic cells and B cells. This may possibly be the reason why activated macrophages are less efficient at presenting antigens to naïve T cells compared to DCs. It must be remembered that the primary role of macrophages, and for which they are better suited, is in elimination of microbes in innate immunity. Additionally, they function as APCs at sites of infection and sustained inflammation where they are present in abundance. At these sites, they present antigens to effector T cells which on activation deliver signals to macrophages to kill microbes residing intracellularly (CMI).

B Cells

Other than dendritic cells and macrophages, B cells, which constitutively express high levels of class II MHC molecules, also function in presentation of antigen. Their role as APCs for T helper cells is significant during the humoral immune response to a protein antigen which is dependent on T cell help (Fig. 3.16). It is to be noted that B cells must be activated before they express costimulatory B7 molecules. The role of B cells as APCs is discussed in greater detail in Chapter 10.

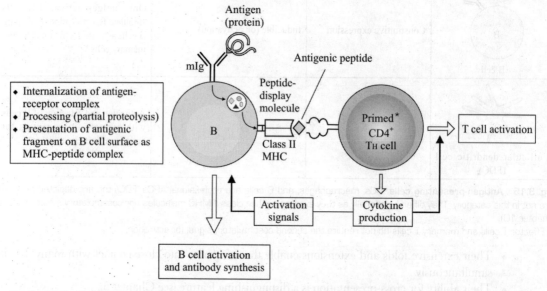

Fig. 3.16   B cells as APCs for T helper cells. B cells display fragments of antigen complexed to class II MHC molecules to primed T_H cells. Costimulatory signals are not shown. T cell–B cell cooperation leads to activation of both B cells and T cells.
* A cell that has seen the same antigen, for which the B cell is specific, on the DC surface.

COLLABORATION BETWEEN INNATE AND ADAPTIVE IMMUNITY

The innate immune system by itself is often able to clear infections, but, if it is unable to do so, the more effective adaptive immune responses are called into play.

The two systems are, however, not completely independent. Rather, there is a high degree of cooperation between innate and adaptive immunity. Innate immunity generates signals that direct subsequent adaptive immune responses. Conversely, innate mechanisms are enhanced by elements of adaptive immunity. This bidirectional cross-talk is important as it helps to optimize defence mechanisms against microbial invasion.

Some ways by which innate and adaptive immune systems work together are briefly described in the following text.

◆ Antibodies by binding to target antigens identify most antigens which enter the host as foreign. Innate immune mechanisms such as phagocytic cells and complements then destroy them.

◆ Macrophages, which represent an important innate defence mechanism, serve as APCs to T cells such as effector T cells and produce cytokines. Activated antigen-specific T lymphocytes, in turn, produce cytokines (IFN-γ) that activate macrophages to kill intracellular microbes (Fig. 3.17).

◆ It is the recognition and uptake of pathogens/antigens by innate mechanisms that leads to development of adaptive immunity. Dendritic cells which occupy a pivotal position at the interface of innate and adaptive immunity can sense danger signals through innate receptors on their surface. They play a major role in antigen uptake and initiation of an adaptive response through expression of costimulatory molecules. The cytokines released by them activate both innate and adaptive immunity.

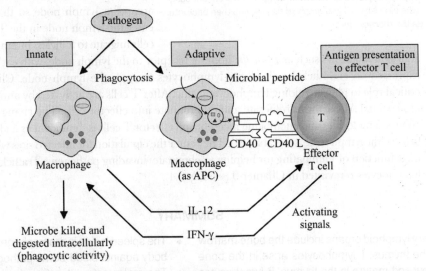

Fig. 3.17 Macrophages link innate and adaptive immunity. Macrophages eliminate infectious microbes and also serve as APCs providing an important link between innate and adaptive immunity (see Fig. 9.5).

LYMPHOCYTE CIRCULATION AND HOMING

Lymphocytes are capable of both entering and leaving tissues. Mature lymphocytes after exit from primary lymphoid organs re-circulate between blood, peripheral tissues, and secondary lymphoid organs, such as lymph nodes and spleen (Fig. 3.18). It should be remembered that none of the other white blood cells can re-enter the circulation once they have migrated into peripheral sites. Re-circulation of lymphocytes is important as it allows the immune system to survey the body for any foreign antigens/pathogens that have gained entry into the body. Circulation through organized lymphoid tissues brings together APCs and T lymphocytes. Besides, it increases the possibility that antigen-specific lymphocytes, which are initially rare, will come in contact with the foreign material and will be activated to clonally expand. This is necessary for mounting an effective immune response against foreign invaders.

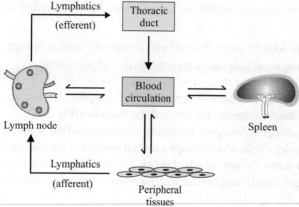

Fig. 3.18 Lymphocyte re-circulation. Lymphocytes continuously traffic from the bloodstream into lymphoid tissues and then back into the blood via the thoracic duct.

Lymphocytes have the unique ability of migrating directly from the bloodstream into lymph nodes. They do this by leaving the blood in HEVs which are specialized blood vessels having a cuboidal endothelium. A smaller proportion of lymphocytes entering a lymph node enter via the afferent lymphatic vessels. The preferential homing of lymphocytes to different lymphoid organs is determined by a particular combination of adhesion molecules expressed on lymphocytes and high endothelial cells. The basic processes involved are similar to those which permit neutrophils to enter sites of inflammation. High endothelial venules are located in the paracortical area of a lymph node so that T lymphocytes enter the lymph node in the T cell area while B cells migrate to follicles. Interaction between cell adhesion molecules such as *L-selectin* (homing receptor to the lymph node) with carbohydrate ligands expressed on endothelial cells allows lymphocytes to enter the lymph node. Chemokines have a critical role to play in guiding lymphocyte traffic. After T cells are activated by antigens displayed on professional APCs, they proliferate and differentiate into effector cells. The change in expression of adhesion molecules and chemokine receptors on effector T cells is significant as it allows lymphocytes to leave the lymph node (see Table 9.1). They enter the circulation for infected sites where they perform their function of eliminating (or helping to eliminate) invading pathogens. Trafficking/homing of T lymphocytes is revisited in Chapter 9 (see Fig. 9.4).

SUMMARY

- Primary lymphoid organs include the bone marrow and the thymus. T lymphocytes arise in the bone marrow and mature in the thymus. B lymphocytes in humans arise and mature in the bone marrow.
- After maturation, lymphocytes migrate to secondary lymphoid organs which include lymph nodes, spleen, and MALT. These are the sites where immune responses are initiated and developed.
- Dendritic cells capture microbial antigens in tissues and transport them to the lymph nodes draining the area. Here, they display antigenic peptides bound to MHC molecules on their surface for recognition by naïve T cells. These are activated to proliferate and differentiate into effector cells and memory cells.
- Mature B cells, too, in response to antigenic stimulation proliferate and differentiate to effector cells (plasma cells) and memory cells. Plasma cells secrete antibodies which enter the circulation from where they can be recruited to sites of infection.

- The spleen is rich in macrophages and protects the body against blood-borne pathogens/antigens.
- The major entry sites for microbes into the body are mucosal linings of the digestive, respiratory, and genitourinary tracts. The digestive tract is guarded by unencapsulated lymphoid tissue and is somewhat structured (Peyer's patches). Diffused cellular collections are present in the lamina propria.
- M cells are specialized antigen-transporting cells which allow antigen to enter mucosal tissues.
- T and B lymphocytes which are involved in adaptive immune responses differ in antigen receptors and other surface molecules. The antigen receptor on T cells is the T cell receptor or TCR. There are two major T cell subsets—T helper cells (TH) and cytotoxic T cells (TC). TH cells are of two types—TH1 and TH2—which differ in functional role.
- T helper cells mediate cell-mediated immunity

which defends against intracellular pathogens. They provide help to B cells to produce antibodies and to macrophages to kill intracellular microbes. Cytotoxic T cells recognize virally-infected cells and tumour cells and kill them. They also are dependent on help from TH cells.

- B cells have surface antibody (monomeric IgM, and IgD) as their antigen receptor. Activated B cells (plasma cells) secrete antibodies which mediate humoral immunity. This provides defence against extracellular microbes. There are two kinds of B cells—B-1 and B-2—which differ in properties.
- Antigen-presenting cells are specialized cells that display antigenic peptides associated with MHC molecules to T cells and provide costimulatory signals. They include dendritic cells, macrophages, and B cells. It is through APCs that T cells respond to antigen.
- The innate and adaptive immune systems cooperate with each other to provide optimal defence against infectious microbes.
- Lymphocytes re-circulate between blood and tissues and are always on the lookout for foreign material. They adhere to endothelial cells of blood vessels with the help of adhesion molecules on their surface. Their migration is guided by specialized homing receptors on the surface of high endothelial venules (HEVs).

REVIEW QUESTIONS

1. Indicate whether the following statements are true or false. If false, explain why.
   (a) T cells in lymph nodes are found primarily in the cortex.
   (b) Spleen responds largely to blood-borne antigens.
   (c) Haematopoiesis occurs in germinal centres.
   (d) Plasma cells in the lamina propria secrete large amounts of IgG.
   (e) Follicular dendritic cells are rich in class II MHC molecules.
   (f) Lymphocytes participate in specific defence.

2. Self-assessment questions
   (a) Cooperation between innate and adaptive immunity provides optimal defence against microbes. Explain some ways by which the working of the two systems is enhanced due to this cooperation.
   (b) Compare antigen recognition by B and T lymphocytes. How can B and T lymphocyte subpopulations be distinguished in a mixed lymphocyte suspension isolated from peripheral blood?
   (c) Why do you think the thymus is considered a primary lymphoid organ? Can you explain why apoptosis is a significant event in the immune system?
   (d) Which antigen-presenting cell is most suited to activate a naïve T cell and what properties of these cells make them unique among APCs?

   (e) Explain why T helper cells are considered central cells of adaptive immunity? What effect would reduction in T helper cells have on immune status of an individual?

3. For each question, choose the *best* answer.
   (a) The medulla of a lymph node comprises mainly of
      (i) plasma cells
      (ii) B cells
      (iii) macrophages
      (iv) T cells
   (b) Which of the following lymphoid organs/tissues is unencapsulated?
      (i) Spleen
      (ii) Thymus
      (iii) Mucosa-associated lymphoid tissue
      (iv) Lymph node
   (c) Antigen-dependent immune responses occur in
      (i) bone marrow
      (ii) lymph nodes
      (iii) spleen
      (iv) both lymph nodes and spleen
   (d) Immature dendritic cells
      (i) kill target cells extracellularly
      (ii) activate naïve T cells
      (iii) mature into efficient APCs
      (iv) release histamine

The Antigens and Antibodies

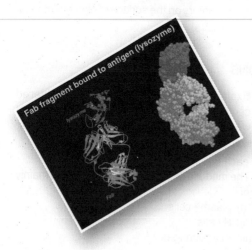

Fab fragment bound to antigen (lysozyme)

LEARNING OBJECTIVES

Having studied this chapter, you should be able to understand the following:

♦ The terms immunogen, antigen, hapten, and epitope, and their features

♦ The types of antigenic determinants and nature of B and T cell epitopes

♦ The basic structure of an antibody and the distinct structural and biological features of the five classes of antibodies

♦ How the antigen-binding site of an antibody molecule determines specificity for an antigen

♦ The nature of isotypes, allotypes, and idiotypes

♦ The distinction between monoclonal and polyclonal antibodies

♦ The theoretical basis of antigen–antibody interactions

♦ Murine, chimeric, and humanized monoclonal antibodies

An immune response arises due to the exposure of the body to foreign substances, referred to as antigens or immunogens, terms which are used interchangeably though functional differences exist. Those active parts of an immunogen to which the immune system responds are called antigenic determinants or epitopes. They are regions that can bind to antigen receptors on lymphocytes (or secreted antibodies), though receptors on B and T cells recognize them in very different ways.

Antibodies are soluble proteins that belong to a class of proteins called globulins, and because they contribute to immunity, they are also called immunoglobulins (Igs). Antibodies exist in both secreted and membrane-bound form, the latter serving as B cell receptor (BCR) for antigen. The structure of Igs allows them to specifically recognize and bind antigen. They exhibit great diversity which enables them to react with a vast array of antigenic determinants. Differences in antibody structure give rise to antibody classes and subclasses. Such differences in structure allow antibody molecules to participate in various types of biological activities.

Although innate immune mechanisms can effectively handle many types of infections, some pathogens have evolved ways that enable them to resist innate responses. For eliminating such microbes, antibodies (and also T lymphocytes) play a critical role. By binding to foreign substances, antibodies mark them for destruction by the immune system.

This chapter begins with a discussion of the nature and properties of immunogenic and antigenic substances and how these properties contribute to activation of the immune response. The types of epitopes, their features, and distinction between B and T cell epitopes is focused on. Antibody structure and the way it enables antibodies to interact specifically with an antigen are described. The link between structural features and functions is briefly introduced, though details of how antibodies function in host defence are described fully in Chapter 11. Polyclonal and monoclonal antibodies (mAbs), and their many applications have been emphasized. The concluding part of the chapter deals with some basic principles underlying antigen–antibody interactions, and also their practical applications.

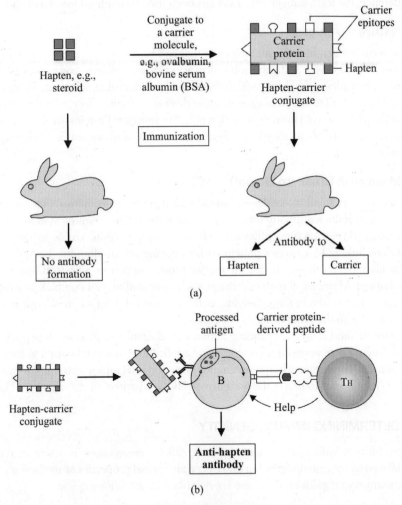

Fig. 4.1 **Haptens.** (a) Hapten-carrier conjugates can be used to raise antibodies to haptens. (b) B cell response to a hapten requires carrier protein and help from T cells. *Note:* In the above figure, hapten is the antigen, whereas the hapten-protein conjugate is the immunogen.

IMMUNOGENS AND ANTIGENS

Certain terms need to be defined before going on to discussions of the acquired immune response in later chapters. An *immunogen* is a substance capable of inducing an immune response (humoral and/or cell-mediated) as well as reacting with components of the immune response. These include soluble antibodies and surface receptors on B and T cells, namely BCR and T cell receptor (TCR), respectively. The term *antigen* was initially used for any molecule that caused *anti*body responses to be *gen*erated in B cells; hence, the name. Although the term is used synonymously with immunogen, a distinction is necessary. This is because not all antigens are capable of inducing an immune response, though they can react specifically with immune system components.

The definitions given in the preceding text imply that all immunogens are antigens, but the reverse is not true, that is, not all antigens are immunogens, for example, *haptens*. Despite this functional difference, the term antigen generally has been used throughout instead of immunogen.

Chemical Nature of Antigens

The term antigen includes all molecules that can be specifically recognized by antigen receptors on T and B lymphocytes. Antigenic substances are chemically diverse and include proteins, carbohydrates, lipids, and nucleic acids. Many self-molecules which induce damaging autoimmune reactions also serve as antigens. While antibodies can recognize diverse molecules, T cells for the most part recognize only small peptides derived from degradation of native proteins. Proteins are the most potent immunogens. Immunogenicity of carbohydrates, lipids, and nucleic acids increases when they are associated with proteins.

Haptens (Meaning in Greek 'to Grasp')

These are very small molecules (or individual antigenic determinants) that can react with antibodies, but cannot induce antibody formation on their own. The immune system apparently is unable to recognize these structures efficiently. However, they become visible to the immune system after covalent linkage to a carrier protein such as bovine serum albumin (BSA) or ovalbumin (Fig. 4.1). This allows a T cell specific for the carrier protein to deliver help to B cells to make antibodies to the hapten. Many small molecule drugs, such as penicillin, can complex to self-proteins and induce antibody formation. In some individuals, this is responsible for severe allergic reactions to subsequent treatment with the same drug.

This method is useful for raising antisera to molecules such as small peptides, steroid hormones, and drugs. These antibodies have practical applications and can be used to assay non-immunogenic substances. For instance, home-pregnancy detection kits employ anti-human chorionic gonadotropin (HCG) antibodies to detect the presence of HCG, a hapten, in the urine (see Fig. A.10).

FACTORS DETERMINING IMMUNOGENICITY

The ability to induce an immune response, called *immunogenicity*, is determined not only by features exhibited by the immunogen, but also by certain special properties of the biological system into which the immunogen gains entry. These are described in the following text.

Foreignness

Immune responses are not generally mounted against molecules of the host itself (self-molecules). Injecting BSA into mice will induce a strong immune response as the protein is foreign to the mouse. However, the same protein injected into cows will be recognized as self and will fail to induce a response. Occasionally, immune attack on self-components does occur. These autoimmune reactions may cause injury and lead to autoimmune diseases.

Molecular Mass

Small compounds (haptens) with a molecular weight < 1000 Da (daltons) such as steroids and penicillin are generally not immunogenic, though some exceptions may be there. Substances with a molecular weight between 5000 and 10,000 Da exhibit weak immunogenicity. The most potent immunogens are large molecules having a molecular mass approaching 1,00,000 Da.

Chemical Complexity

Synthetic molecules containing only a single amino acid, such as lysine, or even a single sugar, lack immunogenicity even though they may be of large molecular size. However, synthetic polymers and also naturally occurring foreign proteins, containing several different amino acids, show increased immunogenicity being chemically complex.

Ease of Antigen Processing (Degradation) and Presentation (Display)

It has been emphasized earlier that T cell recognition of a protein antigen depends on specific interaction of its TCR with a peptide–MHC complex on the surface of an antigen-presenting cell (APC). This requires a process known as *antigen processing* (see Chapter 5). It is only then that small fragments derived from the antigen associate with MHC molecules for display on the APC surface. This activates a specific T cell to clonally expand and differentiate into effector T cells. Substances which are resistant to partial enzymatic degradation in APCs, such as peptides composed of D-amino acids, are not good immunogens. In contrast, large insoluble molecules which are easily phagocytosed and processed are strongly immunogenic. It should be kept in mind that carbohydrate antigens are not susceptible to processing or presentation. They fail to activate T cells on their own, though B cells can be activated.

Besides intrinsic characteristics of the antigen, there are other *host-related factors* that affect immunogenicity. These are considered in the following text.

Genetic Constitution (Genotype) of the Host

MHC molecules which are encoded by genes within the MHC and which function to present antigenic peptides to T cells play a key role in determining immune responsiveness to a particular antigen. An individual will not mount an immune response to an antigen if peptides derived from it are unable to bind to MHC proteins for display on the surface (see Chapter 5).

Besides MHC genes, there are other genes, too, such as those that encode BCRs and TCRs that influence immune responses to antigens.

Dose of Antigen and Route of Administration

The *dose* should not be too large or too small, that is, a certain threshold dose is required at which the response is maximal. Above or below this dose, the response will not be optimal. A small dose may not be capable of activating a sufficient number of lymphocytes. A too high dose may induce a state of unresponsiveness or *tolerance* (inability to respond to an antigen) in responding cells (see Chapter 15). Rather than a single dose, repeated administrations spread over several weeks stimulate robust responses that lead to clonal proliferation and differentiation of antigen-specific B and T cells.

Route of administration is also a critical determinant of immunogenicity as antigens entering the body by various routes are carried to different lymphoid organs. The type and extent of the immune response will depend on the cell populations in that particular location. A subcutaneously (sc) injected antigen elicits a strong immune response. It is taken up by Langerhans cells in the skin and is carried to regional lymph nodes draining the site. Antigens administered via the intravenous (iv) route (for boosters) are transported to the spleen. Orally administered antigens may trigger an antibody response in MALT though they may even favour tolerance induction (see Chapter 15). It is reminded here that MALT is the mucosal lymphoid tissue (a secondary site) located in the gastrointestinal, respiratory, and genitourinary tracts. Intramuscular (im) and intraperitoneal (ip) routes are also common routes of administration.

The use of *adjuvants* along with antigens is another factor that determines the efficacy of the immune response stimulated. Adjuvants act as non-specific stimulators and are generally used along with soluble antigens such as proteins. The different types of adjuvants and their mode of action are described in Chapter 13.

EPITOPES

It is necessary to define first what epitopes are before proceeding to the nature of epitopes recognized by B and T cells. The immune response induced by an immunogen is not directed against the whole molecule as such, but against different parts of the molecule called *antigenic determinants* or *epitopes*. Epitopes are small active parts of the molecule that are recognized and bound by secreted or membrane-bound antibody or TCR. Macromolecules such as globular proteins possess many epitopes on their surface (see Fig. 4.18). Epitopes may be *continuous (linear)* or *discontinuous (conformational/assembled)*. Assembled epitopes are formed when amino acids which are separated in the primary sequence are brought close together in the tertiary structure due to folding of the polypeptide chain. The two types of epitopes are depicted in the folded polypeptide structure of sperm whale myoglobin (Fig. 4.2).

B Cell Epitopes

Epitopes recognized by membrane-bound antibodies on B cells, or secreted antibodies, are typically hydrophilic sequences on the antigen surface which are accessible to both BCR and secreted antibodies. Epitopes hidden inside are inaccessible and so do not function as B cell epitopes. But they may function as epitopes for B cells when they are degraded. However, the antibodies generated do not have a protective role as they fail to bind to an intact antigen.

B cell epitopes may be linear sequential residues or conformational determinants. Denaturation of a protein antigen, such as by heat, leads to unfolding of the protein and loss of conformational determinants. This is the reason why antibodies made against the native (natural) conformation do not, in many cases, react with the denatured molecule even though the primary sequence is unchanged (Fig. 4.3).

Fig. 4.2 Epitopes in the folded polypeptide chain of sperm whale myoglobin. Amino acid residues that contribute to two continuous epitopes (18–22, 56–62) are shown (there are five such epitopes). These are located at bends in the native protein. Amino acids 83, 144, and 145 contribute to a discontinuous epitope, whereas another such epitope is formed from amino acids 34, 53, and 113. The haem group in the protein is not shown.
Source: Based on Benjamin D.C. et al. (1984), 'The antigenic structure of proteins: A reappraisal', *Annual Review of Immunology*, 2, pp. 67–101.

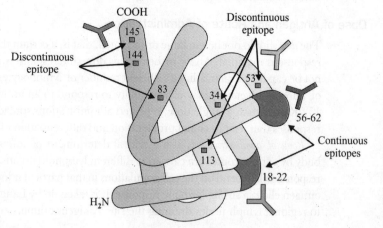

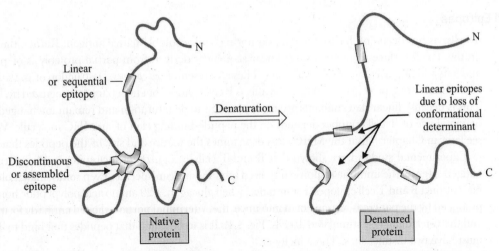

Fig. 4.3   A denatured protein showing loss of a conformational epitope. Antibodies to proteins in the native conformation do not, in many cases, react with the denatured protein. N, amino-terminal end of polypeptide chain. C, carboxyl-terminal end of polypeptide chain.

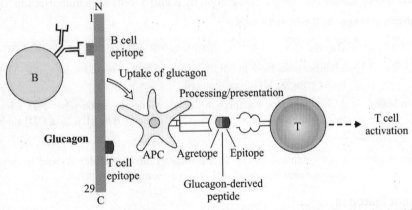

Fig. 4.4   Human glucagon showing B and T cell epitopes. A trimolecular complex involving MHC, TCR, and antigenic peptide forms before a T cell is activated (only signal 1 is shown here).

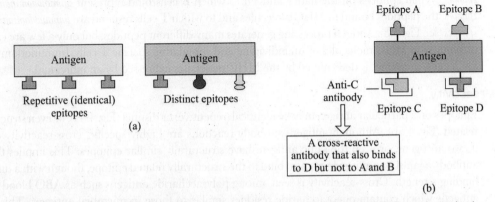

Fig. 4.5   Epitopes on an antigen may be identical, distinct, or structurally related. (a) Two antigens showing repetitive and distinct epitopes. (b) An antigen showing epitopes two of which (C and D) are structurally related. An antibody specific for epitope C also binds to D, though the binding strength (affinity) is lower.

T Cell Epitopes

T cells, as has been emphasized earlier, do not recognize soluble native antigen. Rather, the TCR on the T cell surface recognizes short linear sequences derived from partial proteolysis of protein antigens and displayed on MHC molecules. These represent *T cell epitopes*. Destruction of the shape or conformation of a protein by denaturation affects B cell epitopes but not epitopes recognized by T cells. This is because linear determinants are more resistant to denaturation and remain unchanged. The maximal size of T cell epitopes depends on the peptide-binding cleft of an MHC molecule. We will see later in Chapter 5 that the MHC class determines the nature and size of the peptides that bind.

Experimental studies have shown that B and T cells recognize distinct epitopes on a particular antigen. Hence, the immune response triggered remains antigen-specific. Even some small molecules have distinct B and T cell epitopes. For instance, when glucagon, a 29 amino acid polypeptide hormone produced by the pancreas, was injected into mice, the *N*-terminal portion elicited antibody formation and the *C*-terminal end stimulated T cells (Fig. 4.4). It is to be noted that peptides that bind to T cells must have two distinct sites. These include

- a site that interacts with the TCR called epitope; and
- another site that interacts with the MHC molecule called *agretope*.

Some salient features of antigen recognition by B and T cells are summarized in Table 4.1.

Table 4.1   Recognition of antigen by B cells and T cells.

Feature	B cells	T cells
Antigen interaction	Membrane-bound Ig (BCR) binds native antigen; MHC not required	T cell receptor binds peptide–MHC complex
Nature of antigen bound	Macromolecules, e.g., proteins, polysaccharides, and lipids	Generally peptides, but also lipids and glycolipids presented by MHC-like CD1 molecules
Binding to soluble antigen	Yes	No
Nature of antigenic determinants (epitopes)	Conformational and linear accessible (hydrophilic) sequences	Linear peptides derived from processing of antigen

Immunodominant Epitopes

Those epitopes or sites against which most of the immune response is directed are called *immunodominant epitopes*. While epitopes on the native antigen to which B cells bind represent *immunodominant B cell epitopes*, the peptides bound to MHC molecules and to which T cells respond are *immunodominant T cell epitopes* (see Fig. 5.8). Antigen processing generates many different peptides, but only a few are capable of binding to MHC molecules of an individual and stimulating specific T cells. Immunodominance for T cells, therefore, is determined by the MHC molecules expressed by an individual.

Cross-reactivity

Epitopes on a particular antigen may be identical (repetitive) or distinct (Fig. 4.5a), or even structurally related (Fig. 4.5b). Although antigen–antibody reactions are highly specific, cross-reactivity occurs if two anti-gens, or even the same antigen, have structurally similar epitopes. This implies that an antibody against one epitope may also bind to the structurally related epitope, though with a different binding strength. Cross-reactivity is seen among polysaccharide antigens such as ABO blood group antigens which contain oligosaccharide residues similar to those in microbial antigens. This is the basis for the presence of blood group antibodies which are induced in an individual on exposure to cross-reacting antigens on common intestinal bacteria (see Fig. 10.4).

Many viruses and bacteria have epitopes similar to normal host components. In some cases, these microbial antigens induce antibodies that cross-react with self resulting in tissue-damaging autoimmune reactions. For instance, antibodies produced to streptococcal M antigens in cell wall of streptococci have been shown to react with myocardial proteins leading to rheumatic fever (see Fig. 15.18). Some vaccines also show cross-reactivity, for example, vaccinia virus which causes cowpox expresses cross-reacting epitopes with variola virus, the agent that causes smallpox. This cross-reactivity was the basis of Jenner's method of using vaccinia virus to induce immunity to smallpox.

ANTIBODIES

Antibodies are the secreted form of the B cell antigen receptors and are produced by plasma cells (effector B cells). They are glycoproteins having a globular compact structure. As they confer immunity, they are also called *immunoglobulins* (*Igs*), a common name for antibodies. Early experiments by Tiselius and Kabat in 1939 revealed that most antibodies are found in the γ globulin fraction of serum proteins (Fig. 4.6). Although IgG which represents the major part of serum Igs is mostly found in this fraction, it is now known that antibody molecules of other classes, and IgG too, are found in the α and β fractions also.

There are five classes of Igs which differ structurally in the constant (C) regions of their heavy (H) chains (described in the following text). These are known as *isotypes* and include IgG, IgM, IgD, IgA, and IgE, and their H chains are designated γ, μ, δ, α, and ε, respectively. The salient features of each isotype are described later on in the chapter. The light (L) chains also exist in two forms which differ somewhat in amino acid sequence in their C regions, and are known as *kappa* (κ) and *lambda* (λ) isotypes. A given antibody contains either both κ or both λ chains, but never a mixture of the two. In humans κ chains are more frequent. Functionally, the two chains do not differ.

Fig. 4.6 Most antibodies are found in the γ globulin fraction of serum proteins. Serum from a rabbit immunized with ovalbumin (OVA) when subjected to electrophoresis showed a prominent peak for the γ globulin fraction. The same serum was subjected to electrophoresis after mixing with OVA and removing the precipitated antibody molecules (anti-OVA antibodies). The γ globulin peak declined considerably.
Source: Adapted from Tiselius, A. and E.A. Kabat (1939), 'An electrophoretic study of immune sera and purified antibody preparations', *Journal of Experimental Medicine* 69, pp. 119–131.
Note: The α globulin fraction was later shown to separate into α₁ and α₂ fractions.

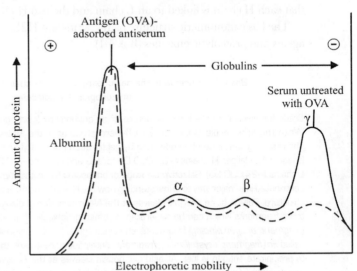

Basic Structure of an Antibody Molecule

The generalized structure of an antibody molecule shown as a Y-shaped symmetrical structure is represented in Fig. 4.7. It is also representative of the structure of IgG1, the most abundant IgG subclass that has been well characterized both structurally and functionally.

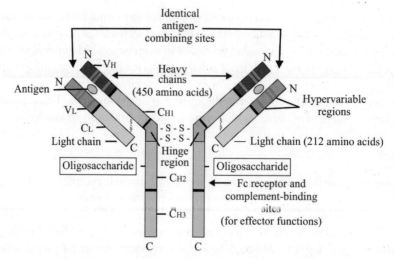

Fig. 4.7 Basic structure of an antibody molecule. The subscripts H and L in VH, CH, VL and CL denote that the variable and constant regions belong to heavy and light chains, respectively.

▮ ▯ variable and constant regions of light chains
▮ ▯ variable and constant regions of heavy chains

The antibody molecule is made up of four disulphide-linked polypeptide chains of which two are identical H chains and two identical L chains. IgG1 depicted in the figure has 450 amino acids in its H chain and 212 amino acids in its L chain. Each antibody chain contains a variable (V) region (which recognizes antigens) and a C region. The chains are joined together by disulphide bridges so that each H chain is linked to an L chain and the two H chains are linked together.

The basic monomeric structure of Igs, written as H2L2, was elucidated with the help of reducing agents and proteolytic enzymes (Box 4.1).

Box 4.1 Elucidating the basic four-polypeptide chain structure in monomeric immunoglobulin molecules

Credit for elucidating the basic structure of an antibody molecule goes to Porter and Edelman (Fig. 4.8). When the Ig molecule is treated with β-mercaptoethanol, the inter-chain disulphide bonds are reduced. The resulting chains can be separated by gel filtration (after alkylation to prevent reformation of disulphide bridges) into larger H chains (~55,000 Da for IgG and IgA, and ~70,000 Da for IgE and IgM), and smaller L chains (~24,000 Da). Selective cleavage of antibodies by proteolytic enzymes, such as papain and pepsin, contributed in a major way to understanding how the H and L chains are assembled to form the Ig monomeric structure. Papain, at neutral pH, cleaves at the N-terminal side of disulphide bonds in the hinge region to give three fragments which can be separated chromatographically. These include two identical monovalent *Fab* (*fragment, antigen binding*) fragments, and one fragment which crystallized at cold temperature and, so, was called *Fc* (*fragment, crystallizable*) fragment. With papain treatment, the ability of an intact antibody molecule to precipitate antigen is lost. At acid pH, pepsin cleaves at the C-terminal side of disulphide bonds to give one *bivalent F*(*ab'*)₂ molecule in which the two Fab fragments are joined by part of the hinge region. It has two antigen-binding sites and, so, can precipitate antigen unlike Fab. The remaining Fc part of the antibody is cleaved into many small fragments.

The above monomeric four-chain structure is present in IgG, IgE, and IgD. IgM is pentameric, whereas IgA exists principally as a dimer.

The Fc region differs in antibodies of different classes, and, so, they are specialized for activating different immune effector mechanisms. Fab, the part of the antibody molecule that recognizes antigen, contains a complete L chain (having one V and one C domain) attached to the V and first C domain (CH1) of the H chain. The two Fab fragments have identical antigen-binding specificity.

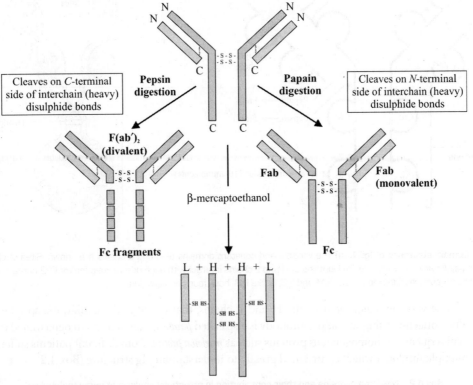

Fig. 4.8   Proteolytic cleavage and reduction of an immunoglobulin molecule.

The amino acids of L and H chains of Igs are not arranged linearly, but are folded to form loops called *domains* which are repeating units of 100–110 amino acid residues (Fig. 4.9).

Each domain is folded into two layers of β pleated sheets (a common element of protein structure) containing antiparallel β strands of amino acids. The structure is stabilized by hydrophobic interactions between the sheets and an intra-chain disulphide bond which encloses a loop of approximately 60 amino acids. The pattern of polypeptide chain folding into a characteristic three-dimensional shape and which is common in each of the domains is referred to as *Ig fold*. This structural feature of antibodies is also shared by other non-antibody proteins which together constitute the so-called *Ig superfamily*.

Both the H and L chains are made up of *variable domains* at their *N*-terminal ends. It is in these domains that amino acid sequence varies in antibodies of different specificities. These are designated V_H and V_L for H and L chains, respectively. The remaining domains are *constant domains* designated C_H and C_L, so-called because the amino acid sequence shows only limited variation in different antibodies.

An L chain has one V and one C domain, whereas an H chain has one V and three/four C domains designated CH1–CH3/CH4. Most of the domains interact with their corresponding domains on adjacent chains, thus, contributing to the tertiary or three-dimensional structure of the molecule. The CH2 domains have branched *N*-linked carbohydrate chains interposed between them and so have limited contact with each other. The *hinge region* is a flexible region rich in proline which lies between the CH1 and CH2 domains of the H chain regions of most antibody molecules. Due to this flexibility, an antibody molecule is able to bind to two determinants that are widely spaced on cell surfaces.

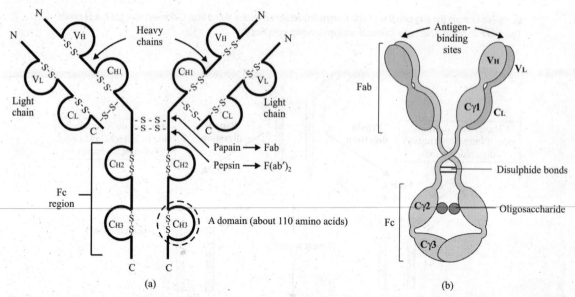

Fig. 4.9 Domain structure of IgG1. (a) The variable and constant domains of H and L chains are shown. Sites of cleavage by pepsin and papain are also indicated. (b) Domains of H and L chains interact with each other excepting for Cγ2 domains which are separated by oligosaccharide side chains. IgM and IgE, unlike IgG, have four constant domains.

The variable region of both the H and L chains, that is, V_H and V_L, bind the specific antigen. The antigen-binding site on the antibody is also called *paratope*. Kabat and Wu determined the amino acid sequence of homogeneous proteins such as *myeloma proteins* from different patients suffering from multiple myeloma which contributed greatly to understanding Ig structure (Box 4.2).

Box 4.2   Myeloma proteins and their contribution in structural analysis of immunoglobulins

Antigen-stimulated B lymphocytes differentiate into plasma cells which represent end-stage cells that secrete antibodies for a few days and then die. But plasma cells in multiple *myeloma patients* are not end-stage cells. In such patients, a single plasma cell undergoes malignant transformation and divides in an uncontrolled manner. This cell, called a *myeloma cell*, secretes large amounts of homogeneous Ig (identical in amino acid sequence) called a *myeloma protein* or *M protein* (Fig. 4.10). Although the plasma cell is abnormal, the product secreted is a normal protein. Myeloma proteins differ from patient to patient and they can constitute about 95 per cent of serum Ig. As this is a non-functional antibody, infections are common in patients.

In most patients, myeloma cells also secrete excessive amounts of L chains which are excreted in the urine. These were first described by Henry Bence Jones in 1847 in the urine of myeloma patients and were named *Bence Jones proteins*. Urine of a myeloma patient, therefore, is a source of a single species of L chain.

As antibodies in antiserum represent a heterogeneous mixture of a wide range of antibody specificities (formed due to exposure of an individual to a wide array of antigens), their use for determining antibody structure posed a big problem. Myeloma proteins and also Bence Jones proteins have helped considerably in deciphering the structure of antibodies as high concentrations of these proteins can be obtained from the serum/urine of myeloma patients.

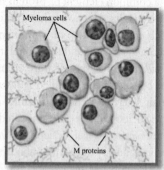

Fig. 4.10   Myeloma (M) proteins are homogeneous proteins secreted by a transformed plasma cell (myeloma cell) in multiple myeloma patients.

Immunologists used these proteins to perform the early amino acid sequencing experiments. Most of our knowledge about Ig structure and the structural basis for diversity of antibodies is based on analysis of these proteins.

It was found that variability was in the *N*-terminal 110 amino acids of both the H and L chains. Within the variable regions are the *hypervariable regions (HVRs)* where amino acid variations in different antibody molecules are most concentrated. Folding of the H and L chains brings together the hypervariable regions to create a surface that is complimentary to the antigen. These regions determine binding specificity to a given antigen and are referred to as *complimentarity determining regions (CDRs)*. There are three CDRs in *VH* and three in *VL*, each having about 10 amino acids. CDR3 exhibits the greatest variability (see Chapter 6). The regions between the hypervariable regions are the *framework regions (FRs)* which do not vary to the same extent as the variable region in different antibody molecules. Figure 4.11 represents the Kabat and Wu plot showing variability in amino acids in H chains of Ig molecules.

Antibody Classes and Subclasses

The salient structural and functional features of the five classes (isotypes) of antibodies (IgG, IgM, IgD, IgA, and IgE) are outlined as follows.

IgG and Its Subclasses

- IgG comprises about 75 per cent of the total Ig in serum. It is also the major Ig in extravascular spaces.
- There are four subclasses of IgG based on small differences in amino acid sequence in H chain C regions. These are designated IgG1, IgG2, IgG3, and IgG4 with IgG1 representing about 70 per cent of total IgG. Their H chains are designated γ1, γ2, γ3, and γ4, respectively.
- The subclasses also differ in the length of the hinge region and in number and position of inter-chain disulphide bonds.

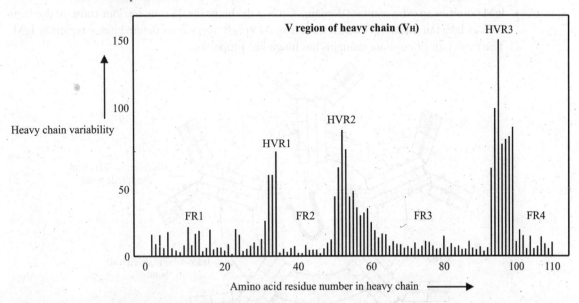

Fig. 4.11 Structure of the V region of the heavy (H) chain. The amino acid sequence of a large number of VH domains was compared. The variability at each position of the heavy chain variable domain is shown. The hypervariable regions (HVRs) are located at regions near amino acid positions 30, 50 and 95. Variable regions of H chains contain three HVRs (HVR1–HVR3) and four framework regions or FRs (FR1–FR4) where variability is low.

Note: Variability = $\dfrac{\text{Number of different amino acids at a given position}}{\text{Frequency of the most common amino acid at that position}}$

- IgG1 and IgG3 are generally superior at mediating effector functions, such as complement activation, phagocytosis, and antibody-dependent cell-mediated cytotoxicity (ADCC) relative to IgG2. IgG4 does not fix complement.

- Macrophages and polymorphonuclear leukocytes, mainly neutrophils (PMNs), carry receptors for the Fc region of IgG (FcγRs). These cells, thus, readily phagocytose IgG-coated targets. Fc receptors are membrane-bound glycoproteins on many cell types to which Fc regions of antibodies can bind. Some biological functions of antibodies are exerted through Fc receptors. There are different Fc receptors for many of the Ig classes. For instance, FcγR binds IgG, FcαR binds IgA, and FcεR binds IgE (see Chapter 11).

- IgG1, IgG3, and IgG4 readily cross the placenta and play an important role in protecting the developing foetus.

IgM

- IgM represents approximately 5–10 per cent of serum antibody with an average concentration of 1.5 mg ml^{-1}.

- In blood, IgM exists as a pentamer (9,00,000 Da) in which the five monomers are cross-linked to each other by disulphide bonds between their Fc regions and by a polypeptide chain called the *J chain* (Fig. 4.12). The J chain is disulphide-bonded to two of the five monomers. It serves to stabilize the pentameric IgM complex.

- IgM does not diffuse well due to its large size and, hence, is mostly intravascular.

- IgM, in monomeric form, serves as an antigen receptor on mature B cells. It is non-covalently associated with membrane proteins (Ig-α/Ig-β) which function as signal transducing molecules (see Chapter 10).

- IgM possesses an extra constant domain, -Cμ2- at the hinge site. It, thus, has four constant domains such as IgE, but unlike IgG which has three. As in IgE, there is no defined hinge region in IgM. The extra pair of constant domains has hinge-like properties.

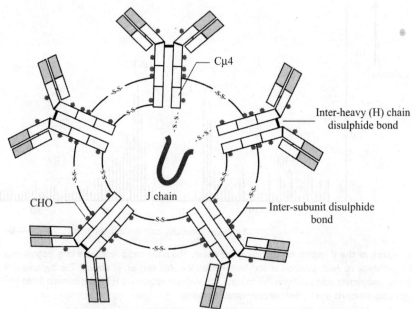

Fig. 4.12 Pentameric IgM. IgM monomers in pentameric IgM are cross-linked by disulphide bonds. The J chain which links two of the five subunits is also present in IgA.

- It is more efficient at activating complement than IgG and is also more effective as an agglutinating antibody. *Agglutination* is the clumping of microorganisms due to cross-linking by antibodies and is an important defence mechanism. Additionally, IgM has an accessory role as a secretory antibody at mucosal surfaces. Unlike IgG, IgM cannot cross the placenta.
- IgM antibodies are the first antibodies to appear after initial exposure to an antigen. Later on, response shifts to IgG antibodies.

IgD

- IgD is present in serum in very low concentration (30 μg ml^{-1}); its role in serum is not certain.
- It is co-expressed with IgM on the B cell membrane where it functions as a receptor for antigen.
- It is monomeric and possesses an extended hinge region and three constant domains.

IgA

- IgA is the second most common antibody in the serum where it exists as a monomer and constitutes about 10–15 per cent of total Ig.
- It is present in saliva, tears, secretions, for example, colustrum and milk, and in mucus as dimers, formed by joining of two monomers by the J chain (Fig. 4.13).
- *The secretory component (SC)*, which is made in epithelial cells, is part of the dimeric structure. It helps in the transport of IgA from the

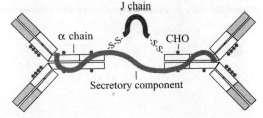

Fig. 4.13 Dimeric IgA. The J chain is attached to each monomer via disulphide bridges. The secretory component (SC) is an additional polypeptide chain present in IgA in mucosal secretions (sIgA).

submucosa across epithelial cells to mucosal surfaces in the alimentary and respiratory tracts where it provides local protection (see Chapter 11). Besides, SC protects IgA from breakdown by proteolytic enzymes present in intestinal secretions.
- There are two closely related subclasses of IgA in humans—IgA1 and IgA2. IgA2 has a shorter hinge region than IgA1 and is more resistant to attack by bacterial proteases.
- IgA cannot cross the placenta but is abundant in colustrum. This protects the newborn infant in the first month of life from gastrointestinal invasion by pathogens.

IgE

- IgE is present in normal serum in extremely low concentrations (0.05 μg ml^{-1}).
- Like IgM, it possesses four constant domains and lacks a hinge region.
- It is found mostly on the surface of blood basophils and also on tissue mast cells bound to Fc receptors (FcεR) even before it has interacted with antigens.
- Levels of IgE are raised in several parasitic diseases and is a protective measure. Binding of eosinophils through their Fc receptors to IgE coating the parasite causes eosinophils to degranulate and release toxic substances directly on the parasite surface causing damage (see Chapters 11 and 12).
- The same reactions that are important for defence can also result in undesirable allergic symptoms by certain antigens. IgE is a mediator of type I hypersensitivity reactions that are responsible for allergic disorders such as asthma, hay fever, and anaphylactic shock (see Chapter 14).
- IgE cannot fix complement.

It is to be remembered that each antibody class and subclass exhibits distinct effector functions. These are described fully in Chapter 11. For the time being, the major ways by which antibodies exert their protective effects are listed as follows:

+ Recruitment of the complement pathway for destruction or removal of pathogens
+ Promoting opsonization, phagocytosis, and killing of microbes by macrophages and neutrophils
+ Neutralization of toxins and viruses
+ ADCC

Some major properties of the different human isotypes are listed in Table 4.2.

Table 4.2 Human immunoglobulins.

Isotype	Subclass	Serum concentration (mg ml^{-1})	Half-life (days)	Major molecular form(s)	Biological function
IgG	IgG1	9	23	Monomer (γ2, L2)	Complement activation, neonatal immunity, opsonization for phagocytosis, ADCC
	IgG2	3	23		
	IgG3	1	8		
	IgG4	0.5	23		
IgA	IgA1	3	6	Monomer (α2, L2) Dimer (α2, L2)$_2$, J Secretory (α2, L2)$_2$, J, SC	Immunity at mucosal surfaces, present in tears, milk, and colustrum
	IgA2	0.5	6		
IgM	–	1.5	10	Pentamer (μ2, L2)$_5$, J	Complement activation, B cell antigen receptor
IgE	–	0.00005	2	Monomer (ϵ2, L2)	Protection against parasites by ADCC, (also mediates allergic reactions, type I hypersensitivity)
IgD	–	0.03	3	Monomer (δ2, L2)	B cell antigen receptor

Secreted and Membrane-associated Forms of Antibody

Immunoglobulins can be produced both in secreted soluble form and as membrane-bound form on B cells. The two forms differ in amino acid sequence at the *C*-terminal end (Fig. 4.14). In the secreted form found in blood and other extracellular fluids, the *C*-terminus has hydrophilic amino acid sequences that allow secretion. In the membrane-associated form of antibody found on plasma membrane of B cells, the *C*-terminus has a hydrophobic membrane-anchoring sequence of approximately 25 amino acids which extends across the lipid bilayer of the plasma membrane. The interaction of side chains of terminal basic amino acid residues of the antibody, which are located in the cytoplasm, with phospholipid head groups on the cytoplasmic surface of the membrane serves to anchor the antibody to the membrane. Secreted IgG and IgE and all membrane Ig molecules, regardless of isotypes, are monomeric, whereas secreted forms of IgM and IgA (sIgA) form pentameric and dimeric complexes, respectively. Membrane-bound Ig molecules expressed on B lymphocytes can be detected by immunofluorescence microscopy (see Fig. 3.14).

ANTIBODY VARIANTS—ISOTYPES, ALLOTYPES, AND IDIOTYPES

There are three types of Ig variants, namely *isotypes*, *allotypes*, and *idiotypes* (Fig. 4.15).

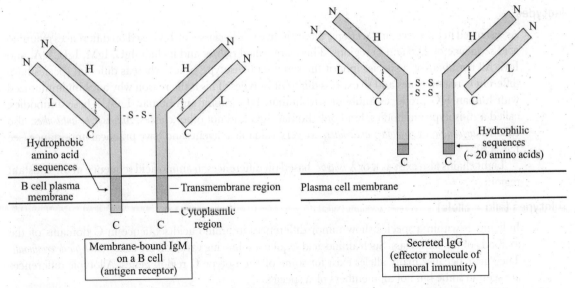

Fig. 4.14 Membrane-bound and secreted forms of immunoglobulins. A mature naïve B cell produces only the membrane-bound form, whereas plasma cells produce secreted antibodies.

Note: The membrane-bound form of IgM is associated with Ig-α/Ig-β which function as signal transducing molecules (not shown).

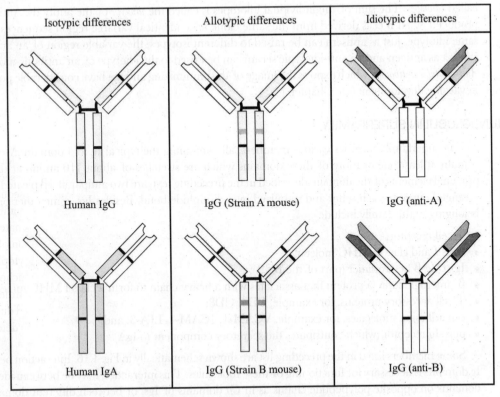

Fig. 4.15 Isotypic, allotypic, and idiotypic variations in antibody molecules.

Isotypes

As discussed in the preceding sections, there are five major classes of Igs based on differences in amino acid sequence of H chain C regions. These are called *isotypes* and include IgG, IgM, IgD, IgA, and IgE. All members of a species inherit the same set of isotype genes, whereas different species have different C region genes and so express different isotypes. This is the reason why a rabbit immunized with human IgG produces antibodies to human IgG (rabbit anti-human IgG). These antibodies, called anti-isotype antibodies, bind only human IgG and not other classes. *Anti-isotype antibodies*, also called *antiglobulins* or *secondary antibodies*, are very valuable reagents and have practical importance (see Fig. A.8).

Light chains also exist as κ or λ *isotypes* based on differences in amino acid sequence in the constant region.

Allotypes (allo = allele)

Individuals within a species show minor differences in amino acid sequence in C domains of the antibody of the same class. Such amino acid sequences showing variation are called *allotypic determinants*. They arise because many alleles exist for some of the isotype C region genes. Allotypic differences are seen in some but not all members of a species.

In man, allotypes have been identified in IgG for all four classes and also for IgA and IgM.

Idiotypes

The unique amino acid sequences in the variable region of L and H chains of an antibody are called *idiotopes*. The sum of the individual idiotopes is called the *idiotype* of the antibody. Antibodies produced by all B cells derived from the same clone have identical variable region sequences or the same idiotype. Just as antisera can be raised to different isotypes, the variable region of an antibody can act as antigen and an anti-idiotypic serum can be raised to the idiotype of an antibody molecule. *Anti-idiotypic antibodies*, which express the image of the immunizing antigen have considerable potential in vaccine development (see Chapter 13).

IMMUNOGLOBULIN SUPERFAMILY

The Ig superfamily includes various members, all containing the typical Ig fold domain. Members contain at least one or more of these domains which are stretches of about 110 amino acids. The principal elements of the domain, described in the preceding text, are two antiparallel β pleated sheets arranged opposite each other and stabilized by a disulphide bond. Besides Igs, some other proteins belonging to this family include

- T cell receptor;
- class I and class II MHC molecules;
- Ig-α/Ig-β heterodimer (part of the BCR);
- β_2 microglobulin (a protein that associates with a heavy chain to form a class I MHC molecule);
- T cell accessory proteins, for example, CD4, CD8;
- cell adhesion molecules, for example, VCAM-1, 1CAM-1, LFA-3; and
- poly-Ig receptor (which contributes the secretory component to IgA).

Some members listed in the preceding list are shown schematically in Fig. 4.16. Interaction between Ig domains is necessary for functioning of these molecules. This interaction may be between identical domains on opposite polypeptide chains as in C_H domains of Igs, or between different domains as in V_H and V_L interaction which forms the antigen-binding site. Similar interactions occur for other members of the Ig superfamily.

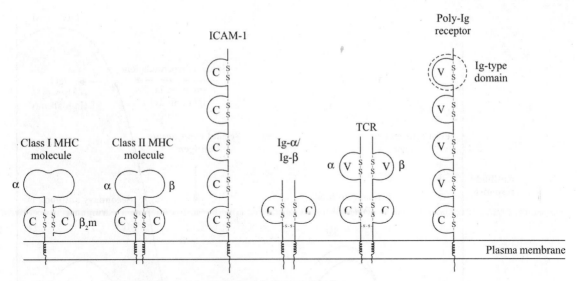

Fig. 4.16   Some selected members of the immunoglobulin superfamily.
C, homology with Ig constant domain. *V,* homology with Ig variable domain.

PRIMARY AND SECONDARY ANTIBODY RESPONSE

As introduced earlier in Chapter 1, the first exposure of an individual to an antigen results in a response called the *primary immune response*, whereas a later exposure to the same antigen activates a *secondary immune response*. Several features summarized in the following text distinguish a primary and secondary antibody response to an antigen (Fig. 4.17).

◆ The primary immune response has an initial latent or lag phase before the antibody can be detected in the serum, whereas the secondary response is much faster.

◆ The secondary immune response is more intense and persists for a longer period.

◆ The major antibody in the primary response is IgM, whereas IgG predominates in the secondary response.

◆ Antibodies produced in the secondary response are of higher affinity due to a phenomenon called *affinity maturation* (see Chapter 10).

The reason for the relatively slow primary response is that naïve lymphocytes are seeing antigen for the first time and many events need to be activated. On the other hand, the secondary response is faster as on second or subsequent antigen encounter, memory cells induced in the primary response are rapidly stimulated.

POLYCLONAL AND MONOCLONAL ANTIBODIES

A large molecule, such as a protein antigen, generally contains multiple distinct epitopes. Hence, when injected into an animal, it stimulates many B cell clones, each specific for a particular epitope to proliferate and differentiate into antibody-secreting plasma cells (Fig. 4.18).

This polyclonal response generates a heterogeneous mixture of antibodies in serum, some of which bind to the antigen with high-affinity, whereas others do not. Such a serum is called a *polyclonal antiserum*. A polyclonal response in vivo has obvious advantages in protecting against pathogens which have a wide variety of antigenic structures on their surface. Polyclonal antibodies can be generated by

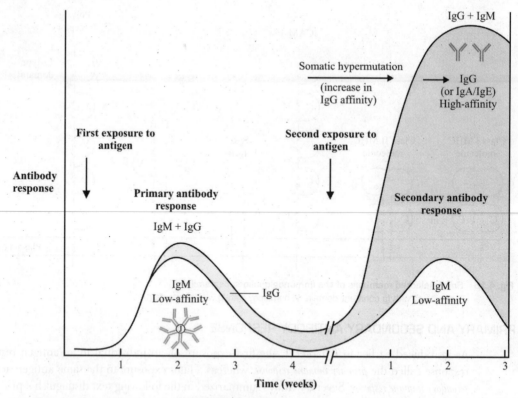

Fig. 4.17   Primary and secondary antibody response.

repeated immunization with the relevant antigen (see Fig. A.1). Without an adjuvant, immunization with an antigen (soluble) alone is not effective (see Chapter 13). Monoclonal antibodies are derived from a single B cell clone and are, therefore, specific for a single epitope. They are homogeneous antibodies with identical antigen-combining sites and are of the same isotype. Monoclonal antibodies are produced by the *hybridoma technology* which is described in detail in Appendix 1 (see Fig. A.3). In this fascinating technology, a single antibody-secreting cell and a transformed plasma cell (myeloma cell) are fused to give a *hybridoma*. This fused product, besides being immortal, produces antibodies of the required specificity.

Important Applications of Monoclonal Antibodies

Antibodies are important research tools and have numerous practical applications. As reagents, monoclonals have striking advantages over polyclonal antibodies. Although antisera raised in different animals are quite distinct from each other and lack consistency, mAbs can be obtained in reproducible batches and in unlimited

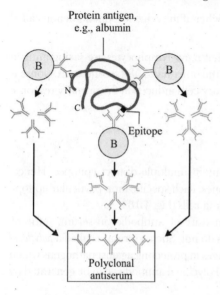

Fig. 4.18   A globular protein antigen activates many B cell clones. Antiserum raised to a large protein antigen having many epitopes, such as albumin, contains many different types of antibodies (anti-albumin antibodies) varying in specificity and affinity and is called *polyclonal antiserum*. A microbe with several antigenic determinants on its surface will produce a similar response.

amounts. Also, a polyclonal antiserum contains antibodies against the immunizing antigen and also many other antibodies of varying specificity. These can interfere in assays and yield results that are often misleading, a problem that is avoided by the use of a monoclonal preparation. With the added advantages of homogeneity and unique specificity, mAbs are used in research laboratories all over the world.

Some practical uses of mAbs include identification of proteins using Western blot method, in affinity purification of antigens, in epitope analysis of proteins for identification of B and T cell epitopes, in distinguishing between cell types, and many more.

Besides the many practical uses of mAbs, they have a major role in clinical laboratories as diagnostic tools. They are used for diagnosis of infectious diseases based on detection of particular antigens or antibodies in the circulation. Radiolabelled mAbs find use in imaging techniques for tumour detection, both primary and metastatic growth. As the labelled antibody is specific for the tumour, it concentrates at the tumour site which can be traced by use of body scanners. In addition, they are being used for early detection of pregnancy and for detection of various hormones in blood or urine samples. Typing of blood group antigens and human leukocyte antigen (HLA) typing are other important applications.

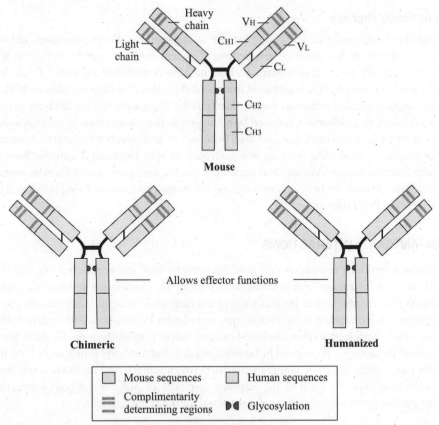

Fig. 4.19 Chimeric and humanized antibodies. Variable regions of murine monoclonals fused to human Ig constant regions generate chimeric antibodies. Grafting the six mouse CDRs onto a constant and variable domain framework provided by human Ig produces humanized antibodies.
Source: Adapted from Cartier, P. (2001), 'Improving the efficacy of antibody-based cancer therapies', *Nature Reviews Cancer*, 1, pp. 118–129.

The use of *Rhogam*, an antibody to the RhD antigen, which is given to Rh negative mothers to protect against haemolytic disease of the newborn (HDN), has been a significant development in immunology. Other noteworthy successes of the use of mAbs are highlighted at relevant places in the book.

Although mAbs have tremendous potential as immunotherapeutic agents, their use is not without limitations. As these antibodies are commonly raised in mice (murine monoclonals), they are seen as foreign proteins by the human immune system and induce an immune response (see Chapter 18). This gives rise to complications due to formation of large quantities of immune complexes in the circulation. To overcome this, murine antibodies are being genetically engineered to produce *chimeric antibodies* in which mouse variable regions are fused to C regions of human Igs. Mouse sequences can be reduced still further to produce *humanized antibodies* for use in therapy. The hypervariable region or CDRs of murine products are transplanted onto the C regions and framework provided by human antibodies (Fig. 4.19). As foreign sequences are reduced, the immune response is minimized.

Some mAbs have been approved for clinical use, mostly for immunotherapy of cancer (see Chapter 18) and for rheumatoid arthritis, an autoimmune disorder (see Chapter 15). Many others are undergoing clinical trials.

Passive Antibody Therapy

Administering preformed antibody (passive immunization) affords protection, although temporary, against infection. It is also used in treatment of patients with immunodeficiencies in which circulating antibodies are reduced or absent, such as in *X-linked agammaglobulinemia* (*X-LA*). Immunoglobulin for passive immunization is prepared from pooled plasma of a large number of healthy donors. This preparation is called *intravenous immune globulin* (*IVIG*). Recipients of such antibody preparations receive a sample of the antibodies produced by many people to a broad range of pathogens (see Chapter 16).

Specific Ig is also used. It is prepared from sera of individuals who have been recently immunized or who are convalescing from an infection, such as with Hepatitis B virus, or from *Clostridium tetani* which causes tetanus. Monoclonal antibodies specific for a particular infectious agent and which are humanized would be better therapeutic agents. Some products are being developed and will be able to replace IVIG therapy.

ANTIGEN–ANTIBODY INTERACTIONS

Antigen–antibody complexes can be dissociated by high salt concentrations and extremes of pH. Hence, the interaction is non-covalent in nature. The association involves the same non-covalent forces that are involved in protein–protein interactions in general. They include electrostatic forces, hydrogen bonds, hydrophobic interactions, and van der Waals forces. Although individual interactions are weak, many interactions combined can give rise to firm binding. As the above forces operate over a small distance (~1 Å), a good fit between antigen and antibody is necessary for a firm interaction. For this, a high degree of complimentarity between antigen and antibody is required (Fig. 4.20). It is this that forms the basis of the exquisite specificity of antigen–antibody interactions, and makes antibodies extremely valuable as reagents and for other applications.

Antigen–Antibody Interaction—A Reversible Reaction

The antigen–antibody interaction is a reversible reaction. This can easily be demonstrated by placing a mixture of hapten and its specific antibody in a dialysis bag. Hapten–antibody complexes form and spontaneously dissociate depending on the binding strength. After a period of time, when equilibrium

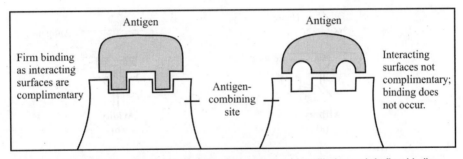

Fig. 4.20 Complimentary interacting surfaces in antigen and antibody result in firm binding.

is attained, rate of complex formation and dissociation is equal. If the dialysis bag is placed in a container filled with fluid, the hapten diffuses out of the bag into the surrounding fluid. By changing the fluid continuously, all the hapten will diffuse out of the bag demonstrating that binding of hapten with antibody is reversible in nature.

Antibody Affinity

This is the strength of binding of a single epitope to the antigen-binding site of an antibody and includes strength of all non-covalent interactions involved. For determination of affinity of a single antigen-binding site, a small antigen, such as a hapten with a single epitope is required (Fig. 4.21a). The association called a *primary interaction* (described in the following text) can be represented by the following equation:

$$Ag + Ab \rightleftharpoons Ag - Ab$$

As the reaction is reversible, it follows the Law of Mass Action and chemical equilibrium according to which

$$K = \frac{[Ag - Ab]}{[Ag][Ab]}$$

where K is the equilibrium constant represented as Ka or association constant and the square brackets indicate the concentration of the reactants. Ka, also called *affinity constant*, measures affinity and can be calculated. Its value varies for different antigen–antibody complexes. High-affinity antibodies bind antigen relatively tightly and so remain bound longer than do the low-affinity antibodies. The affinity of antibodies is of importance physiologically as a toxin or a virus in the body must be neutralized by rapid and firm binding with its specific antibody. Antibodies formed after primary immunization with an antigen are of much lower affinity than antibodies generated later on subsequent immunization (boosters).

Antibody Avidity

This is the firmness of association of a multideterminant antigen (having many epitopes) and a bivalent/multivalent antibody. The strength of the interaction with an antibody having more binding sites will be greater as more bonds will be formed with antigens and the antibody is less likely to dissociate (Fig. 4.21b and c).

Although IgM antibodies (pentameric) have poor intrinsic affinity for an antigenic deter-minant, they have high avidity due to the large number of antigen-binding sites per molecule. The higher avidity of IgM antibodies compensates for low-affinity. Immunoglobulin M frequently recognizes repetitive epitopes that are commonly present in bacterial cell wall polysaccharides and viral particles. It can bind

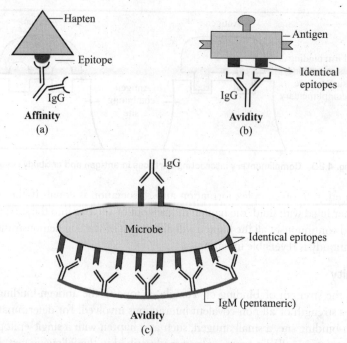

Fig. 4.21 Antibody affinity and avidity.

antigens very firmly and, hence, is more effective than IgG in neutralizing a virus or a bacterial cell, or agglutinating particles. Besides, IgM is efficient at activating complement.

Primary and Secondary Antigen–Antibody Interactions

It is necessary to understand the nature of primary and secondary antigen–antibody interactions as many sensitive assays and techniques included in Appendix 1 are based on them.

The specific recognition and interaction of an antigenic determinant with the binding site of its corresponding antibody usually occurs very rapidly and is not a visible reaction. This is because the immune complex formed is small in size (Fig. 4.21a). Such interactions are *primary interactions* on which sensitive immunoassays, such as *radioimmunoassay (RIA)* and *enzyme-linked immunosorbent assay (ELISA)* are based. As primary interactions are non-visible reactions, the binding of antigen and antibody can only be detected by use of various labels. Commonly used labels include

- radioisotopes,
- fluorochromes, and
- enzymes.

Some other labels include biotin and minute gold particles. The most widely used labels are enzymes.

Secondary interactions are due to interaction between multideterminant antigens and anti-bodies, or even F(ab′)₂ which has two combining sites per molecule. These interactions result in increase in size of the antigen–antibody complex to form a large aggregate or a lattice which is a network of alternating antigen and antibody molecules (Fig. 4.22). Unlike primary interactions, these reactions are visible reactions and take the form of *agglutination* (for particulate antigens; see Fig. 11.3) or *precipitation* (for soluble antigens). Precipitation reactions are slow to develop and may take hours or days to reach completion.

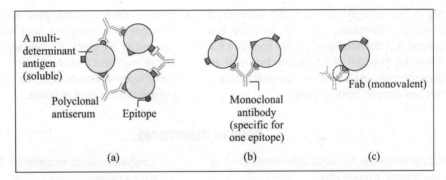

Fig. 4.22 **Secondary interactions.** A multideterminant soluble antigen precipitates well with a polyclonal antiserum (a). With a monoclonal antibody (b) or a monovalent Fab fragment, obtained on papain treatment (c), there is no precipitation as the complex does not grow.

SUMMARY

- An immunogen is a substance that can both induce an immune response as well as react with components of the immune response, whereas an antigen reacts with immune system components. So, all immunogens are antigens, but all antigens are not immunogens.
- Small molecules called haptens are antigens which induce an immune response only when conjugated to a large protein molecule.
- Many factors determine immunogenicity of a substance such as foreignness, molecular mass, chemical complexity, ease of antigen processing, and genetic constitution of the individual. Dose, route of administration of antigen, and adjuvants are also important factors.
- Epitopes or antigenic determinants are those small regions on an antigen against which the immune response is directed. Epitopes may be continuous (linear) or discontinuous (conformational). B and T cells recognize distinct epitopes on a particular antigenic molecule.
- Antibodies, also called immunoglobulins (Igs), basically consist of two light (L) chains and two heavy (H) chains which are disulphide-linked. Each chain contains a variable (V) region (which recognizes the antigen) and a constant (C) region. The heavy chain C region carries out the effector functions of antibodies.
- There are five types of heavy chains based on small amino acid differences in heavy chain constant regions. This gives rise to five types of Ig classes.

- These include IgG, IgM, IgD, IgA, and IgE, and their heavy chains are designated γ, μ, δ, α, and ε. The different classes of Igs differ in properties and biological activities.
- Immunoglobulin domains have a characteristic structure called the immunoglobulin fold. This structure is present in many other proteins besides antibodies. All proteins with this structure are members of the immunoglobulin superfamily.
- Antigens are recognized and bound by Fab regions of antibodies. These regions contain highly variable amino acid sequences called CDRs which differ in different antibody molecules. As these are the regions which contact antigens, antibody molecules produced by different clones bind to distinct antigens. Remaining regions in the variable part show less variation and are the framework regions.
- Antibodies exist in two forms. The soluble form is secreted by plasma cells and is the effector molecule of humoral immunity. The membrane-bound form on the B cell surface (mIgM) is the B cell receptor for an antigen or BCR. The two forms show structural differences.
- The secondary immune response is swifter and more intense than the primary immune response.
- Polyclonal antibodies are generated from many B cell clones and represent a heterogeneous mixture, whereas monoclonal antibodies arise from a single B cell clone and are homogeneous.
- An antigen–antibody interaction involves non-covalent forces. Covalent links are not involved.

- Affinity is the strength of interaction between a single antigen-combining site of an antibody and an epitope. It is defined by an affinity constant Ka. Avidity is the strength of interaction between an antigen with multiple epitopes and an antibody with at least two antigen-binding sites.

- Primary interactions are non-visible reactions. Many sensitive immunoassays, such as ELISA and RIA are based on them. Secondary interactions are visible reactions and are due to increase in size of the antigen–antibody complex. They manifest as precipitation or agglutination.

REVIEW QUESTIONS

1. Indicate whether the following statements are true or false. If false, explain why.
   (a) Agretope is the part of an antigenic peptide that interacts with the T cell receptor.
   (b) IgE has four constant region domains in its heavy chain.
   (c) Antibody avidity defines the binding strength of a single antigen-binding site of an antibody molecule with an epitope.
   (d) A Fab fragment is produced by cleavage of an antibody molecule by pepsin.
   (e) Idiotype of an antibody is found in the variable region of both light and heavy chains.
   (f) A paratope is that part of the antigen surface that is in contact with an antibody.

2. Self-assessment questions
   (a) An animal is immunized with antigen X and then re-exposed to the same antigen 3 weeks later. How would you explain differences in the immune response activated on the first and second encounter with the antigen?
   (b) What is the major obstacle in the use of murine monoclonals for therapeutic purposes? Can you explain ways by which this obstacle is overcome?
   (c) Which regions contribute to antigen-binding in an antibody molecule and determine its specificity. Where are these sites located?
   (d) An antigen entering the bloodstream is bound by IgG, the major Ig isotype in serum. Would the same antigen gaining access to the body by the oral route be bound by IgA, the abundant isotype in mucus secretions? Give reasons for your answer.
   (e) Monoclonal antibodies to a globular protein antigen failed to react with the antigen when it was subjected to heat. What, in your opinion, could be the reason for this? Would T cells respond to the denatured protein?

3. For each question, choose the *best* answer.
   (a) A F(ab')$_2$ fragment
      (i) is divalent
      (ii) lacks light chains
      (iii) is produced by papain cleavage
      (iv) lacks inter-chain disulphide bonds
   (b) Binding of antibody to Fc receptors on phagocytic cells depends on
      (i) variable region of heavy chain
      (ii) constant region of heavy chain
      (iii) light chain
      (iv) hinge region
   (c) Which of the following is not true for IgM?
      (i) heavy chain has four constant domains
      (ii) is good at agglutinating particles
      (iii) neutralizes pathogens in tissues
      (iv) can fix complement
   (d) Antigenic determinants found in the variable region domains of antibodies are described as
      (i) allotypic
      (ii) isotypic
      (iii) idiotypic
      (iv) complimentarity determining regions

Major Histocompatibility Complex (MHC)

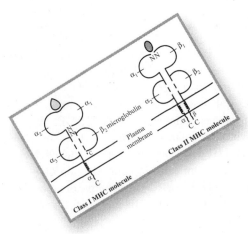

LEARNING OBJECTIVES

Having studied this chapter, you should be able to understand the following:

- How the MHC is organized and the inheritance pattern of MHC genes
- Major structural features of the two types of MHC molecules and their role
- The nature of peptides that bind to MHC class I and class II molecules
- The unique polymorphism of MHC genes and its significance
- How endogenous and exogenous antigens are processed and presented for activation of an immune response
- Cross-presentation by dendritic cells
- A third pathway of antigen presentation by which lipid antigens are presented by class I MHC-like molecules

The major histocompatibility complex (MHC) is a closely linked cluster of genes located on chromosome 6 in humans. The region codes for cell surface proteins called the major histocompatibility complex molecules (from *histo*, a Greek word meaning 'tissue'). The MHC molecules in humans are also referred to as human leukocyte antigens (HLA) as these antigens were first detected on leukocytes. Early studies identified these highly polymorphic molecules as the major barrier to organ/tissue transplantation (the term polymorphism refers to the existence of a gene in many different allelic forms). It is due to differences in amino acid sequence of MHC proteins between individuals that tissue grafts are recognized as foreign by T cells. Activation of a very strong T cell-mediated immune response to foreign MHC molecules on the graft causes graft rejection. This role of MHC proteins in graft rejection is incidental. Their major physiological role is to present antigenic peptides to T cells for initiation of an immune response. It should be recalled from preceding chapters that there is a very important distinction between B and T lymphocyte receptors. While antibodies recognize native, unmodified antigen (e.g., on the surface of a bacterium or free in solution), T cell receptors (TCRs) recognize protein antigens only after they have been processed (degraded) into peptides inside cells and presented on the surface in context of self-MHC molecules. This is known as *self-MHC restriction of T lymphocytes* and is a very important and fundamental feature of the immune system.

The crucial role of MHC molecules is evident from the immunodeficiency disorder *bare lymphocyte syndrome* (*BLS*), a congenital defect in which antigen-presenting cells (APCs) do not express class II MHC molecules (see Chapter 16). CD4$^+$ T cells fail to be activated due to inability of APCs to present antigenic peptides. All T helper cell functions are affected, such as B cell activation, cytotoxic T lymphocyte (CTL) generation besides others.

This chapter commences with a brief description of the general organization and inheritance pattern of MHC genes, and the structure and function of MHC class I and class II molecules that are encoded within it. The advantage the high degree of MHC polymorphism exhibited by these specialized molecules confers on individuals, and the link between certain MHC genes and disease susceptibility is described. The sequence of events in processing and presentation pathways for endogenous and exogenous antigens is briefly reviewed. Cross-presentation of exogenous antigens and also presentation of non-peptide antigens are outlined in the concluding part of the chapter.

ORGANIZATION OF MAJOR HISTOCOMPATIBILITY COMPLEX

The MHC in humans, also known as the HLA complex, is organized into three distinct regions which include class I, class II, and class III MHC gene loci. The class I MHC genes were the first to be discovered. They are sometimes designated as *classical class I MHC genes* or *class IA*. Some class I genes were identified subsequent to discovery of classical class I MHC genes. These are referred to as *class IB* or *non-classical class I MHC genes*. Their products in humans include HLA-E, HLA-F, HLA-G, and others also. These class I-like MHC molecules are limited in distribution and some have specialized functions to perform. For instance, HLA-G and HLA-E molecules expressed by cells at the foetal–maternal interface have a role in protecting the foetus from being recognized as foreign.

Mouse MHC located on chromosome 17 is known as the H-2 *complex*. The genomic organization of human and mouse MHC genes are diagrammed in simplified form in Figs 5.1 and 5.2, respectively.

Class I MHC Genes

The three genes in human class I region are designated *HLA-A*, *HLA-B*, and *HLA-C*. These encode class I MHC molecules which are expressed on almost all nucleated cells. There is one gene in each locus which codes for the α chain (described in the following text). It pairs with β_2 *microglobulin* (β_2m) which is non-MHC encoded. This pairing is essential for expression of MHC class I molecules on the cell surface. The gene for β_2m lies on chromosome 15 in humans. In mice, the three class I MHC genes are named *K*, *D*, and *L*. A noteworthy feature is that the class I region in mouse is split into two. Also, the D region encodes class I MHC molecules, unlike the D region in humans which codes for class II molecules as described in the following text.

Class II MHC Genes

The genes in the class II MHC region in humans are designated *HLA-DP*, *HLA-DQ*, and *HLA-DR*. These genes encode proteins which are expressed mostly on APCs where they function to present antigenic peptides to CD4$^+$ T helper cells. Additionally, the class II MHC locus has genes which encode molecules having specialized roles. Products encoded include peptide transporter proteins TAP-1 and TAP-2 (these are involved in class I MHC antigen processing pathway), *HLA-DM* (an HLA class II-like molecule which facilitates loading of antigenic peptides into class II molecules), and others also.

In mice, H-2 contains two class II MHC regions (unlike humans where there are three class II regions) named *I-A* and *I-E*. These encode I-A αβ and I-E αβ molecules, respectively.

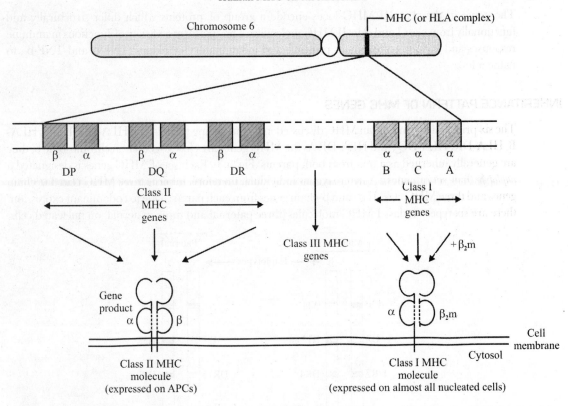

Fig. 5.1 Organization of MHC genes in humans. Each class II subregion codes for α and β chains of an MHC class II protein.
Note: Distances between various genes and regions are not drawn to scale.
β₂m, β₂ microglobulin.

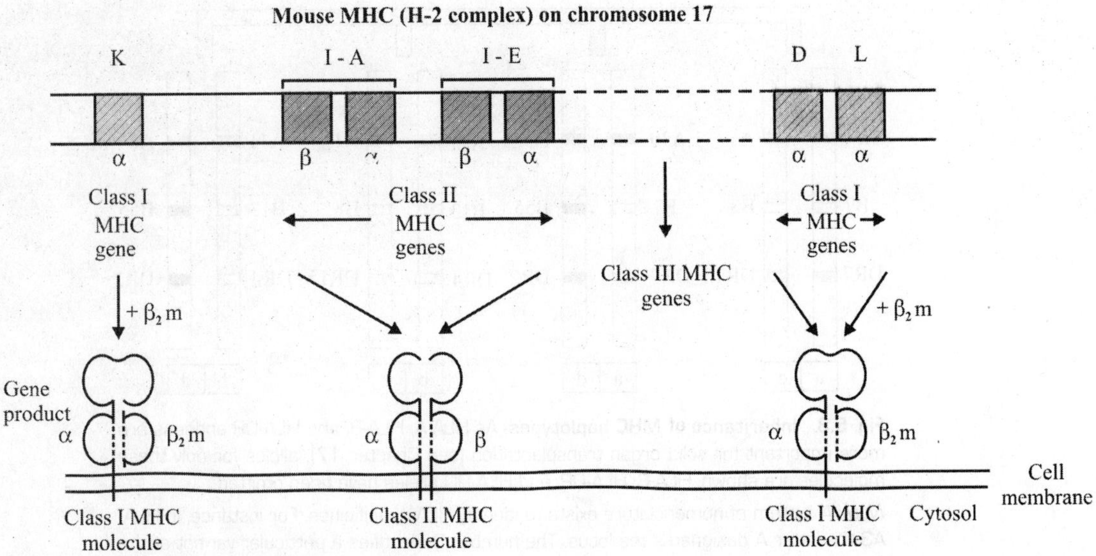

Fig. 5.2 Organization of MHC genes in mouse.

Class III MHC Genes

The genes in the class III MHC locus encode a group of proteins which differ structurally and functionally from class I and class II MHC molecules. They perform a variety of functions in immune responses and include complement proteins, and inflammatory cytokines (TNF-α and TNF-β), to name a few.

INHERITANCE PATTERN OF MHC GENES

The six principal loci in human MHC discussed in the preceding text include HLA-A, HLA-C, HLA-B, HLA-DR, HLA-DQ, and HLA-DP. As the MHC genes are close together on chromosome 6, they are generally inherited as a unit from both parents (Fig. 5.3). Each set of MHC genes is designated a *haplotype* (half set of genes). A heterozygous individual, therefore, inherits three MHC class I α-chain genes and three MHC class II α- and β-chain genes from each parent. Due to codominant expression, there are six types of class I MHC molecules (three paternal and three maternal) on nucleated cells,

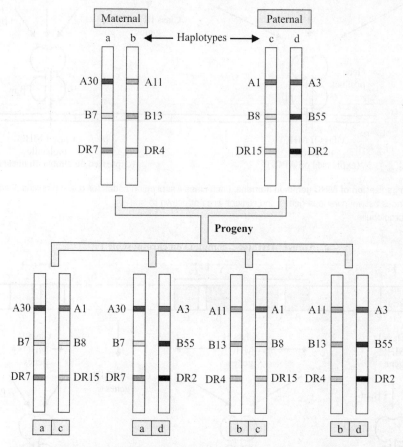

Fig. 5.3 Inheritance of MHC haplotypes. As HLA-A, HLA-B, and HLA-DR antigens are more important for solid organ transplantation (see Chapter 17), alleles for only these molecules are shown. HLA-C, HLA-DP, and HLA-DQ alleles have been omitted.

Note: A system of nomenclature exists to identify HLA specificities. For instance, in HLA-A3 the letter A designates the locus. The number 3 identifies a particular variant at the HLA-A locus.

and at least six different class II molecules on APCs. This is because α- and β-chains from different chromosomes may pair to generate different α- and β-chain combinations . The advantage of this is evident and needs to be emphasized. It maximizes the number of different MHC molecules available to bind peptides allowing a wide range of peptides to be presented to T cells. The pattern of expression of MHC molecules in an individual is genetically determined and is unique to that individual. This is the reason why it is rare to find identical sets of HLA genes in two individuals who are unrelated.

CLASS I AND CLASS II MHC MOLECULES

Class I and class II MHC molecules are membrane-bound glycoproteins that form stable complexes with antigenic peptides. These complexes are displayed on the surface for recognition by antigen-specific T lymphocytes. The structural features of class I and class II MHC molecules are shown in Fig. 5.4.

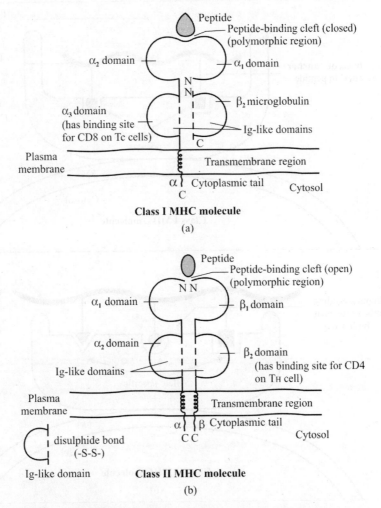

Fig. 5.4   Schematic diagram of structure of (a) Class I MHC molecule and (b) Class II MHC molecule.

Class I MHC Molecules

Class I MHC molecules consist of two polypeptide chains. These include a glycosylated α chain, which is the heavy chain, and a light chain called β_2 microglobulin, which is identical in all cells and, as mentioned in the preceding text, is not encoded within the MHC. The α chain is a transmembrane protein organized into three extracellular domains α_1, α_2, and α_3. The α_1 and α_2 domains which form the peptide-binding cleft are extremely polymorphic and have a sequence unique to that allelic form. As the ends of the cleft are closed, bound peptides are short having 8–9 amino acid residues (Fig. 5.5a). These peptides have two or three key *anchors* which bind to *allele-specific pockets* in the binding cleft. *The peptide fits into the pocket in a position which allows it to be recognized by the TCR.*

Due to variations in shape and charge of amino acids in the peptide-binding cleft, different class I MHC molecules differ in the peptides they bind. In the absence of key anchors, binding will not occur and the peptide fails to be presented to a T cell. This explains why certain antigens fail to evoke an

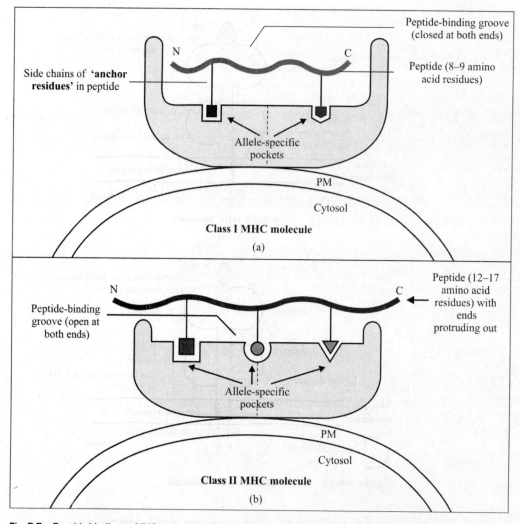

Fig. 5.5 **Peptide binding to MHC molecules.** Class I and class II MHC molecules differ in the nature of the peptides they bind, as specificity of their allele-specific pockets varies.

immune response. It is also the reason why certain MHC profiles determine susceptibility or resistance of an individual to a particular disease. It would not be out of place to mention here again that MHC molecules can only bind peptides derived from proteolysis of protein antigens inside the cell. Unlike the B cell receptor, they do not bind non-protein antigens such as carbohydrates and lipids.

The invariant (similar among various alleles of a particular gene) α3 domain contains the binding site for CD8 T cell accessory molecule present on cytotoxic T lymphocytes. CD8$^+$ T cells, therefore, only respond to peptides displayed by class I MHC molecules (*class I MHC restriction*).

The β_2m chain has no transmembrane region and is non-covalently bound to the heavy chain of class I MHC molecule. In Daudi tumour cells which are unable to synthesize β_2m, class I MHC molecules are not expressed on the cell surface. Cytokines, for example, interferons discussed in the following text, can alter expression of MHC class I molecules on the cell surface.

Class II MHC Molecules

These are transmembrane glycoproteins composed of two non-covalently associated α and β polypeptide chains. Each chain has two domains—β_1 and β_2 domains in the β chain and α_1 and α_2 domains in the α chain. The polymorphic residues are located in α_1 and β_1 domains. The ends of the peptide-binding cleft, unlike class I molecules, are open so that longer peptides with 10–30 amino acids (optimal size 12–17 amino acids) can be accommodated with their ends projecting beyond the groove (Fig. 5.5b). Three or four anchor residues need to be present in peptides which fit in allele-specific pockets in the binding cleft of MHC class II molecules.

The invariant α_2 and β_2 segments of class II MHC molecules are folded into immunoglobulin domains. The CD4 accessory molecule which is associated with the TCR on T helper cells interacts with the non-polymorphic β_2 domain. This explains why CD4$^+$ T helper cells only respond to peptides presented by class II MHC molecules (*class II MHC restriction*).

The salient features of class I and class II MHC molecules are summarized in Table 5.1.

Table 5.1   Salient features of class I and class II MHC molecules.

Features	Class I MHC	Class II MHC
Polypeptide chains	α, β_2m	α, β
Peptide-binding domains	α_1 and α_2	α_1 and β_1
Nature of peptide-binding groove	Closed at both ends	Open at both ends
Size of peptide-binding groove	Binds peptides of 8–11 amino acid residues	Binds peptides of 10–30 amino acid residues
Presentation of peptides	To CD8$^+$ T cells	To CD4$^+$ T cells
Binding site for T cell co-receptor	CD8 contacts α_3 domain	CD4 contacts β_2 domain
Nomenclature (human)	HLA-A HLA-B HLA-C	HLA-DP HLA-DQ HLA-DR

Distribution of MHC Molecules on Cells

The distribution of MHC molecules on all cells of the body is not the same. Class I molecules are constitutively expressed on almost all nucleated cells. This is essential as viruses can infect almost any nucleated cell in the body, and these cells need to be recognized by CD8$^+$ CTLs for elimination. It is reminded here that CD8$^+$ CTLs require recognition of viral peptide–MHC class I complexes displayed on the surface of infected cells to execute their function. Class II MHC molecules, on the other hand, are more restricted in distribution. They are normally expressed only on specialized APCs, such as dendritic cells (DCs), B lymphocytes, and macrophages. They may be expressed on some non-immune cell types on stimulation by IFN-γ.

Effect of Cytokines on MHC Molecule Expression and Presentation

Type I interferons (IFN-α/IFN-β) which are produced during the innate immune response to viral infections increase expression of class I MHC proteins on most cell types. Overall, this increases display of viral peptides to appropriate T cells—a good example of the way innate immunity promotes adaptive immune responses. Type II IFN (*IFN-γ*) is the major cytokine that upregulates class II MHC expression on APCs, such as macrophages. It should be recalled that resting macrophages express low levels of class II MHC molecules. Another relevant and important function of IFN-γ is to promote transcription and synthesis of immune-specific subunits of the proteasome which replace its constitutive subunits. This enhances antigen presentation by class I MHC molecules. IFN-γ is produced by

- natural killer (NK) cells during innate immune responses; and
- activated T cells during adaptive immune responses.

MHC Polymorphism and Disease Susceptibility

It is once again reminded here that the genes for class I and class II MHC molecules exist in a large number of allelic forms, that is, they are highly polymorphic. Several hundred different allelic variants at each locus have been identified in humans. Due to allelic differences, individuals vary in their ability to present antigenic peptides and, hence, in immune responsiveness. In other words, a particular microbial peptide that binds to MHC molecules in an individual may not bind to the MHC molecules expressed by another individual. This fails to activate a T cell and initiate an immune response. Such individuals are susceptible to infection by that pathogen. In this context, the extensive polymorphism of the MHC system, along with the tremendous diversity in TCRs, has an obvious advantage. It increases the range of processed antigens with which MHC molecules can interact. This ensures that there will always be some individuals in the population who are equipped to fight almost any infection. Interestingly, a link between the class I MHC molecule HLA-B53 and protection against severe malaria has been recognized.

Besides the link of MHC with microbial infections, many diseases, mainly autoimmune diseases and allergic diseases, are also associated with particular HLA types. In such individuals, frequency of certain MHC alleles is much higher than in the general population. The link between MHC and susceptibility to autoimmune disease will be revisited in Chapter 15.

The MHC profile of an individual is determined by HLA typing (see Chapter 17). It is necessary for

- matching donor and recipient for organ/tissue transplantation; and
- studying the role of MHC in determining susceptibility to autoimmune and allergic diseases.

ANTIGEN PROCESSING AND PRESENTATION BY MHC MOLECULES

As T cells recognize protein antigens only in the form of peptides displayed on the surface of APCs by self-MHC molecules, native proteins must be converted into MHC-associated peptides in a process called *antigen processing*. Exogenous (extracellular) protein antigens, which are endocytosed by APCs into intracellular vesicles, or endogenous antigens synthesized in the cytosol, are proteolytically degraded into peptides which bind to MHC molecules. The display of antigenic peptides by class I MHC and class II MHC molecules on cell surfaces for recognition by T cells is termed as *antigen presentation*.

APCs have to sample both exogenous and endogenous antigens (unlike target cells which sample endogenous antigens); hence, the need for two distinct pathways of antigen processing. These include

- *Cytosolic pathway for endogenous antigens*—Class I MHC molecules bind to peptides derived from these antigens.
- *Endocytic pathway for exogenous antigens*—Here, the peptides generated bind to class II MHC molecules.

Both the source of the peptide and the route taken to bind MHC proteins are fundamentally different in the two pathways, which are described in the following sections.

The Cytosolic Pathway for Endogenous Antigens

The sequence of events in the processing and presentation of endogenous antigens is outlined in the following text and depicted in Fig. 5.6.

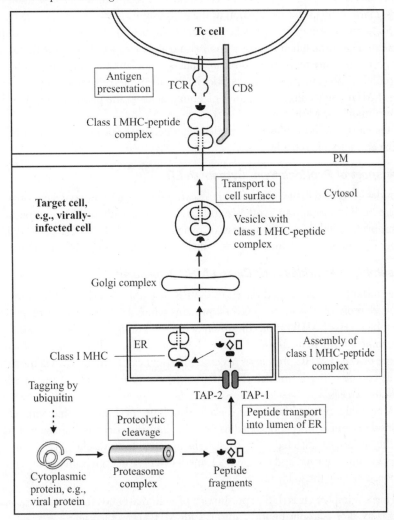

Fig. 5.6 Class I MHC pathway of processing and presentation of endogenous antigen in a virus-infected cell.
TAP, transporter associated with antigen processing.

Proteolytic Degradation of Cytosolic Proteins in Proteasomes

Some proteins targeted for proteolytic degradation include

- viral proteins synthesized in the cytoplasm of virally-infected cells;
- antigenic proteins of phagocytosed microbes (e.g., *Listeria monocytogenes*) which escape from vesicles into the cytoplasm;
- products of mutated host genes as in tumours; and
- cytoplasmic proteins that are no longer useful.

The proteasome found in the cytoplasm of most cells is a large multiprotein enzyme complex with proteolytic activity. It has an important physiological role. It degrades cytosolic and nuclear proteins during the normal process of protein turnover in healthy uninfected cells. Faulty proteins synthesized in cells have a similar fate. Peptide fragments derived from these self-proteins bind to class I MHC molecules and are displayed on the cell surface. Tagging by *ubiquitin*, a small protein in eukaryotic cells, marks proteins for destruction in the proteasome.

Some proteasomes are specialized to generate peptide fragments that can bind to MHC class I proteins. During an inflammatory response, and also in response to IFN-γ, three constitutive subunits of the proteasome are replaced by three immune-specific subunits. This substitution alters the processing of proteins and generates short peptides having the preferred anchor residues suitable for binding to class I MHC molecules. The nature of amino acids in the peptides and their length are important determinants for MHC binding.

The next step shows how the peptides generated by the proteasome bind to class I MHC molecules in the endoplasmic reticulum (ER).

Transport of Peptides from Cytosol to ER

Peptides generated in the cytosol need to be translocated into the rough endoplasmic reticulum (RER) where MHC molecules are synthesized. This transport is with the help of a specialized ATP-dependent transporter called *TAP* which consists of two proteins TAP-1 and TAP-2. TAP has highest affinity for peptides containing 8–9 amino acids, which is the optimal peptide length for class I MHC binding.

Assembly of Peptides with Class I MHC Molecules

The α and β_2m chains synthesized in the ER assemble into class I MHC molecules. This involves *chaperone* molecules, a special class of proteins which facilitate folding of polypeptide chains. The assembled class I MHC molecules then acquire an antigenic peptide. As the process is a complex one, some intermediate steps are omitted here for simplicity. The presence of a peptide in the binding groove of class I MHC proteins is necessary for their exit from the ER via the secretory pathway. The stable complex travels through the Golgi to the cell surface where it can present antigenic peptides to $CD8^+$ T cells.

Amazingly, certain viruses have evolved unique mechanisms that interfere with MHC class I molecule assembly and peptide loading (see Fig. 12.6). By reducing expression of MHC class I molecules on the surface of infected cells, these cells are unable to display MHC–viral peptide complexes. They go unrecognized and escape CTL-mediated destruction. Some viruses that evade the immune response include the following:

- Herpes simplex virus (HSV) produces a protein that binds to the TAP transporter. This prevents transport of cytosolic peptides into ER for MHC class I loading.
- Human cytomegalovirus (CMV) produces a protein that binds to β_2m. This prevents assembly of class I MHC molecules and transport to the plasma membrane.

Endocytic Pathway for Exogenous Antigens

The processing and presentation of an exogenous antigen is depicted in Fig. 5.7. The sequence of events is outlined in the following text.

Uptake and Processing

APCs, such as DCs, macrophages, and B cells, play a major role in the processing and presentation of exogenous material. It is through endocytosis that APCs ingest macromolecules, particulate matter, and

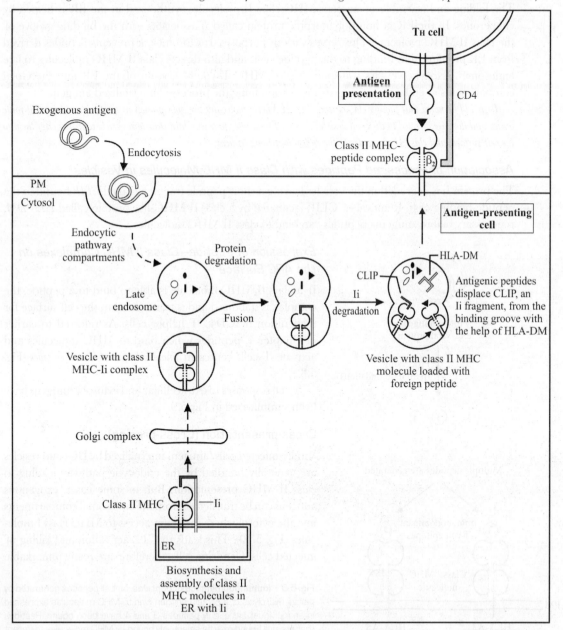

Fig. 5.7 Class II MHC pathway of processing and presentation of exogenous antigens. B cells internalize antigens by receptor-mediated endocytosis. CLIP, class II-associated invariant chain peptide; Ii, invariant chain.

even other cells. The ingested material is enclosed in intracellular membrane-bound endocytic vesicles. Their size varies depending on how the material is endocytosed (by phagocytosis or pinocytosis). In the compartments of the endocytic pathway, progressive acidification facilitates enzymatic degradation of protein antigens to peptides by proteases. Some of the peptides generated may be appropriate in length and binding motifs for association with class II MHC molecules.

Biosynthesis and Transport of Class II MHC Molecules to Endosomes

The folding and assembly of nascent MHC class II molecules synthesized in the ER is helped by chaperones. In the ER, a non-polymorphic protein called *Ii* associates with the binding groove of the class II MHC molecule. This serves various purposes. For instance, it prevents peptides derived from ER proteins from binding to the peptide cleft, and also directs class II MHC molecules to late endosomes. Exocytic vesicles transport class II MHC–Ii complexes out of the ER and the Golgi compartments to endosomal compartments containing the processed internalized antigen.

It should be noted that though class I and class II MHC molecules are both present in the Golgi, subsequent route varies and they are directed to different vesicles—class I molecules to a standard transport vesicle which carries them to the cell surface, and class II molecules to the endosomal compartment.

Association of Processed Peptides with Class II MHC Molecules in Vesicles

The protein Ii is degraded in the vesicles leaving a short peptide fragment called *CLIP* bound to the peptide-binding cleft. Removal of CLIP, facilitated by a class II MHC-like protein called *HLA-DM*, is necessary before antigenic peptides can bind to class II MHC molecules.

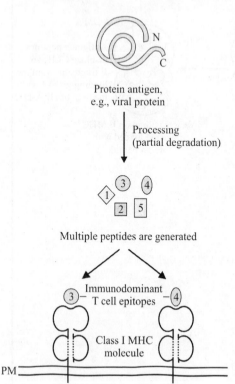

Protein antigen,
e.g., viral protein

Processing
(partial degradation)

Multiple peptides are generated

Immunodominant
T cell epitopes

Class I MHC
molecule

PM

HLA-A3   HLA-A5
Cytosol

Expression of Peptide—Class II MHC Complexes on the APC Surface

If a class II MHC molecule is able to bind to a peptide, the complex is stabilized and is transported to the cell surface for recognition by CD4$^+$ T helper cells. As referred to earlier in Chapter 4, peptides which bind to MHC molecules and activate T cells represent *immunodominant T cell epitopes* (Fig. 5.8).

T cell responses to extracellular and cytosolic antigens have been summarized in Fig. 5.9.

Cross-presentation (Cross-priming)

Virally-infected cells/antigens internalized by DCs into vesicles are generally handled by the endocytic pathway leading to class II MHC presentation. But, in some cases, exogenous antigens can be transferred from the endosomal compartments into the cytosol where they gain access to MHC class I molecules (Fig. 5.10). This leads to CTL activation and killing of infected cells. Dendritic cells, therefore, are really remarkable

Fig. 5.8   Immunodominance of peptides. Not all peptides generated by partial hydrolysis of a protein antigen bind to MHC molecules expressed in an individual. Here, only peptides 3 and 4 have been bound. Peptides that are not bound may be selectively bound by MHC molecules (different allelic forms) expressed in another person.

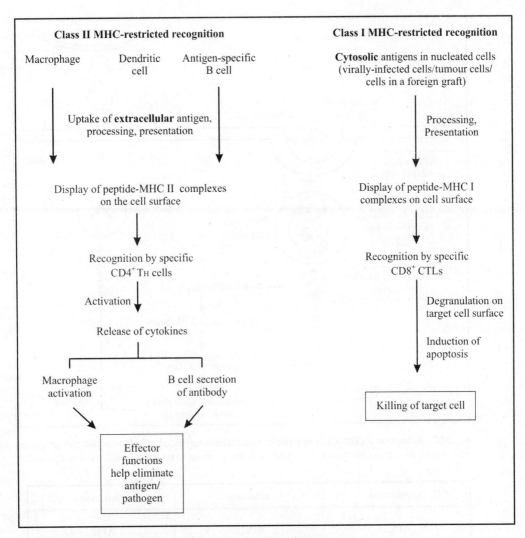

Fig. 5.9   T cell responses to extracellular and cytosolic antigens.

cells. They can present peptides derived from exogenous antigens on both class I and class II MHC molecules. This process by which DCs present exogenous antigens to CD8+ CTLs specific for the antigen and activate them is referred to as *cross-presentation* (*cross-priming*). This feature enables DCs to present antigens from microbes that may not infect DCs. Using the same mechanism, DCs are able to present tumour antigens to CD8+ CTLs and activate them (see Chapter 18). The way internalized proteins are transferred across membranes of the endocytic pathway compartments to the cytosol for proteasomal degradation needs to be fully understood.

Significance of MHC-associated Antigen Presentation

As antigen processing and presentation occur routinely inside cells independent of the immune system, class I and class II MHC molecules on cell surfaces are occupied by self-peptides. Self-peptide–MHC complexes have an important role to play in T cell developmental processes in the thymus (see Chapter 8). These complexes do not stimulate autoreactive T cells which may have escaped into the

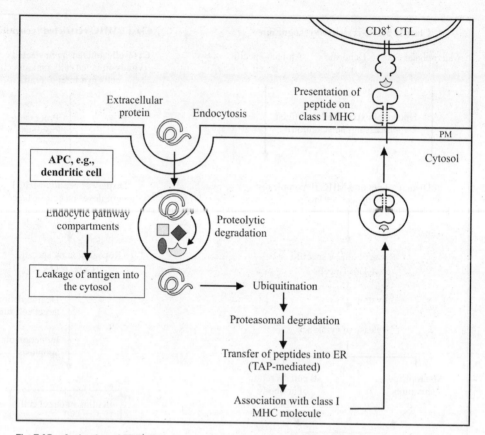

Fig. 5.10 **Activation of CD8$^+$ CTLs by cross-presentation.** Internalized antigens may be transferred from vesicles into the cytosol. Sequence of events that follow is similar to those for endogenous antigens.

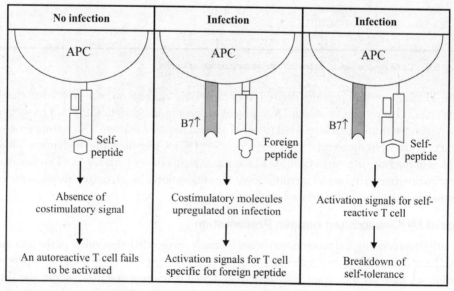

Fig. 5.11 **Association of MHC molecules with self and non-self peptides.**

periphery from the thymus. This is because APCs in absence of infection do not express costimulatory molecules (Fig. 5.11). In an infection, a small fraction of the total MHC molecules expressed on the APC surface are occupied by foreign peptides. As T cells are extremely sensitive, these complexes along with costimulatory molecules which have been upregulated due to infection, are sufficient to deliver activation signals to antigen-specific T cells. It may even enable APCs to stimulate self-reactive T cells which may have spilled over into the periphery resulting in breakdown of T cell tolerance to self-antigens.

AN ADDITIONAL PATHWAY OF PRESENTATION OF NON-PROTEIN ANTIGENS

In addition to the processing of protein antigens and their presentation by classical class I and class II MHC molecules, some T cells expressing the $\gamma\delta$ TCR, and also NKT cells, recognize non-protein antigens, namely lipids derived from infectious microbes such as *Mycobacterium tuberculosis*. These lipid antigens are presented by non-classical class I-like molecules which belong to the CD1 family. Some details about this third pathway of antigen processing and presentation are presented in Box 5.1.

Box 5.1   Presentation of lipid antigens

In addition to the classical MHC class I and class II molecules that present peptide antigens to T lymphocytes, there is a third system that is specialized to present pathogen-derived lipid/glycolipid antigens. This system involves non-MHC class I-like molecules called *CD1 molecules* which are comprised of a heavy chain non-covalently associated with β_2m (Fig. 5.12). CD1 molecules are encoded by genes outside the MHC. The CD1 genes are located on chromosome 1 in humans and chromosome 3 in mouse. In man, five CD1 genes have been identified including CD1A, CD1B, CD1C, CD1D, and CD1E. These correspond to five CD1 proteins which are designated CD1a–CD1e. The limited allelic variation of CD1 genes is in striking contrast to the extreme polymorphism of MHC class I and class II genes.

CD1 molecules are expressed on a variety of professional APCs predominantly DCs, and also on B cells and epithelial cells in the intestine. Their antigen-binding groove is deeper than that of classical class I molecules and is accessible through a narrow entrance. There are still many unknown facts about the intracellular trafficking pattern followed by CD1 molecules. They can present both exogenous (and endogenous) lipids in such a way that the polar or charged head groups of the lipids are exposed for recognition by TCR of CD1-restricted T cells, such as NKT cells (see Chapters 2 and 3). These are unusual lipid antigen-specific cells that are non-MHC restricted, that is, they do not recognize MHC-bound peptide. Besides the novel NKT cells, some $\gamma\delta$ T cells, too, recognize lipid antigens presented by CD1 molecules (see Chapter 3). The physiological role of these cell types in host defence against microbes is as yet not fully understood.

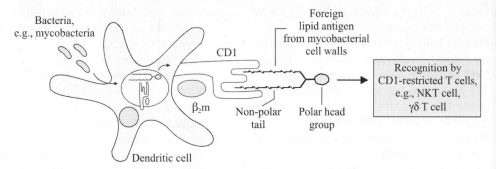

Fig. 5.12   Presentation of lipid antigens by CD1 molecules. CD1-restricted T cells recognize pathogen-derived lipid antigens presented on the surface of APCs bound to CD1 molecules.

SUMMARY

- The major histocompatibility complex (MHC), a tightly linked cluster of genes on chromosome 6 in humans, encodes proteins which have a critical role to play in the T cell response to antigens.
- The class I and class II MHC genes in humans encode two types of cell surface transmembrane proteins. There are three major types of class I molecules (HLA-A, HLA-B, and HLA-C), and three major class II molecules (HLA-DP, HLA-DQ, and HLA-DR).
- The class III MHC region encodes molecules that have diverse roles to play in the immune response. They have no role in antigen presentation.
- Each heterozygous individual inherits three MHC class I α-chain genes and three MHC class II α- and β-chain genes from each parent.
- Class I and class II MHC molecules are membrane-glycoproteins. Class I molecules are expressed on almost all nucleated cells. Class II molecules are expressed constitutively only on professional APCs, such as DCs, B cells, and macrophages.
- Cytokines released during an immune response to a foreign agent can induce expression of MHC molecules on many cell types.
- Both class I and class II MHC genes are highly polymorphic (many allelic forms exist). Variation in MHC profile of individuals explains why differences

exist amongst them in immune responsiveness to a particular antigen.
- An individual's MHC haplotype affects susceptibility to disease. Certain MHC alleles are linked to increased susceptibility to autoimmune diseases.
- Conversion of a native protein into peptides that can associate with MHC molecules is known as antigen processing. Display of peptide–MHC complexes on the cell surface for recognition by T cell antigen receptors is referred to as antigen presentation.
- The source of antigenic peptides bound to class I and class II MHC molecules differs. Class I MHC molecules bind to peptides derived from intracellular cytosolic proteins (cytosolic pathway). The complex is presented on the cell surface where it interacts with CD8$^+$ T cells. In contrast, class II molecules bind to peptides derived from extracellular proteins that have been phagocytosed or pinocytosed (endocytic pathway). The peptide–MHC II complex is displayed on the cell surface where it interacts with a specific CD4$^+$ T helper cell.
- Presentation of peptides derived from exogenous antigens on class I MHC molecules by DCs is called cross-presentation.
- CD1 molecules are class I MHC-like molecules which present lipid and glycolipid antigens to non-MHC restricted T cells, such as NKT cells and $\gamma\delta$ T cells.

REVIEW QUESTIONS

1. Indicate whether the following statements are true or false. If false, explain why.
   (a) Class II MHC molecules are constitutively expressed on all nucleated cells.
   (b) Peptides that fail to bind to MHC molecules do not trigger a T cell response.
   (c) MHC genes are codominantly expressed.
   (d) The processed peptide, which binds to the groove of class I MHC molecule, is generally more than 11 amino acids in length.
   (e) Human leukocyte antigens (HLA) are expressed only on leukocytes.
   (f) Peptides from an exogenous antigen associate with class II MHC molecules in the endoplasmic reticulum.

2. Self-assessment questions
   (a) What do you understand by immunodominance of peptides? Is there any advantage conferred on individuals by the high degree of MHC polymorphism?
   (b) MHC molecules are constantly presenting self-peptides as they cannot discriminate between them and microbial peptides. Why is it that autoimmune reactions are generally not triggered in individuals?
   (c) List structural and functional differences between class I and class II MHC molecules. What is meant by self-MHC restriction of T cells?
   (d) Explain the following terms:

(i) Antigen processing

(ii) Antigen presentation

(iii) Exogenous and endogenous antigens

(e) Justify the statements given below:

  (i) Lipid and glycolipid antigens, too, can activate T cells but not in the conventional way.

  (ii) Exogenous peptide antigens can be presented by class I MHC molecules.

3. For each question, choose the *best* answer.

(a) Binding site in class I MHC molecules for T cell co-receptor CD8 is

  (i) $\alpha 1$ region

  (ii) $\alpha 2$ region

  (iii) $\alpha 3$ region

  (iv) β_2 microglobulin

(b) The processing of exogenous proteins does not involve

  (i) proteasomal cleavage

  (ii) transport into late endosomes

  (iii) HLA-DM-catalyzed displacement of CLIP

  (iv) peptide binding to class II MHC groove

(c) CD1 molecules

  (i) are non-MHC class I-like molecules

  (ii) structurally resemble class II MHC molecules

  (iii) present antigens only to $\gamma\delta$ T cells

  (iv) are encoded in the MHC region on chromosome 6

(d) The major histocompatibility complex (MHC) does not code for

  (i) tumour necrosis factor

  (ii) complement proteins

  (iii) β_2 microglobulin

  (iv) both chains of class II MHC molecules

Generation of Antibody Diversity and B Lymphocyte Development

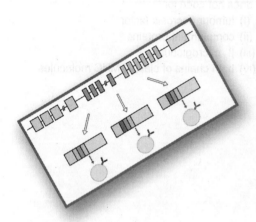

A unique feature of the immune response is the exquisite specificity with which antibodies, the secreted form of the B cell receptor (BCR) for antigen, and also T cell receptors (TCR), recognize and react with antigen. Each individual is equipped with a vast collection of antibody specificities referred to as the *antibody repertoire* which consists of over 10^7 different types of antibody molecules. This tremendous diversity ensures that whatever the nature of the invading organism/antigen, a suitable antibody is available to bind specifically with it. As the amount of genetic material is far too small to account for this enormous diversity, immunologists remained puzzled for many years. The long-time puzzle cleared when Susumu Tonegawa in 1976 discovered the nature of the genes that encode immunoglobulins (Igs), an achievement which won him the Nobel Prize for Physiology or Medicine in 1987. Subsequently, the continued work of several investigators made it clear that B cells (and also T cells) use an amazing strategy to generate the huge diversity in antigen receptors from a large but limited number of antibody genes. Understanding the mechanisms by which antigen receptor genes are expressed was a very significant breakthrough in immunology.

The expression of antibody receptor genes is an essential feature of B lymphocyte maturation in the bone marrow. A substantial part of the vast repertoire of antigen-binding sites of antibodies is generated during the process of B lymphocyte development from precursor cells which lack antigen receptors and, hence, cannot respond to antigen. Various sequential stages are involved in B cell development, which finally lead to selection of the mature B cell repertoire. Checkpoints during B cell development ensure that lymphocytes entering the peripheral tissues express useful receptors that respond to foreign antigens but not self-antigens. However, sometimes, some autoreactive B cells may also leak into peripheral sites.

This chapter focuses on the germline organization of Ig genes and the unique genetic mechanisms that contribute to receptor diversity. Somatic hypermutation and its significance, and how B cells are able to switch to a different antibody class are described. The sequential events in B lymphocyte maturation in the bone marrow, and how the various stages are linked to the generation of B cell antigen receptors are briefly reviewed.

GERMLINE ORGANIZATION OF IMMUNOGLOBULIN GENES AND THEIR RECOMBINATION

Before describing events in recombination of antigen receptor genes in B cells that result in the creation of functional genes, it is essential to understand some salient features of germline (unrearranged) Ig genes and how they rearrange.

General Features of Immunoglobulin Genes

Some major features regarding antibody genes and their rearrangement are highlighted in the following text.

- There are no complete antibody genes in the germline that encode heavy (H) or light (L) polypeptide chains of an antibody molecule. Instead, each type of antibody chain—kappa (κ) L chain, lambda (λ) L chain and H chain—has a separate pool of scattered gene segments that encode the variable (V) and constant (C) regions of the antigen receptor.
- Immunoglobulin genes (the term genes and gene segments are sometimes used interchangeably) for κ and λ L chains, and H chains are located on separate chromosomes (Table 6.1).

Table 6.1   Chromosomal location of Ig genes in human and mouse.

Gene	Chromosome	
	Human	Mouse
Lambda (λ) light chain	22	16
Kappa (κ) light chain	2	6
Heavy chain	14	12

- Some germline *V* genes are pseudogenes (non-functional genes) that are not capable of being expressed.
- Antibody genes are widely separated in germ cells and all somatic cells, but in developing B lymphocytes, they undergo rearrangement and are brought together by enzymatic deletion of intervening DNA, and then ligation. This creates complete functional genes that are transcribed and translated to H and L chains of an antibody molecule (Fig. 6.1).
- The process of rearrangement of gene segments to create functional antigen receptor genes, known as *somatic recombination*, occurs randomly in developing B lymphocytes. This is an irreversible

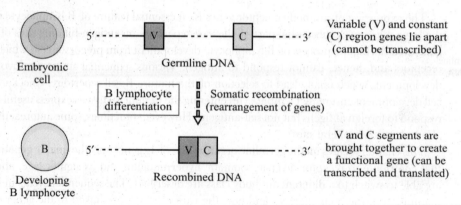

Fig. 6.1 **Antibody genes in an embryonic cell and in a developing B lymphocyte.** The figure is shown in simplified form with other gene segments in the V region omitted.

process that occurs differently in each precursor B cell during development. Every cell, thus, forms a unique gene for the variable region of H and L chains, and all its progeny inherits genes encoding receptors of the same specificity. The process generates a large part of the diversity in antigen receptors, though there are other processes too that contribute significantly.

♦ Only differentiating lymphocytes undergo the process of gene rearrangement; no other vertebrate cell type undergoes these rearrangement events.

With this brief background, the chapter proceeds to a discussion of how unrearranged or germline genes, which cannot be transcribed into mRNA, undergo somatic recombination that makes appropriate gene segments contiguous. Rearrangement of Ig germline genes is the initial step in B cell maturation (the terms recombination and rearrangement are used synonymously in B lymphocytes). It occurs prior to antigen exposure and in a precise order, H chain genes rearranging before L chain genes. The mechanism by which antibody genes rearrange is described in the following text in the same sequence.

Heavy Chain Genes and Their Assembly

The sequence of H chain genes from the 5′ to 3′ end of chromosome 14 as occurs in human germline and how they rearrange into functional genes is depicted schematically in Fig. 6.2.

There are four gene segments that code for an H chain, namely *V* (variable), *D* (diversity), *J* (joining), and *C* (constant). The *D* genes which are present in Ig H chain locus but are absent in the L chain locus create additional diversity.

The joining process for H chain variable region genes (*V, D,* and *J*) occurs in an ordered sequence in which two recombinational events are involved. The process is initiated when one of many D gene segments moves adjacent to one of several *J* segment genes to form a *DJ* combination. This encodes the *C*-terminal part of the H chain variable region. A V gene segment is then randomly chosen and rearranged with the *DJ* combination to create a *VDJ* DNA sequence. This combination contains only one of several *V* genes, one of *D* genes, and one of *J* genes, and encodes a complete H chain V region. This process, called *V-D-J recombination*, is mediated by enzymes which together constitute the *V (D) J recombinase*, some components of which are unique to developing lymphocytes. It occurs mainly via looping out (excision) of the intervening DNA between the joining gene segments followed by their ligation. The above recombination process is controlled by special sequences located at the joining ends and which are described later in the chapter. As is depicted in the figure, D2 has joined to J5

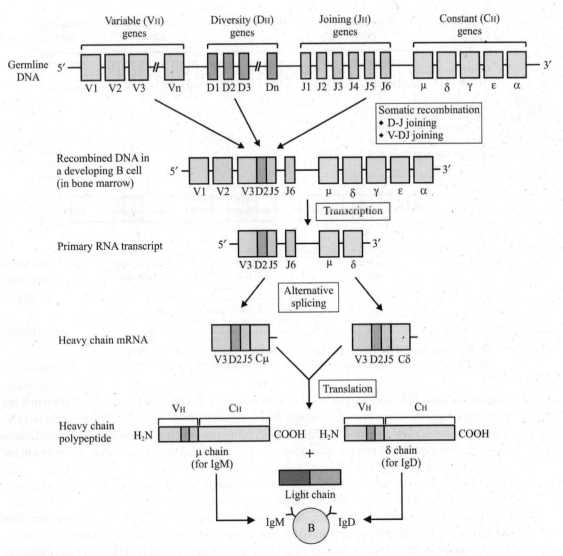

Fig. 6.2 Germline organization of heavy (H) chain genes and assembly. In a developing B cell, one each of the many V, D, and J genes are brought together to form a sequence, in this case *V3D2J5*, which ligates to a constant region gene. This is expressed to produce an H chain. The blocks in the figure represent coding sequences (exons), whereas intervening lines represent non-coding sequences (introns). Each V gene has its own leader sequence. For simplicity, it has been omitted. The figure is not drawn to scale.

followed by joining of V3 to D2J5 to form V3D2J5. *V, D, and J genes are combined differently in different clones of lymphocytes which as a result (along with other mechanisms that contribute to antibody diversity) differ in the antigen receptors they express* (Fig. 6.3).

Once a functional Ig V region gene has been produced by *V-D-J* recombination, a B cell cannot express a different variable region gene—a phenomenon called *allelic exclusion*, significance of which will be described in the following text.

In the next step, V3D2J5 ligates with constant region genes Cμ and Cδ which lie closest to the *VDJ* DNA sequence. There are nine functional C region genes in the H chain gene locus located

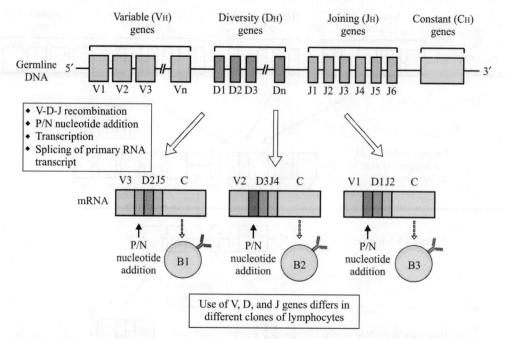

Fig. 6.3 Diversity in B lymphocyte antigen receptors. Combinatorial association of gene segments and addition (and also deletion) of nucleotides during recombination contribute to antigen receptor diversity.

downstream from V, D, and J segments. These include Cμ, Cδ, Cγ1–4, Cε and Cα1–2. This is unlike the κ and λ L chains where there are one and four C region genes, respectively. The rearranged DNA sequence is transcribed to give the primary RNA transcript which contains both Cμ and Cδ gene segments. Subsequent alternative splicing of the primary RNA transcript yields the final mature mRNA: VDJ-Cμ and VDJ-Cδ. Splicing of RNA is the process by which *introns*, non-coding pieces of DNA that separate coding sequences, or *exons*, are removed from the primary transcript. Although introns are transcribed and are present in the primary transcript, they are not present in mRNA. After processing, the mature RNA is exported from the nucleus to the rough endoplasmic reticulum (RER) where it is translated to give μ and δ H chain polypeptides having identical antigenic specificity. These associate with L chains following which they are co-expressed as IgM and IgD on the mature B cell surface. As described in the following text, membrane or secreted forms of IgM molecule are produced by altering the RNA splicing.

Light Chain Genes and Their Assembly

Rearrangement at the H chain locus is followed by sequential rearrangements at the *κ L chain gene locus* which lies on chromosome 2. The organization and assembly of κ L chain genes is depicted in Fig. 6.4.

There are three gene segments that code for an L chain, namely, V, J, and C. As D genes which are present in the H chain gene locus are absent, a complete variable L chain gene is constructed from V and J genes only. There are, thus, a total of seven gene segments that encode a complete antibody molecule. Events involved in recombination for L chain synthesis are similar to those for H chains and occur randomly. In the figure, V3 has joined to J3. The V3J3 rearranged DNA sequence of the variable region of the L chain then ligates with the single constant region gene to give the V3J3C

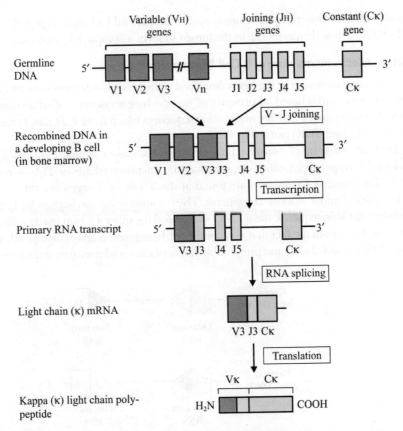

Fig. 6.4 Germline organization of kappa (κ) light (L) chain genes and assembly. A single recombination event occurs as compared to two for the H chain. In the figure, Vκ3 has joined to Jκ3 by gene rearrangement. This then ligates to a Cκ unit.

unit. This is then transcribed to give the primary RNA transcript from which the intervening introns are spliced to form mature mRNA for the κ L chain.

It is the κ L chain genes which undergo rearrangement events before λ chain genes rearrange. Rearrangement is initiated at the λ locus only when κ L chain gene rearrangements are non-productive on both chromosomes. Kappa L chains are more frequent in antibody molecules than the λ L chains.

The organization of the λ *L chain gene locus* located on chromosome 22 differs somewhat from the organization of the κ gene locus. There are fewer λ *V* and *J* gene segments than for the κ chain. Another noteworthy difference is that each *J* λ segment, of which there are four, is associated with a distinct *C* λ gene. Therefore, there are four different types of *C* λ polypeptide chains in humans. DNA rearrangement events, similar to those involved for synthesis of κ chains, are involved in λ chain synthesis.

A short hydrophobic sequence called *leader* (*L*) or *signal sequence* is found at the 5′ end of each V region exon. It encodes a *signal peptide* which is a common feature of all secreted proteins. Signal peptides are the first part of the protein to be synthesized (the *N*-terminus) and function to direct proteins that are newly synthesized to proper cellular compartments. After translation of H and L chain mRNA, the signal peptide is cleaved from the newly synthesized H and L chain polypeptides in the lumen of the cell's RER. These then associate in the lumen to form a complete Ig molecule.

Recombination Mechanisms during B Cell Maturation

The recombination of gene segments described in the preceding text occurs only between appropriate gene segments and is based on presence of specific base sequences called *recombination signal sequences* (*RSSs*) at joining sites. These are non-coding sequences which flank *V*, *D*, and *J* genes, and are a unique feature of Ig (and TCR) genes (Fig. 6.5).

They are made up of conserved heptamer and nonamer sequences (a block of seven and nine nucleotides, respectively) which are separated by unconserved 12- or 23-base pairs (bp) of 'spacer' DNA. The conserved sequences are found at the 3′ side of *V* segments, the 5′ side of *J* segments, and on both 5′ and 3′ sides of *D* segments. The recombination mechanism for Ig genes operates only when one flanking sequence has a 12-bp spacer and the other a 23-bp spacer called the *12/23 bp rule*. This rule arises from the fact that this number of base pairs roughly corresponds to one or two turns of the DNA double helix, and presumably the heptamer and nonamer sequences are brought into a

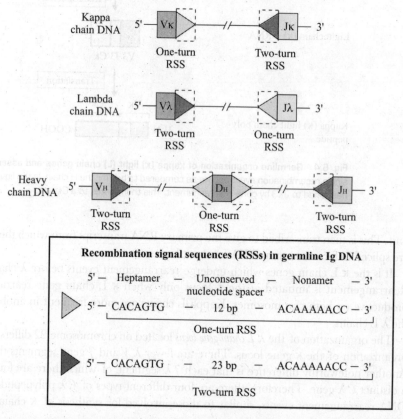

Fig. 6.5   Recombination signal sequences (RSSs) direct recombination of gene segments. For appropriate gene recombination, a segment with a two-turn RSS (23-bp) must join a segment with a one-turn RSS (12 bp). Location of two-turn and one-turn RSS varies with the Ig gene. RSSs with a 12-bp spacer flank DH, Vκ, and Jλ gene segments, whereas RSSs with a 23-bp spacer flank VH, JH, Jκ, and Vλ gene segments.

position where both sequences can be recognized by recombinase enzymes that mediate recombination (described in the following text).

V$_L$, V$_H$, or D$_H$ sequences are followed by heptameric and nonameric sequences that are complimentary to those preceding the J$_L$, D$_H$, or J$_H$ segments, respectively, with which they combine. Note that for H chains, V segments cannot recombine directly with the J segments, as both are flanked by RSSs with 23-bp spacers.

V(D)J recombinase is an enzyme complex that recognizes these conserved sequences and mediates recombination of *V* and *J*, or *V*, *D*, and *J* gene segments. Recombination activating genes RAG-1 and RAG-2 encode proteins which are components of the *V(D)J* recombinase. Although RAG-1 and RAG-2 genes are present in all cell types, their expression is lymphocyte specific and is seen only in immature cells of the B and T lymphocyte lineage. Other components of the *V(D)J* recombinase, such as the enzymes involved in DNA repair are expressed in many cell types. Mutations in RAG genes are the cause of some forms of *severe combined immunodeficiency* (*SCID*; see Chapter 16).

The process of recombination is guided by RSSs and involves bringing together appropriate gene segments by the RAG components of the *V(D)J* recombinase. In brief, the recombinase generates double-stranded breaks in the DNA that lies between the RSS and the adjacent *V-*, *D-*, or *J-*coding sequence. This forms temporary hairpin loop structures by which the parallel DNA strands on either side of the break remain connected. After the intervening DNA is excised as a circle, the broken ends are ligated by DNA repair enzymes, which are also components of *V(D)J* recombinase. This results in joining of the coding sequences to create genes that can be transcribed. It is to be noted that the recombinase is enzymatically active only in immature B (and also T) lymphocytes and not mature cells which express functional antigen receptors.

GENERATION OF ANTIBODY DIVERSITY

In the foregoing discussion, we have seen that H and L chains of Igs are encoded by multiple gene segments and how these rearrange randomly to generate functional H and L chain genes. This contributes substantially to antibody diversity, though it is limited by the number of available gene segments. There are other mechanisms, too, that magnify the diversity of the antibody repertoire but their precise contribution is not clear. Overall, mechanisms by which diversity is generated include

♦ multiple germline gene segments,
♦ combinatorial *V-J* and *V-D-J* joining,
♦ combinatorial association of H and L chains,
♦ junctional diversity, and
♦ somatic hypermutation.

The way these mechanisms generate diversity is briefly examined in the following text.

Multiple Germline Gene Segments and Combinatorial V-J and V-D-J Joining

The contribution of multiple germline gene segments and combinatorial *V-J* and *V-D-J* joining to diversity generation is shown in Table 6.2. It is seen that in humans, there is the potential to generate 8,262 H chain genes and 320 L chain genes as a result of variable region gene rearrangements.

Combinatorial Pairing of Heavy and Light Chains

This is the pairing of a particular H chain rearrangement with any L chain rearrangement. As seen in the foregoing discussion, H and L chain variable region genes rearrange independently in each

Table 6.2 Combinatorial antibody diversity in humans.

Germline gene segments	Heavy (H) chain	Light (L) chains	
		Kappa (κ)	Lambda (λ)
Estimated number of gene segments in humans*			
V	51	40	30
D	27	0	0
J	6	5	4
Combinatorial V-D-J and V-J joining (possible number of combinations)	51×27×6 = 8,262	40×5 = 200	30×4 = 120
Combinatorial association of heavy and light chains (possible number of combinations)	8,262×(200 + 120) = 2.64×10^6		

* Minor differences in the number of gene segments may be seen in individuals; the figures shown represent only functional gene segments.

Note: Junctional diversity and somatic hypermutation magnify considerably the combinatorial antibody diversity.

B cell. It is possible that two B cells may, by coincidence, have identical VH domains. But if these associate with L chains having different VL domains, it creates a different antigenic specificity for the two B cells. As almost any H chain may pair with any L chain in a B cell, the potential number of H and L chain combinations possible is $2.64×10^6$ (see Table 6.2).

The numbers for combinatorial diversity depicted in the table are in all probability far higher than the actual diversity generated in an individual, as all gene segments may not be used with the same frequency and some may not be used at all. It should be noted that these figures do not represent the total potential diversity because other mechanisms described in the following text also contribute.

Junctional Diversity

The variability in nucleotide sequences created at junctions of V and D, D and J, and V and J gene segments during recombination is called *junctional diversity*. This variability is generated by either removal of nucleotides from V, D, and J gene segments by an exonuclease or by addition at junctions of two types of nucleotides (insertional diversity) not present in the germline. These include *P-nucleotides* and *N-nucleotides*. Combinatorial diversity is restricted by the number of available gene segments, whereas junctional diversity is almost unlimited and makes the maximum contribution to antigen receptor diversity.

P-nucleotide Addition

RAG-1 and RAG-2 enzymes which mediate the recombination process recognize recombination signal sequences and bring a 12-bp and a 23-bp RSS into a synaptic complex where they are in close proximity. Asymmetric cleavage at junctions of RSSs and coding sequences by RAG-1 and RAG-2 enzymes in an intermediate stage during $V(D)J$ recombination events results in one DNA strand that is shorter than the other and which needs to be filled up before the joining of gene segments. Addition of nucleotides complimentary to the longer strand by repair enzymes extends the shorter strand and results in a *P (palindromic) sequence*. This addition is called *P-addition* and the short lengths of template-mediated nucleotides that are filled in at the $V–D–J$ junctions are called *P-nucleotides*. These introduce further variability in the antigen-binding surface of antibodies.

N-nucleotide Addition

Rearranged H chain genes contain short nucleotide sequences in their variable region-coding joints which are not coded for by H chain germline DNA. These non-coded nucleotides, called *N-nucleotides*, are added randomly during the joining of D_H to J_H and V_H to $D_H J_H$ in a reaction catalyzed by the terminal deoxyribonucleotidyl transferase (TdT) enzyme forming *N-regions*. The additional amino acids encoded by *N*-region nucleotides magnify further the variability of the antigen-combining site of the antibody.

It is due to junctional diversity that a large number of diverse new sequences are created at *V–D–J* (and also *V–J*) coding joints. This is the reason why the greatest variability is concentrated in these regions. Also, as these regions encode amino acids that form the third hypervariable or complimentarity determining region (CDR3) of both the V_H and the V_L segments of the antigen receptor, the CDR3 region is the most important region that determines specificity of antigen binding. Different antibodies, and also TCRs, differ from each other in nucleotide sequences particularly at *V–J* and *V–D–J* coding joints and, thus, in CDR3.

The variability in amino acid sequence of the first and second hypervariable regions (CDR1 and CDR2) is due to multiple V region germline genes in both H and L chains, which is unlike CDR3 where diversity is generated by recombination events (Fig. 6.6).

Heavy (μ) chain of membrane-bound antibody (IgM)

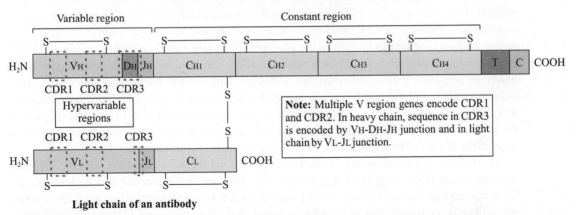

Fig. 6.6 Generation of diversity in hypervariable regions in Ig H and L chain domains. A single L and H chain of a membrane-bound Ig—molecule are shown here C, cytoplasmic region; T, transmembrane region.

SOMATIC HYPERMUTATION

All the mechanisms described in the preceding text for generation of diversity in antibodies operate during development and differentiation of bone marrow stem cells when specific variable region gene rearrangements occur. Additional antibody diversity is generated in mature B cells in their rearranged V regions by *somatic hypermutation* (see Chapter 10). Although the precise mechanism is not well understood, it involves point mutations (single nucleotide substitutions that occur during DNA replication/cell proliferation) rather than deletions or insertions. Somatic hypermutation, which introduces these substitutions in a largely random fashion, occurs at a much higher frequency than the spontaneous mutation rate for other cellular genes (hence, the name hypermutation). This alters individual nucleotides in *VJ* and *VDJ* units as a result of which the affinity of the encoded Ig undergoes a change. This may generate a receptor with a higher affinity for antigen. In mature B cells, somatic hypermutations are concentrated within the CDRs of V_H and V_L

sequences. The process normally occurs within *germinal centres* during maturation of an ongoing immune response. Germinal centres are structures that form in secondary lymphoid organs in response to protein antigens which require help from T cells to stimulate a B cell response. As B cells bearing high-affinity receptors are preferentially selected for survival, efficiency of the immune response is increased. This process of generating antibodies with higher binding affinity for antigen and which occurs in mature B cells is called *affinity maturation*.

Somatic hypermutation is the only form of antibody diversity that is generated after antigen stimulation. This, combined with mechanisms that operate before antigen exposure generates a vast B cell repertoire, such that whatever the nature of the foreign substance, a complimentary antibody is available to bind to it. Although precise diversity calculations for these mechanisms are not possible, in view of the many variations that can occur, the potential for combinatorial diversity is magnified enormously to a huge number that may exceed 10^{10}. However, considering that many B cells do not pass through selection processes that are an essential part of maturation (described in the following text), actual numbers of antigenic specificities in an individual at any particular time may be lower ($\sim 10^7$ combinations).

CLASS-SWITCHING IN B CELLS

Maturation of a primary antibody response to a secondary response is closely linked to switching of antibody isotypes, a process which allows a B cell to produce different classes of antibodies. In this process, the constant region of the H chain of an antibody can be changed without a change in its unique antigen-binding specificity (i.e., the idiotype). This phenomenon is known as *class-switching* or *isotype switching*. It depends on an antigenic stimulus and is regulated by cytokines produced by T cells which are activating B cells to produce antibodies (see Chapter 10). For instance, interleukin (IL)-4 induces switching to IgG4 and IgE, whereas transforming growth factor (TGF)-β promotes switching to IgA. The phenomenon of isotype switching involves rearranging H chain DNA and depends on the presence of specific DNA sequences called *switch (S) regions* at the 5′ end of each constant region gene of the H chain. However, the δ gene has no S region and is an exception (Fig. 6.7).

These switch regions allow any of the CH genes (but not δ gene) to associate with the *VDJ* unit, the intervening DNA being deleted in the process. Although details are not well understood, it is likely that appropriate switch sequences become accessible to a switch recombinase which facilitates recombination by recognizing and binding to switch sites. The rearranged *VDJ* segment initially lies next to the 5′ end of the μ gene segment. In the case of protein antigens, which require T cell help, signals are delivered that direct a second rearrangement of H chain DNA. In this, the rearranged *VDJ* segment is moved such that it is brought adjacent to an S region in front of another C region gene such as Cγ1. This shifts the response from IgM (the first isotype to be produced by a B cell) to IgG isotype. The signals necessary for isotype switching are elaborated in Chapter 10.

Further rearrangement of the H chain DNA, directed by T cells and their cytokines, moves the *VDJ* segment adjacent to the S region of the ε segment or the α segment, thereby shifting the response to IgE or IgA. A cell which has switched to making IgA antibody cannot revert to making IgE or IgG antibody molecules. This is because when ligation occurs during rearrangement, the intervening C region DNA is deleted and eventually broken down. The *activation-induced cytidine deaminase* (*AID*) enzyme has been shown to be essential for class-switch recombination and also for somatic hypermutation which has been described in the preceding section.

It should be remembered that *VDJ* or *VJ* segments join to C region gene segments at the RNA level and not at the DNA level, both during classical gene rearrangements and isotype switching.

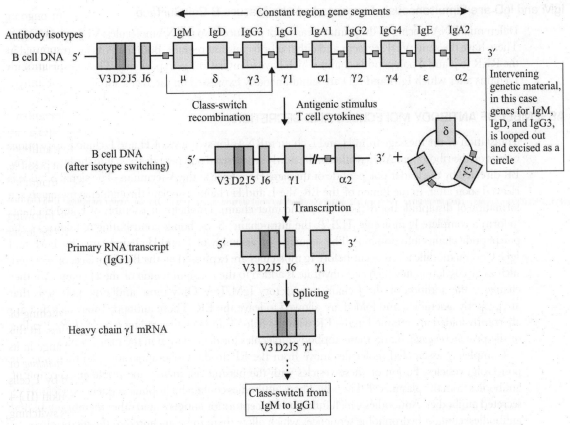

Fig. 6.7   Class-switching in B cells.

DIFFERENTIAL RNA PROCESSING OF IG HEAVY CHAIN PRIMARY TRANSCRIPTS

Alternative processing of the Ig H chain primary RNA transcript in a single B cell results in

- expression of membrane-bound antibody (in mature B cells) or secretion of antibody (by plasma cells); and
- production of both membrane IgM and membrane IgD (in mature B cells).
  This is considered in the text that follows.

Membrane-bound and Secreted Forms of Antibodies

After synthesis, antibodies are either bound to the membrane (IgM as B cell antigen receptor) or secreted into the extracellular environment. The two forms differ in the amino acid sequence of their H chain C-terminal domain. An antibody is destined to be bound to the membrane if a hydrophobic sequence that serves to anchor the antibody in the lipid bilayer is present. On the other hand, absence of the hydrophobic sequence allows the antibody to be released from the cell surface (see Fig. 4.14). The constant region genes have coding sequences for C-termini of both membrane and secreted forms of Igs. Differential splicing of the same primary RNA transcript generates mRNA for the membrane or secreted form of the antibody. A naïve B cell produces only the membrane-bound form of IgM, whereas plasma cells produce only the secreted form. As the membrane-bound form is unable to associate with the J chain, it exists in monomeric form and not as a pentamer.

IgM and IgD are Simultaneously Expressed on the Mature B Cell Surface

Differential RNA splicing of the primary transcript produces two mRNA molecules: VDJ-μ and VDJ-δ. These have the same VDJ segment and either μ or δ constant regions. Both mRNAs are translated in the RER to μ and δ polypeptide chains which have identical antigen specificity. These associate with L chains after which IgM and IgD are simultaneously expressed on the B cell surface.

ASSEMBLY OF ANTIBODY MOLECULES AND SECRETION

Translation of the message from H and L chain mRNAs for synthesis of H and L chain polypeptides occurs on the ribosomes. After synthesis, the newly synthesized polypeptides pass into the lumen of the ER directed by the leader polypeptide or the signal sequence at the *N*-terminus. The signal peptide is cleaved soon after. In the lumen of the ER, the L and H chains associate through enzyme-catalyzed formation of disulphide bonds (both intra- and inter-chain). This helps in assembly of L and H chains to form a complete Ig molecule (H2L2), the intra-chain –S–S– bonds contributing to folding of the polypeptide chains into domains. The sequence of assembly of L and H chains varies for IgM and IgG. Certain modifications occur before Ig molecules are expressed on the B cell surface, or secreted, such as glycosylation in which carbohydrate is added to the constant region of the H chain. Another change is the addition of the J chain to secretory IgM/IgA. Only those antibody molecules that are properly assembled and folded are allowed to leave the ER. Those antibody molecules that are aberrantly folded are retained in the ER with the help of an H chain-*bi*nding *p*rotein (*BiP*). Binding of the protein *ubiquitin* marks these antibody molecules for degradation in the proteasomes.

Completely assembled molecules move from the ER to the Golgi apparatus and then into the post-Golgi vesicles. Fusion of these vesicles with the plasma cell membrane results in secretion of antibodies from the plasma cell (Fig. 6.8). These antibodies contain hydrophilic sequences, a feature of secreted antibodies. Antibodies which function as receptors for antigens (and other membrane-bound antibodies) contain hydrophobic sequences which allow them to be anchored to the membrane.

Allelic Exclusion

Although every B cell has two copies of each chromosome, one set from each parent, a B cell does not produce two different H chains or two different L chains. If this did occur, a single cell would form antibodies of different specificities. Expression of only one of the two parental alleles of Ig in a B cell is referred to as *allelic exclusion*. This is the reason why each B cell expresses receptors of only a single specificity formed from combination of a single L and H chain.

The two H chain rearrangements that occur (*DJ*, and *V* to *DJ* to form a *VDJ* unit) can either be productive (produces a functional protein) or non-productive (produces a non-functional protein). A productive rearrangement that produces an H chain polypeptide shuts down H chain rearrangement on the other chromosome. But sometimes, when the rearrangement on the first chromosome is non-productive, as may happen due to mutations/deletions or other causes, the H chain gene locus on the other chromosome is allowed to go through similar recombination events. If this too is non-productive, the B cell does not differentiate further to become a mature B cell. It follows that in an antibody-producing B cell, the rearrangement of one allele is productive, whereas the other allele is either not rearranged or is rearranged aberrantly. It is to be noted that rearrangement is initiated on the λ locus only when gene rearrangements for κ L chain synthesis are non-productive on both chromosomes.

In the preceding text we saw how Ig genes are rearranged to functional genes. The chapter now goes on to describe various developmental stages in B cell maturation and how these stages are linked to generation of antigen receptors.

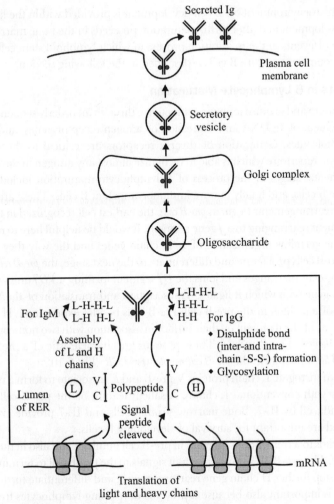

Fig. 6.8 Assembly and secretion of immunoglobulins.
Note: Membrane-bound antibody contains a hydrophobic sequence at the
C-terminal end which anchors it in the membrane of a mature B cell when
a vesicle fuses with the plasma membrane (not shown here).

B LYMPHOCYTE MATURATION AND SELECTION

B cell developmental processes in vertebrates involve three stages:

- B cell maturation
- B cell activation and proliferation
- B cell differentiation

This chapter covers the sequence of events in B cell maturation. Subsequent events, namely, B cell activation, proliferation, and differentiation are covered in Chapter 10. These late events occur when mature B cells exit the bone marrow and populate peripheral lymphoid organs, such as lymph nodes and spleen. Here, they are activated when they interact with antigens and proliferate in response. This is the antigen-dependent phase of B cell development, unlike maturational events which occur in absence of antigen.

The microenvironment for B cell development is provided within the liver in early foetus. Late in foetal development and after birth, maturation proceeds in the bone marrow for the rest of life. The sequence of events in the maturation process in which lymphoid stem cells (LSCs) differentiate into immunocompetent mature B cells is described in the following section.

Sequential Events in B Lymphocyte Maturation

B cells mature and acquire immunocompetence through an orderly sequence of events which include rearrangement of Ig DNA and expression of antigen receptor genes, and acquisition of important surface molecules. Generation of diverse receptors are critical to the development of a vast B lymphocyte repertoire which is able to recognize almost any antigen in the environment. The various developmental stages in the process of B lymphocyte maturation include pro-B cells, pre-B cells, immature B cells, and finally mature immunocompetent B cells. These are illustrated in Fig. 6.9.

Gene rearrangements begin in *pro-B cells,* the earliest cell recognized in the B cell lineage, with a *D* gene segment rearranging to a *J* gene segment. It would be helpful here to refer back to Fig. 6.2 which depicts the germline organization of Ig H chain genes and the way they rearrange into functional genes. Pro-B cells proliferate and differentiate to the next stage, the *pre-B cell stage.* During this stage, a *V* gene segment rearranges and joins the *DJ* segment forming a *VDJ* unit which is then brought close to the Cμ gene with which it ligates. Transcription and translation of the VDJCμ gene unit leads to synthesis of a μ chain in the pre-B cell. Pre-B cells besides expressing μ H chains in their cytoplasm express some of the μ protein on their surface in association with two non-covalently associated *surrogate (pseudo) L chains—Vpre-B* and *λ5.* These proteins are characteristic of a pre-B cell and along with the *Ig-α/ Ig-β heterodimer* form the *pre-B cell receptor (pre-BCR)* (Fig. 6.10).

The two surrogate L chain proteins V pre-B and λ5 associate to form a molecule having structural homology with conventional L chains. A salient feature of the pre-B cell stage is the high mitotic activity induced by IL-7. Bone marrow stromal cells and IL-7 provide critical signals in the initial stages, and are important for survival of developing B cells.

This leads to a tremendous increase in pre-B cell numbers and also in the diversity of the antibody repertoire. The pre-BCR is important as it signals to the pre-B cell to terminate synthesis of surrogate L chains, stop further H chain gene rearrangements, and differentiate further. Signalling through the pre-BCR is important also because it prevents developing lymphocytes from undergoing apoptosis. This serves as a critical checkpoint to ensure that expression of one chain of the antigen receptor (the first somatic recombination) was successful.

Immature B cells, the next stage in development, undergo L chain *VJ* gene rearrangement to form a κ or a λ chain which associates with the cell's μ chain to form monomeric IgM. This inserts in the lipid bilayer forming the BCR for antigen. As described in the following text, immature B cells which have potential to react with self-components undergo selection processes, so that only those cells with useful receptors exit the bone marrow for peripheral lymphoid organs. An immature B cell progresses further to develop into a *mature B cell* which, in addition, expresses IgD having an antigenic specificity identical to IgM. Expression of both IgM and IgD on the surface is a feature that marks the B cell as a functionally competent mature B cell.

It should be borne in mind that expression of recombinase enzymes RAG-1 and RAG-2 is increased during those stages of B cell development when H and L chain rearrangement events occur. Also, each B cell expresses receptors of only a single specificity. This is because only one of two inherited parental H chain alleles is rearranged and expressed (*allelic exclusion*). When the rearrangement on the first chromosome is productive, signals from the pre-BCR inhibit rearrangement of the Ig H chain locus on the second chromosome. Non-productive recombinations in both alleles in a B cell are common

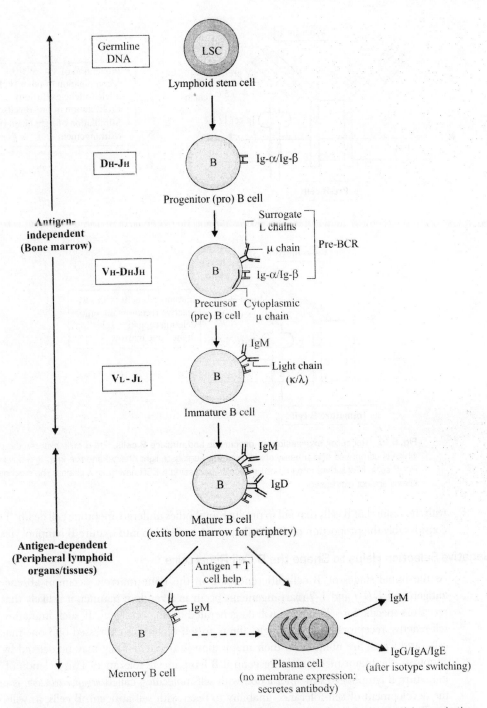

Fig. 6.9 Differentiation pathway of B lymphocytes. The figure depicts the sequential steps in the maturation of B lymphocytes. The various stages are characterized by specific Ig gene rearrangements and appearance of surface molecules. Read the main text for details.

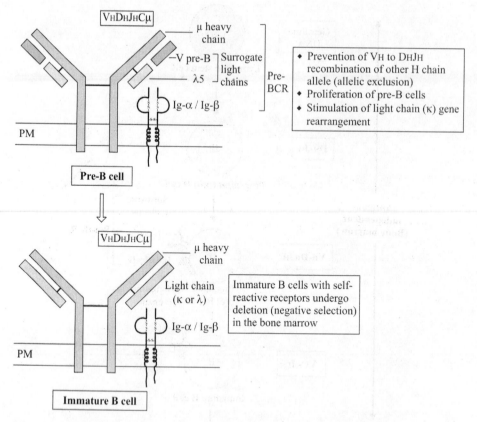

Fig. 6.10 Receptor expression on precursor and mature B cells. Pre-B cells express the pre-BCR which is comprised of a μ heavy chain, invariant surrogate light chains, and the Ig-α/Ig-β heterodimer. Pre-B cells differentiate into immature B cells expressing a BCR having κ/λ chains. The surrogate light chains are not expressed.

with the result that B cells that fail to produce antibodies undergo apoptotic cell death. This decreases considerably the proportion of B cells that go on to develop into mature B lymphocytes.

Negative Selection Helps to Shape the B Cell Repertoire

As the initial stages of B cell differentiation in the bone marrow occur in absence of specific antigen and *V-D-J* and *V-J* rearrangements occur in a random manner, it is likely that B cells with receptors specific for self-antigen will be generated during ontogeny. If such immature B cells with self-reactive receptors bind with high-affinity to self-molecules expressed on bone marrow stromal cells, and which are ubiquitous, their maturation is arrested. They may be deleted by undergoing apoptosis, the major mechanism for central B lymphocyte tolerance. This deletion of self-reactive immature B lymphocytes by interaction with self-molecules, called *negative selection*, is important for the development of self-tolerance (inability to react with self-antigen). B cells, as will be explained for T cells in Chapter 8, also undergo positive selection, in which cells with functional receptors are preserved but the phenomenon is poorly understood. Also a process called *receptor editing* may occur in which immature B cells with self-reactive receptors change receptor specificity for a receptor that lacks self-reactivity. Additional V and J gene segments recombine to produce a new L chain. The process is dependent on reactivation of RAG genes (see Chapter 15).

The majority of B cells (more than 75%) die by apoptosis during development in the bone marrow following which they are cleared by bone marrow macrophages. As we will learn in Chapter 8, developing T cells in the thymus undergo similar negative selection that is marked by tremendous apoptosis.

The developmental events in the bone marrow, briefly reviewed in the preceding text, occur in the absence of antigens, and lead to the generation of mature immunocompetent B cells. The generation of a vast B cell repertoire having antigen specificities directed against a wide array of antigens is amazing. Further stages in B cell development are dependent on antigens and occur in secondary lymphoid organs, such as lymph nodes and spleen. When an antigen enters the body, it interacts specifically with an existing B cell clone resulting in clonal proliferation and differentiation to plasma cells (see Fig. 1.18). Antibodies produced have specificity identical to that of membrane-bound IgM on the selected B cell. This concept which is central to the clonal selection theory of antibody production has been focused on in detail in Chapter 1.

The pathways of B cell differentiation are different if TH cell–B cell interactions are involved and include germinal centre events, such as affinity maturation, isotype switching, and development of memory cells. These events are described in detail later in Chapter 10.

B-1 B AND CONVENTIONAL B-2 B CELLS

There are two B cell subsets—B-1 and B-2. B-1 B cells appear earlier than the conventional B-2 B cells and represent a minority (5%) of the B cell population. Some of their attributes are listed in the following points:

- Self-renewal (new B-1 B cells are generated by division of existing B-1 B cells); this is unlike B-2 B cells which are generated from precursor cells in the bone marrow
- Major cell type found in the peritoneum
- Little or no surface IgD expression
- Secrete low-affinity IgM antibodies
- Do not require T cell help
- Respond well to carbohydrate antigens but poorly to protein antigens (B-2 B cells respond well to protein antigens and to polysaccharides also)
- Display little or no memory
- No somatic hypermutation
- Produce anti-RBC blood group antibodies
- V region diversity is restricted

SUMMARY

- Immunoglobulin H chains are encoded by V, D, J, and C gene segments, whereas L chains are encoded by V, J, and C segments. Recombination of a limited number of V, D, and J (and V and J) gene segments generates a vast antibody repertoire.
- Random rearrangement events in variable region gene segments in germline DNA generate functional heavy chain and light chain genes, heavy chain genes rearranging before light chain genes.

- Recombination signal sequences (RSSs) direct joining of different gene segments. They contain conserved heptamer and nonamer sequences and either a 12-bp (one-turn RSS) or 23-bp (two-turn RSS) spacer.
- Gene segments flanked by one-turn spacers can only combine with gene segments flanked by two-turn spacers allowing appropriate V_H–D_H–J_H and V_L–J_L joining (12/23 bp rule).

- Somatic recombination of gene segments is mediated by a recombinase enzyme complex. RAG-1 and RAG-2 are lymphocyte-specific components of the complex.
- Besides the diversity generated due to multiple germline gene segments and the combinatorial joining of different V, D, and J genes (or V and J genes), other mechanisms include random association of H and L chains, junctional diversity, and somatic hypermutation.
- Junctional diversity is generated by P-nucleotide addition, and by random addition of nucleotides not coded for by germline DNA (N-nucleotide addition) during pairing between H chain V, D, and J segments.
- Somatic hypermutation occurs in variable regions which further adds to diversity. Both somatic hypermutation and selection allow survival of cells with high-affinity receptors for antigens.
- Isotype switching generates antibodies of different classes and subclasses in which the variable region which determines antigen specificity is same but constant regions on which effector functions depend differ.
- Differential RNA processing of the heavy chain primary transcript generates membrane-bound antibodies (in mature B cells) and secreted antibodies (in plasma cells), and allows simultaneous expression of IgM and IgD in mature B cells.
- B cells express receptors of only a single antigenic specificity due to allelic exclusion.
- B cell development which occurs in the bone marrow is closely linked to Ig-gene rearrangements. The various stages include pro-B cells, pre-B cells, immature B cells, and finally mature immunocompetent B cells.
- Selection processes during B lymphocyte maturation help to eliminate B cell precursors that express receptors for self-antigens present in the bone marrow (negative selection).
- Receptor editing helps to replace a self-reactive receptor with a receptor that does not react with self.
- There are two types of B cells. The major B cell population is represented by the conventional B-2 cells, whereas B-1 cells arise earlier than B-2 cells and represent a minority.

REVIEW QUESTIONS

1. Indicate whether the following statements are true or false. If false, explain why.
   (a) The heavy chain variable region of all classes of antibodies are encoded by V, D, and J gene segments.
   (b) Somatic hypermutation occurs early in the B lymphocyte differentiation process.
   (c) Re-expression of RAG-1 and RAG-2 genes in mature B cells allows receptor editing.
   (d) Help from T cells directs the switch from IgM isotype to the IgG isotype.
   (e) Vpre-B is part of the surrogate IgM receptor on pre-B cells.
   (f) Immature B cells develop in the germinal centres of lymph nodes and spleen.

2. Self-assessment questions
   (a) Which mechanisms contribute to non-germline generation of diversity? Allelic exclusion is a critically important feature in antibody production. Why is it so?
   (b) A V_H gene segment is unable to join directly with a J_H gene segment during rearrangement of Ig heavy chain genes. Can you explain why?
   (c) What would be the number of different antibody specificities potentially generated from germline DNA that contains 50 V_H, 25 D_H, and 5 J_H gene segments and 40 V_L and 5 J_L gene segments? Consider only the combinatorial generation of antibody diversity.
   (d) What is the mechanism behind isotype switching? Can you suggest advantages for switching from IgM heavy chain gene to IgG, IgA, or IgE heavy chain genes?
   (e) (i) Of the three CDRs present in heavy and light chains of antibody molecules, CDR3 shows the most variability. Why is there greater diversity in CDR3? (ii) Would B cell maturation proceed in knockout mice having no μ chain or the surrogate light chain λ5? Give reasons in support of your answer.

3. For each question, choose the *best* answer.
   (a) The surrogate light chains in a developing B cell
       (i) consist of Vpre-B
       (ii) are expressed in pro-B cell stage
       (iii) consist of Vpre-B and λ5
       (iv) are expressed in immature B cells
   (b) The antigen-binding site of a B cell changes after antigenic stimulation by
       (i) alternative splicing of primary RNA transcripts
       (ii) somatic hypermutation
       (iii) allelic exclusion
       (iv) junctional diversity
   (c) Which of the following class-switches does not occur?
       (i) IgM to IgG
       (ii) IgM to IgA
       (iii) IgA to IgG
       (iv) IgM to IgE
   (d) VH genes begin to rearrange during
       (i) pro-B cell stage
       (ii) pre-B cell stage
       (iii) differentiation of pre-B cells to mature B cells
       (iv) class-switching

Cytokines

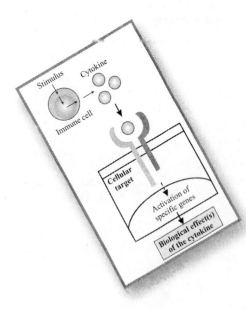

LEARNING OBJECTIVES

Having studied this chapter, you should be able to understand the following:

- Common features of cytokines and their important role in immune and inflammatory responses
- The functional classification of cytokines not being absolute as some cytokines function in both innate and adaptive immune responses
- The role of some major cytokines in innate and adaptive immunity, and the functional importance of cytokines designated chemokines and haematopoietic cytokines
- The five types of receptors through which cytokines act
- The signal transduction pathway commonly used by cytokines
- The pathophysiology that is associated with excess cytokine production
- The therapeutic value of cytokines, which are useful clinically for treatment of inflammatory disorders, besides other uses

Cytokines represent a functionally diverse group of chemical messengers secreted by leukocytes and many other cell types in the body. They are regulatory proteins/glycoproteins produced in response to a stimulus, for example, foreign material, and have important roles to play in immune and inflammatory responses. Their functioning, however, is not limited to the immune system. For instance, some cytokines are involved in wound healing, for example, transforming growth factor (TGF)-β. Cytokines produced by lymphocytes were earlier collectively called *lymphokines*, and those produced by monocytes/macrophages came to be known as *monokines*. But as the same proteins may be secreted by various other cells, such as epithelial cells and endothelial cells, the term *cytokine* came into use. In this book, the preferred name cytokine has been used throughout. Since many cytokines are released by leukocytes and act on other leukocytes, the term *interleukin (IL)* was coined. This term has helped to maintain a standard system of nomenclature because, as new cytokines are being characterized, they are assigned a number, for example, IL-1, IL-2, and so on. Numbers have been assigned to about 33 interleukins and it is very likely that the list will grow as more are identified.

There are some cytokines that are known by their common names, such as tumour necrosis factor (TNF) and TGF-β.

This chapter focuses on the general properties of cytokines, functional categories of cytokines based on their major biologic actions, and their receptors. Some individual cytokines are discussed and signal transduction mediated by cytokine receptors is briefly outlined. The role of cytokines in disease pathogenesis and use of cytokines and their receptors for therapy are summarized.

GENERAL PROPERTIES OF CYTOKINES

Of the various cytokines described to date, some are shown in Table 7.1.

Table 7.1 **Major cytokine families.** Only selected cytokines are listed with their principal sources.

Major cytokine families	Members	Cellular source
Interferons (IFNs)	IFN-α	Macrophages, dendritic cells, lymphocytes
	IFN-β	Fibroblasts, dendritic cells, some epithelial cells
	IFN-γ	TH1 cells, CD8$^+$ T cells, NK cells
Interleukins (ILs)	IL-1	Monocytes/macrophages, dendritic cells, stromal cells
	IL-2	TH1 cells
	IL-3	TH1 cells, TH2 cells, mast cells, NK cells, macrophages
	IL-4	TH2 cells, mast cells, NKT cells
	IL-5	TH2 cells
	IL-6	Macrophages, TH2 cells, stromal cells, fibroblasts, endothelial cells
	IL-7	Bone marrow and thymic stromal cells, fibroblasts
	IL-8*	Macrophages, fibroblasts, endothelial cells
	IL-9	TH cells
	IL-10	TH cells, macrophages
	IL-11	Bone marrow stromal cells
	IL-12	Macrophages, dendritic cells
	IL-13	TH2 cells
Tumour necrosis factors (TNFs)	TNF-α	Macrophages, endothelial cells
	TNF-β (lymphotoxin)	TH1 cells
Transforming growth factor (TGF)	TGF-β	TH3 cells, macrophages, fibroblasts
Colony stimulating factors (CSFs)	GM-CSF	TH cells , macrophages, endothelial cells, fibroblasts, stromal cells
	G-CSF	Fibroblasts, endothelial cells, macrophages, stromal cells
	M-CSF	Fibroblasts, endothelial cells, macrophages, epithelial cells, stromal cells
Chemokines	MCP-1	Macrophages, fibroblasts, keratinocytes, TH1 cells
	RANTES	T cells
	MIP-1 β	Monocytes/macrophages, endothelial cells, PMNs

* IL-8 (original designation) is a CXC chemokine. Its systematic name is CXCL8 (L stands for ligand). MCP, monocyte chemotactic protein; MIP, macrophage inflammatory protein; CSF, colony stimulating factor; RANTES, regulated on activation, normal T cell expressed and secreted

Cytokines as a group have several features in common (Box 7.1).

Box 7.1 Common features of cytokines

- Cytokines are antigen non-specific low molecular weight (<30 kDa) proteins/glycoproteins.
- They are highly potent and often induce their biological effects at femtomolar (10^{-15} M) concentrations.
- Most are soluble but some exist as both secreted and membrane-bound forms, for example, tumour necrosis factor (TNF).
- They are usually not stored and are synthesized and rapidly secreted on cellular activation.
- Their production is transient and tightly regulated. This is essential considering their role in immune and inflammatory responses which need to be strictly under control.
- They have short half-lives.

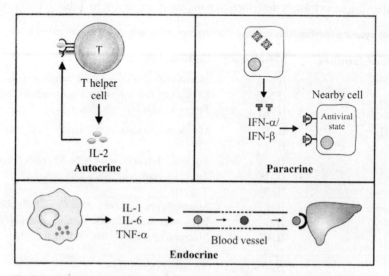

Fig. 7.1 Cytokine action. Most cytokines act locally (paracrine), whereas some are autocrine or, like classical hormones, endocrine in action.

Cytokines act over both short range and long range (Fig. 7.1). Most act locally on cellular targets that are close to the producer cell (*paracrine*). A cytokine may sometimes even act on the cell which synthesizes it (*autocrine*) or on distant cells and organs to which it is carried via the circulation (*endocrine*) like most hormones.

Some additional important features of cytokines shown in Fig. 7.2 are listed here:

- Many cytokines act on many cell types and so mediate diverse roles; this action is called *pleiotropy*.
- Cytokines may inhibit biological activities of other cytokines, referred to as *antagonism*.
- Another property is *synergism*, a term used when the biological effect of two cytokines is greater than the summation of their individual effects.
- Although each cytokine has its unique functions, many exhibit similar or overlapping functions, a feature called *redundancy*.
- Cytokine action on cellular targets induces release of cytokines which, in turn, release still other cytokines from other cell types. One such *cytokine cascade induction* is presented in Fig. 7.3.
- Cytokine action is mediated through interaction with specific receptors on cell surfaces (Fig. 7.4). To respond to a particular cytokine, a cell must express a receptor for it. Signals transduced lead to changes in expression of genes which modify various aspects of cell behaviour.

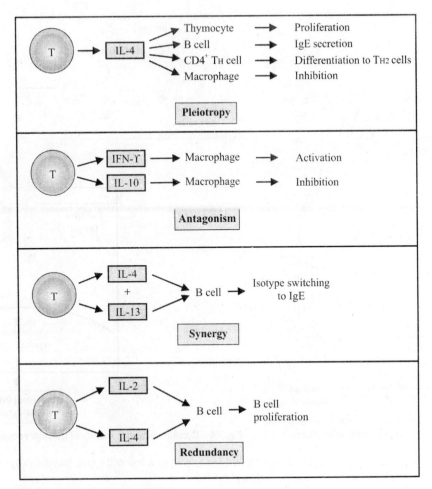

Fig. 7.2 Features of cytokines.
Note: The T cells shown in the figure are activated CD4$^+$ T helper cells.

In vivo, cytokines are rarely produced alone and rarely act alone. Since the cells in the body are exposed to different cytokines produced by many cell types, interactions may yield synergistic, cooperative, or antagonistic effects. This is referred to as the *cytokine network*. Its complexity makes it difficult to understand fully the in vivo role of these molecules.

Cytokines and hormones have many properties in common:

- They are highly potent secreted proteins that elicit various biological effects by binding to specific receptors on target cells.
- Their production is induced in response to a stimulus and is transient.

However, some important differences exist:

- Hormones generally act over long distances (endocrine). On the other hand, cytokine action is mostly paracrine, but sometimes autocrine or endocrine.
- While hormones are secretions of ductless glands, cells that produce cytokines are not organized into discrete glands. In other words, there is no single organ source for each cytokine.

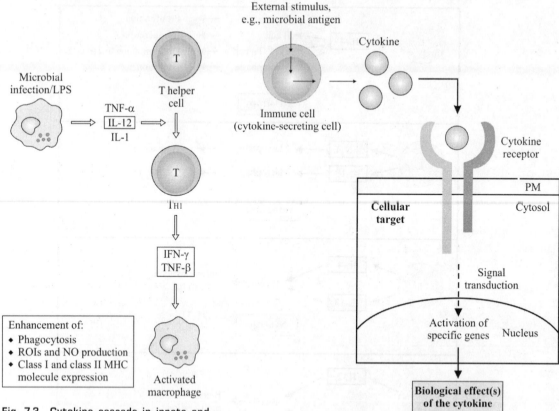

Fig. 7.3 Cytokine cascade in innate and adaptive immune response to infection.

Fig. 7.4 Cytokine action is mediated through receptors.

♦ Cellular targets of hormones are limited to one or a few cell types, but the range of target cells on which cytokines act on is much wider.

Some major roles of cytokines include

♦ inflammation,
♦ chemotaxis,
♦ phagocyte activation,
♦ haematopoiesis,
♦ isotype switching,
♦ apoptosis,
♦ lymphocyte proliferation and differentiation, and
♦ viral resistance.

FUNCTIONAL CLASSIFICATION OF CYTOKINES

Functionally, cytokines can be grouped into the following major categories:

♦ Cytokines of innate immunity
♦ Cytokines of adaptive immunity
♦ Chemokines
♦ Haematopoietic cytokines

The classification given in the preceding text is not absolute as many cytokines overlap in function. Moreover, the key cytokine IFN-γ is produced both by natural killer (NK) cells (innate) and T cells (adaptive) on activation.

Cytokines of Innate Immunity

Some important cytokines of innate immunity and their functional roles are considered in the following section. It is to be remembered that macrophages are the major producers of cytokines during innate immune responses.

Interleukin-1

Interleukin-1 has a broad range of targets and performs multiple diverse roles (Fig. 7.5). It is a major proinflammatory cytokine and plays a critical role in synthesis of acute-phase proteins by the liver. Some other cytokines in this category include TNF-α and IL-6.

Tumour Necrosis Factor-α

Tumour necrosis factor-α was initially identified as a substance that caused necrosis of tumours when injected into tumour-bearing animals. It is produced mainly by macrophages when they are activated by certain bacterial products, for example, lipopolysaccharide (LPS). It is the major mediator of acute inflammatory reactions, and promotes recruitment of neutrophils and monocytes to peripheral sites of infection. Besides, it activates these cells to eliminate microbes. Some effects of TNF-α which are critical for acute inflammation include the following:

- It increases expression of adhesion molecules on vascular endothelial cells which facilitates adhesiveness of neutrophils and monocytes to the endothelium.
- It stimulates secretion of chemokines by macrophages and endothelial cells, thereby promoting leukocyte chemotaxis.

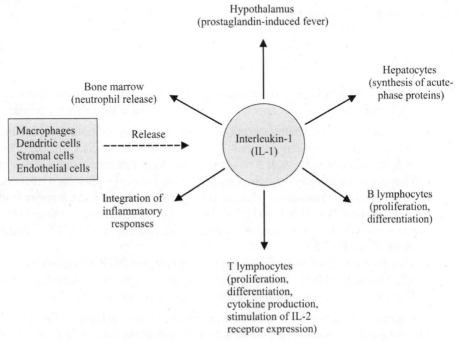

Fig. 7.5   Role of IL-1 in amplification of immune responses.

◆ It induces fever by acting on the hypothalamus. This effect of TNF-α is mediated through prostaglandins synthesized by hypothalmic cells.
◆ Along with IL-1 and IL-6, it induces synthesis of acute-phase proteins by the liver (see Fig. 2.4).

Production of excessive amounts of TNF-α in persistent infection can lead to pathological consequences; symptoms include fall in blood pressure and shock (described in the following text). High levels in the circulation of tumour-bearing animals causes thrombosis in blood vessels (see Chapter 18).

Interferons

Interferons (IFNs), which are the antiviral proteins introduced in the early chapters, include the following:

◆ IFN-α and IFN-β called type I IFNs
◆ IFN-γ called immune or type II IFN

In humans, there are at least 20 closely related types of IFN-α, one IFN-β, and one IFN-γ. Some new members have also been included in the IFN family. The major cellular sources of IFNs and some of their features are shown in Table 7.2.

Table 7.2 Interferon types—a comparison. Additional names for interferons are indicated in brackets.

Interferon type	Major cellular source	Cell activated	Antiviral activity	HLA expression
IFN-α (leukocyte interferon)	Macrophages/Monocytes Lymphocytes Dendritic cells	NK cell	+++	Class I ↑
IFN-β (fibroblast interferon)	Fibroblasts Epithelial cells (some) Dendritic cells	NK cell	+++	Class I ↑
IFN-γ (immune interferon)	T lymphocytes NK cells	Macrophage	+	Class I Class II ↑

Both *IFN-α* and *IFN-β* have an important role to play in early innate immune defence against viral infections. Some of their important features are listed in the following points:

◆ They are secreted by virally-infected cells and other cell types into the extracellular fluid.
◆ The most potent stimulus for their production includes dsRNA produced by viruses during replication in infected cells. It is recognized as a distinct pattern by toll-like receptor (TLR)-3.
◆ They act on virally-infected cells (autocrine) to inhibit viral replication in that cell.
◆ They also act on uninfected adjacent cells (paracrine) making them resistant to viral infection (antiviral state). Both IFN-α and IFN-β bind to the same cell surface receptor. The antiviral effect is due to synthesis of new enzymes, which overall, degrade viral mRNA and inhibit viral protein synthesis (see Fig. 12.4).
◆ They increase class I major histocompatibility complex (MHC) molecule expression on infected cells making them better targets for killing by effector cytotoxic T lymphocytes (CTLs) (Fig. 7.6). The way CTLs induce apoptotic death in target cells is described in Chapter 9.

Interferon-γ is secreted both by NK cells in innate defence and also by TH1 subset of T cells when adaptive immune responses are activated. It performs various roles and is considered under cytokines of adaptive immunity.

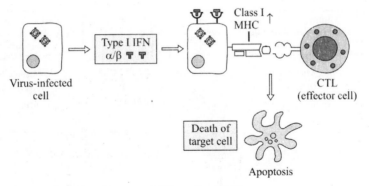

Fig. 7.6 Type I interferons and CTL-mediated killing.

For the biologic roles of some key cytokines involved in innate defence, refer to Fig. 2.8.

Cytokines of Adaptive Immunity

Cytokines that stimulate adaptive immune responses are produced mainly by antigen-activated CD4$^+$ T lymphocytes. They are depicted in Fig. 7.7.

There are two major T helper cell subsets: TH1 and TH2. These two subsets produce different cytokines and have different functions to perform (Fig. 7.8). The type of microbe and the cytokine environment established during innate responses determines which subset predominates.

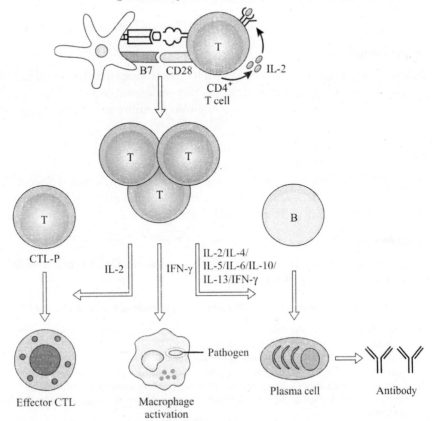

Fig. 7.7 Some key cytokines of adaptive immunity.

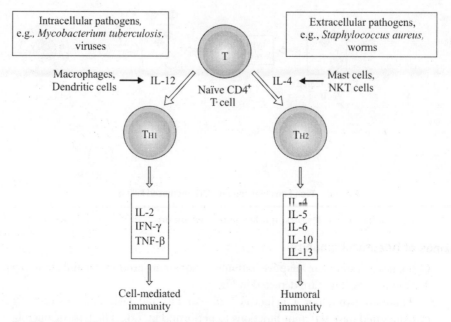

Fig. 7.8 **TH1 and TH2 subsets and their cytokine profile.** Cytokines produced by the two T cell subsets determine the course of the immune response.

The important biologic roles of IL-2 and IFN-γ are highlighted in the following text.

Interleukin-2

When T cells recognize specific peptide–MHC class II complexes on the antigen-presenting cell (APC) surface and receive a costimulatory signal, they undergo activation and release IL-2. Interleukin-2 is vital for T cell proliferation and was originally identified as a T cell growth factor. Other major biological roles of IL-2 include

- enhancement of IFN-γ and IL-4 production by T cells
- proliferation and differentiation of cytotoxic T lymphocytes
- growth and enhancement of cytotoxic activity of NK cells. Activated NK cells called lymphokine-activated killer cells or *LAK cells* have potential for cancer therapy (see Chapter 18).
- stimulation of B cell proliferation and antibody synthesis

Interferon-γ

In the course of an adaptive immune response, activated CD4$^+$ T cells release IFN-γ. It has multiple important functions to perform (Box 7.2).

Box 7.2   The diverse roles of IFN-γ secreted by stimulated T lymphocytes and NK cells.

- Enhances transcription of genes encoding MHC proteins (increases antigen presentation), immune-specific proteasome subunits, and TAP (see Chapter 5).
- Promotes killing of virally-infected cells by effector CTLs.
- Induces TH1 and inhibits TH2 responses; this activates macrophages.
- Endothelial cell activation; induces adhesion molecules and chemokines on endothelium.
- Stimulates antibody production and modulates class-switching to opsonizing and complement-fixing antibodies.
- Has weak antiviral activity.

Chemokines

Chemotactic cytokines are designated chemokines. They are produced by monocytes/macrophages, endothelial cells, T cells, neutrophils, fibroblasts, and some other cell types. When produced in response to infection/injury, their major role is in chemoattraction of leukocytes, primarily neutrophils, monocytes, and lymphocytes, to sites of infection where inflammatory reactions have been initiated. They are also produced constitutively in absence of inflammation in which case they are involved in house-keeping functions, such as regulation of cell-trafficking through peripheral lymphoid organs and tissues. Of the four chemokine families, the two major ones include CC chemokines and CXC chemokines.

CC Chemokines

These chemokines induce migration of monocytes into tissues where they transform into macrophages, for example, monocyte chemotactic protein-1 (MCP-1) or CCL2. Some of these chemokines are also chemotactic for T cells.

CXC Chemokines

A familiar example is IL-8 or CXCL8. It acts preferentially on neutrophils and induces chemotaxis (see Fig. 2.14). Overall, chemokines perform diverse roles including

- inflammation
- cell-trafficking
- wound-healing
- angiogenesis
- lymphoid organ development
- cell compartmentalization in lymphoid organs/tissues

Haematopoietic Cytokines

Haematopoietic cytokines produced by stromal cells, fibroblasts, macrophages, T cells, and also other cells, are involved in differentiation of stem cells into various formed elements of blood in a process called haematopoiesis (Fig. 7.9). *Granulocyte-colony stimulating factor (G-CSF)* increases growth of granulocytes. It also enhances production of neutrophils from the bone marrow, particularly at times of infection to replace neutrophils consumed during inflammation. *Monocyte-colony stimulating factor (M-CSF)* is a growth and differentiation factor selective for monocytes. It stimulates production of monocytes from precursor cells in the bone marrow. *Granulocyte–monocyte-colony stimulating factor (GM-CSF)* besides promoting growth of granulocytes, stimulates maturation of bone marrow cells into dendritic cells and monocytes. It is also a macrophage-activating cytokine.

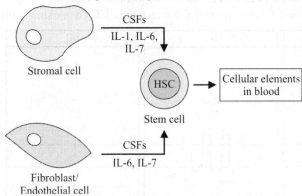

Fig. 7.9 Cytokines control haematopoiesis in bone marrow.

CYTOKINE RECEPTORS AND SIGNAL TRANSDUCTION

Cytokines which are small protein communication molecules of the immune system act through high-affinity cell-surface receptors to transduce signals into the cell. Various changes in protein synthesis occur in the cells they act on, thereby modifying various aspects of cell behaviour.

Cytokine Receptors

Receptors for cytokines are classified on the basis of structural properties into five families listed in the following text:

1. Class I cytokine receptor family (haematopoietin receptor family). There are three subfamilies of class I cytokine receptors:
    - GM-CSF receptor subfamily
    - IL-6 receptor subfamily
    - IL-2 receptor subfamily
2. Class II cytokine receptor family
3. Immunoglobulin superfamily cytokine receptors
4. Tumour necrosis factor receptor family
5. Chemokine receptor family

Some selected cytokine receptors are depicted in Fig. 7.10.

Ligands for the IL-2 receptor subfamily of class I cytokine receptors include IL-2, IL-4, IL-7, IL-9, IL-15, and IL-21. Their receptors share a common γ (γc) chain which functions in signalling. The complete high-affinity IL-2 receptor comprises three chains: α, β, and γc chains (IL-15 receptor, too, is trimeric, whereas other receptors in this subfamily are dimers). High-affinity binding to IL-2 requires all the three chains. Resting (naïve) T cells (and also NK cells) express the intermediate-affinity receptor IL-2 R$\beta\gamma$c. The IL-2Rα chain (CD25) is expressed only when T cells are stimulated by antigen/mitogen and other signals (costimulatory) resulting in the formation of the complete high-affinity IL-2 R$\alpha\beta\gamma$c complex (Fig. 7.11).

Expression of the functional IL-2 R only on activated T cells ensures that it is only antigen-activated T cells that proliferate in response to IL-2 (autocrine). CD25 is a marker for T cell activation and can be identified by monoclonal anti-CD25. It should be borne in mind that Tregs also express high levels of CD25 (see Chapter 15).

Chemokine receptors have a unique structure, distinct from the other cytokine receptors. They are also designated serpentine receptors as their hydrophobic transmembrane domains, of which there are seven, traverse back and forth through the membrane several times. Chemokine receptors are grouped according to the type of chemokine they bind: CC receptors (CCRs) recognize CC chemokines, and

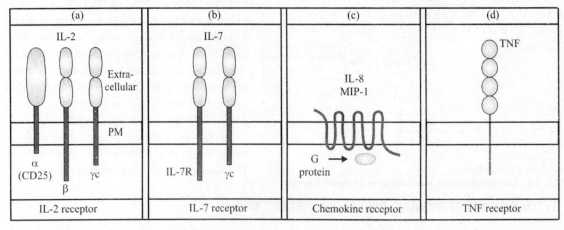

Fig. 7.10 Some selected cytokine receptors. Two receptors [(a) and (b)] belonging to the IL-2 receptor subfamily are shown. Interleukin-2 receptor is a trimer, whereas IL-7 receptor is dimeric. Note the common γ (γc) chain in both receptors. It is involved in signalling. Chemokine (c) and TNF (d) receptors are also shown.

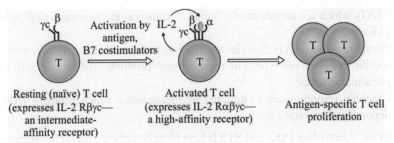

Fig. 7.11 Interleukin-2 receptor on naïve and activated T cells. Natural killer cells, too, express the intermediate-affinity receptor IL-2 Rβγc.

CXC receptors (CXCRs) recognize CXC chemokines. Some chemokine receptors act as co-receptors for HIV; these include *CCR5* and *CXCR4* (see Chapter 16). Chemokine ligands for these receptors block infection by HIV by competing with the virus for receptor binding.

Cytokine Receptor-mediated Signal Transduction

After a cytokine has interacted specifically with its receptor on the cell membrane, signals are transmitted to the interior across the membrane. These signals translocate to the nucleus resulting in activation of specific genes. Many proteins, some of which function as second messengers, are implicated in downstream signalling events. There are four types of signalling pathways, and most is known about the *JAK/STAT pathway* of signal transduction. This pathway is used by cytokines which are ligands for type I and type II cytokine receptors. *Janus kinases (JAKs)* are a novel family of cytosolic protein tyrosine kinases named after Janus, a two-headed Roman God. They have two functional sites—one serves as the binding site to the cytokine receptor subunit and the second is a catalytic site which exhibits tyrosine kinase activity.

The sequence of events in the JAK/ STAT signalling pathway depicted in Fig. 7.12 is outlined in the following text:

- Inactive JAK kinases spontaneously associate with the cytoplasmic tails of type I and type II cytokine receptors.
- Cytokine binding induces clustering of receptors at the cell surface. JAK kinases which are brought close together activate each other by transphosphorylation.
- Activated JAKs phosphorylate the receptors at specific tyrosine residues in the cytoplasmic domains. These serve as docking sites for cytosolic *signal transducers and activators of transcription (STAT)* proteins and binding occurs.

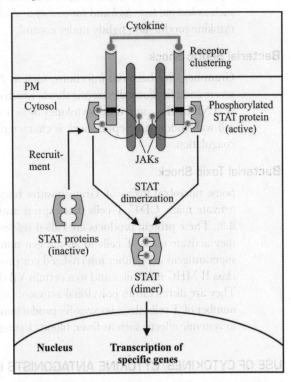

Fig. 7.12 Class I and class II cytokine receptor-mediated signalling.

- STATs, which are members of a family of transcription factors, are phosphorylated by activated JAKs.
- Phosphorylated STATs dimerize and migrate to the nucleus where they activate gene transcription specific to a given cell type. The resulting gene products mediate effects that are attributed to that particular cytokine.
- Cytokine responses are terminated by mechanisms which suppress JAK activity and STAT-dependent transcription.

Many mammalian JAKs and STATs have been described, and each receptor can activate a specific JAK-STAT combination. However, due to a common signalling subunit in receptors for some cytokines, more than one cytokine may activate a particular pathway. This is the basis for *redundancy* of cytokines which has been referred to in the early part of the chapter.

Some rare immune defects designated *severe combined immunodeficiencies* (*SCID*) arise due to defects in cytokine signalling pathways underscoring the important role of cytokines (see Chapter 16). For instance, a mutation in γc chain of receptors for IL-2, IL-4, IL-7, IL-9, IL-15, and IL-21 is seen in *X-L SCID*. Normal cytokine signalling which results in activation of JAKs fails to occur and resultant downstream signalling for all the above cytokines is blocked. In another rare defect, expression of a dysfunctional JAK protein due to a mutation results in failure to phosphorylate STAT molecules.

CYTOKINE-ASSOCIATED PATHOPHYSIOLOGY

Cytokine overproduction can be detrimental to the host and can lead to life-threatening conditions, such as *bacterial toxic shock* and *bacterial septic shock*. Hence, there is necessity as mentioned earlier to keep cytokine produc-tion tightly under control.

Bacterial Septic Shock

Gram-negative bacterial infections, such as *Pseudomonas aeruginosa* and *Escherichia coli* can lead to a severe complication called septic shock, which can sometimes be fatal. It is due to excessive production of TNF-α, IL-1, and other cytokines by activated macrophages and is induced by LPS, a bacterial cell wall endotoxin. Septic shock is characterized by fall in BP, fever, and widespread intravascular coagulation.

Bacterial Toxic Shock

Some microbial toxins of Gram-positive bacteria, such as enterotoxins of *Staphylococcus aureus*, can activate many CD4$^+$ T cells that express antigen receptors with a particular Vβ domain (see Fig. 8.9). These protein products are called *superantigens*. They differ from conventional antigens in that they activate many T cells in an antigen non-specific manner. Another point of difference is that superantigens are neither internalized nor processed. They exhibit unique binding to the α chain of class II MHC molecules and to a certain Vβ domain of the TCR, outside the peptide-binding cleft. They are distinct from polyclonal activators which stimulate all T cells. Due to activation of a large number of T cells, there is excessive production of IL-1 and TNF (proinflammatory cytokines) leading to systemic effects, such as fever, blood clotting, drop in BP, and shock.

USE OF CYTOKINES/CYTOKINE ANTAGONISTS IN THERAPY

Therapies based on cytokines/cytokine receptor antagonists/soluble receptors offer hope for the future and are being exploited for clinical use in various types of immune disorders. Some examples of these biological therapeutic agents and the conditions in which they have shown benefit are briefly considered in the text that follows.

Cytokines

Some cytokines including IFNs, IL-2, GM-CSF, and G-CSF have shown therapeutic value and are useful clinically. Since the genes for these cytokines have been cloned, recombinant products are available in unlimited amounts and at low costs, making them desirable for therapeutic purposes.

♦ *IFNs*—Hairy cell leukaemia patients and patients suffering from Kaposi's sarcoma respond well to *IFN-α* therapy. Kaposi's sarcoma, a tumour of small blood vessels caused by human herpes virus 8 (HHV 8), affects mostly those infected by HIV-1. Interferon-α has also found use in Hepatitis B and C treatment. Therapy with *IFN-β* has shown a good response in patients suffering from the autoimmune disorder multiple sclerosis. *Interferon-γ* is used to treat chronic granulomatous disease (CGD) in which, though phagocytosis is normal, bacteria engulfed are not killed. Side effects of IFNs are much milder than other cytokines and include flu-like symptoms.

♦ *IL-2*—Treatment of advanced melanoma and renal cell carcinoma with IL-2 has shown benefit in patients. Activation and expansion of NK cells and CTLs from tumour patients with IL-2 in vitro and subsequent re-infusion into patients has potential in tumour therapy (*adoptive cellular immunotherapy*; see Chapter 18). But in high doses, IL-2 can have severe toxic effects.

♦ *CSFs*—Two CSFs having considerable clinical importance include *G-CSF* and *GM-CSF*. They help to restore functioning of the bone marrow after cancer chemotherapy and bone marrow transplantation.

Some difficulties in exploiting cytokines for safe and successful clinical use include

♦ short half-life, for example, rIL-2 has a half-life of only 7–10 minutes when given intravenously

♦ undesirable side effects ranging from mild ones such as fever, chills, diarrhoea to more serious ones such as anaemia, thrombocytopenia, shock, respiratory distress, and coma

In spite of problems, efforts are going on to develop safe cytokine-related therapeutic strategies for inflammatory and allergic disorders , cancer, organ transplantation, and infectious diseases besides others.

Cytokine Antagonists

These are proteins that inhibit the biological action of cytokines and include cytokine receptor antagonists, soluble cytokine receptors, and anti-cytokine antibodies. *Interleukin-1 receptor antagonist (IL-1Ra)* is a naturally occurring inhibitor produced by mononuclear phagocytes that binds to IL-1R on CD4$^+$ T cells and prevents IL-1 from binding. Activation signals in CD4$^+$ T cells are thus blocked (Fig. 7.13). The recombinant product is being investigated for treatment of chronic inflammatory diseases.

Soluble cytokine receptors interact with the cytokine ligand, reducing the concentration of cytokine available to bind to the receptor. For instance, *soluble TNF receptors* (see Chapter 15) have been successfully used in treatment of rheumatoid arthritis, which is an autoimmune disorder characterized by pain and stiffness in joints due to chronic inflammation (Fig. 7.14).

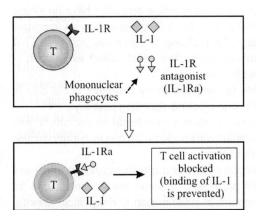

Fig. 7.13 Inhibition of cytokine functions by a cytokine receptor antagonist.

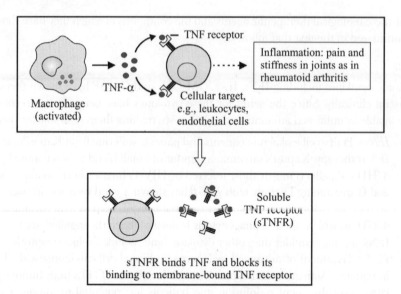

Fig. 7.14   Neutralization of TNF with a soluble receptor.

Anti-cytokine antibodies too are important as they can be used to block biological activity of a cytokine by preventing cytokine binding to its receptor. Inflixinab (anti-TNF-α antibody) is one such example (see Chapter 15). Anti-cytokine antibodies have other applications too. They find practical use in measurement/detection of cytokines by enzyme-linked immunosorbent assay (ELISA), which is also commonly used to measure anti-cytokine antibodies in hybridoma supernatants (Appendix 1).

SUMMARY

♦ Cytokines are low molecular weight regulatory proteins/glycoproteins secreted by leukocytes and other cell types in the body. Most are soluble but a few also exist in membrane-bound form.

♦ They perform important roles in immune and inflammatory responses but functioning is not limited to the immune system.

♦ They are usually not stored and are produced transiently in response to an external stimulus. They have short half-lives.

♦ Cytokines act over both short range and long range. Their action may be autocrine, paracrine, or endocrine.

♦ Some important features of cytokines include pleiotropy, antagonism, synergism, and redundancy.

♦ Based on function, cytokines can be broadly classified into cytokines of innate immunity, cytokines of adaptive immunity, chemokines, and haematopoietic cytokines.

♦ Only target cells expressing receptors for a particular cytokine will respond to it. There are five families of cytokine receptors.

♦ The JAK/STAT signalling pathway triggered by class I and class II cytokine receptors has been well studied. Since cytokine receptors have no kinase activity, JAKs (protein kinases) play an important role in the pathway. The pathway activates STAT transcription factors which affect expression of specific genes.

♦ Rare immunodeficiency diseases occur due to defects in cytokine signalling pathways.

♦ Diseases such as bacterial septic shock and bacterial toxic shock are caused by overproduction of cytokines.

♦ Therapies exploiting cytokines/cytokine receptors hold promise and some are in clinical use for treatment of inflammation in rheumatoid arthritis, an autoimmune disorder.

REVIEW QUESTIONS

1. Indicate whether the following statements are true or false. If false, explain why.
   (a) Activated NK cells express the high-affinity IL-2 receptor as do activated T cells.
   (b) Some chemokine receptors are essential for HIV entry into cells.
   (c) TNF-α blocks synthesis of acute-phase proteins by the liver.
   (d) Increase in class I and class II MHC molecule expression is an immune activity of IFN-γ.
   (e) A receptor antagonist binds to a specific receptor but does not transmit signals.
   (f) IFN-β produces clinical improvement in patients suffering from multiple sclerosis.

2. Self-assessment questions
   (a) T cells stimulated with phytohaemagglutinin (PHA; a mitogen for T cells) and unstimulated T cells were incubated in separate culture dishes in presence of known amounts of IL-2 for a brief period. ELISA assays for IL-2 were then conducted on culture supernatants. It was found that levels of IL-2 remained unchanged in supernatants from unstimulated cells while it declined in supernatants from PHA-stimulated cells. Explain these observations.
   (b) What are superantigens and how do they differ from conventional antigens? Why do they induce damaging effects in the host?
   (c) Which cytokines fall in the category of proinflammatory cytokines? How do they participate in host defence?
   (d) How do cytokines mediate their biologic effects in target cells? Is the short half-life of cytokines of any advantage to the host? If so, explain why.
   (e) Describe some therapeutic approaches based on cytokines and cytokine receptors that find use in clinical practice.

3. For each question, choose the *best* answer.
   (a) The synthesis of the α chain of the IL-2 receptor on T cells is triggered by
      (i) Signal 1
      (ii) Signal 1 + costimulatory signal
      (iii) IL-4
      (iv) IFN-γ
   (b) The cytokine which functions also as a long range mediator is
      (i) IL-6
      (ii) TGF-β
      (iii) IL-12
      (iv) IL-10
   (c) The cytokine that controls trafficking of immune cells is
      (i) IFN-γ
      (ii) IL-8
      (iii) IL-1
      (iv) GM-CSF
   (d) The action of a cytokine on many cell types to produce diverse effects is a feature referred to as
      (i) Redundancy
      (ii) Synergism
      (iii) Pleiotropy
      (iv) Antagonism

T Lymphocyte Maturation and Activation

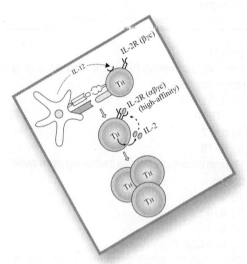

LEARNING OBJECTIVES

Having studied this chapter, you should be able to understand the following:

- The salient features of germline organization of αβ TCR genes and generation of receptor diversity
- T cell maturation events in the thymus, and selection of cells with useful receptors and its significance
- The structural and functional features of the T cell receptor and its associated proteins
- APC and T lymphocyte interactions in peripheral lymphoid organs and how T cells clonally expand into effector T cells
- The importance of costimulatory signals in T cell activation
- The different roles of the two major T cell subsets: T$_{H1}$ and T$_{H2}$
- How superantigens differ from conventional antigens
- The signalling cascades triggered on T cell activation by antigen and how T cell activation is controlled

Antigen receptors on lymphocytes, which are the central cells of adaptive immunity, are highly diverse and can recognize a wide range of foreign substances/pathogens. This diversity in T cell antigen receptors is generated after progenitor T cells enter the thymus from the bone marrow. These early developing T cells, called early thymocytes, undergo a process of maturation in which germline T cell receptor (TCR) genes are rearranged and various surface molecules are expressed. The developmental pathway generates an enormous T cell repertoire which exits the thymus for peripheral lymphoid tissues.

T cells, unlike B cells, afford protection against those microbes which reside intracellularly (cell-mediated immunity) and which are protected from antibody and complement-mediated attack. T cells also participate in adaptive humoral immunity by releasing cytokines that stimulate B cell antibody synthesis (see Chapter 10). To perform the various activities of adaptive cell-mediated immunity, T cells need to undergo activation, proliferation, and differentiation to effector cells. It is in the peripheral lymphoid organs that naïve T cells initially encounter antigen and are activated to clonally expand, an event which increases the number of cells having identical specificity that can cope effectively with the foreign invader. Both processes, namely, maturation in thymus and activation of mature T cells in the periphery are highly dependent on major histocompatibility complex (MHC) molecules. Knockout mice lacking expression of class I or class II MHC molecules fail to develop mature CD8$^+$ or CD4$^+$ T cells, respectively.

This chapter focuses on the structural aspects of the T cell antigen receptor and its associated proteins. The germline organization of TCR genes and generation of receptor diversity are briefly outlined. The sequential stages in T cell maturation that lead to development of the mature T cell repertoire, the process of antigen-induced activation of naïve T cells in peripheral lymphoid organs, and also the essential steps in receptor-induced signalling are described.

T CELL RECEPTOR COMPLEX

Cell-mediated immune responses depend on direct contact of T lymphocytes with antigen-presenting cells (APCs) or target cells. Hence, the antigen receptor made by T cells, unlike the receptor made by B cells, exists only in membrane-bound form and is not secreted. Another major difference highlighted in Chapter 1 is that while the TCR has a single antigen recognition site, the B cell receptor (BCR) has two such sites which are identical.

There are two distinct types of TCR for antigen, the most common form of which is *TCR2*. It is a disulphide-linked heterodimer comprised of α and β glycoprotein chains (*αβ TCR*). *TCR1*, a second less-abundant form of the receptor, is composed of γ and δ glycoprotein chains (*γδ TCR*). It appears earlier than αβ TCR during thymic ontogeny and is expressed on only 1–2 per cent of the total T cell population. The structure of αβ TCR is depicted in Fig. 8.1.

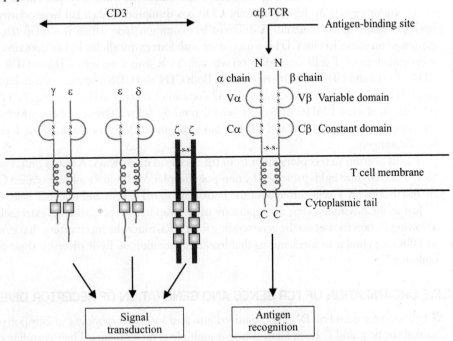

Fig. 8.1   Structure of αβ T cell receptor complex. The T cell receptor and associated CD3 proteins form the T cell receptor complex. While TCR recognizes antigen, signals are delivered to T lymphocytes by CD3 proteins.

▭ : immunoreceptor tyrosine-based activation motif

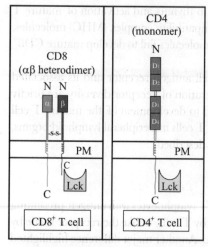

Fig. 8.2 Schematic representation of CD8 and CD4 co-receptors.

It should be noted that the structure is very similar to the Fab fragment of the Ig molecule. Each chain consists of an *N*-terminal variable (V) domain and a constant (C) domain at the *C*-terminal end. The Vα and Vβ segment of each chain contains three *hypervariable regions* or *complimentarity determining regions* (*CDRs*) (see Chapters 4 and 6); these recognize complexes of processed protein antigens and MHC molecules. The greatest diversity in amino acid sequence among different TCRs is in CDR3. There are five invariant (identical in all cells) polypeptide chains (γ, δ, ε, ζ, and η) that are non-covalently associated with the TCR. These proteins also associate with each other to form three dimers, namely, εδ, εγ, and ζζ or ζη. These together constitute the *CD3 complex* which functions in signal transduction during T cell activation. Approximately 90 per cent of CD3 complexes incorporate ζζ disulphide-linked homodimers, whereas the rest have ζη heterodimers. The TCR and associated CD3 proteins form the *TCR complex*. A typical T cell has about 30,000 receptor complexes on its surface. The cytoplasmic tails of CD3 chains contain conserved *immunoreceptor tyrosine-based activation motifs* (*ITAMs*) which function in signal transduction and initiation of T cell activation. Phosphorylation of tyrosine residues in ITAMs creates docking sites for elements involved in signalling (Fig. 8.11).

CD4 and *CD8* are accessory molecules/co-receptors which associate with the TCR and are essential for T cell activation (Fig. 8.2). They are transmembrane glycoproteins and are members of the immunoglobulin (Ig) superfamily. CD8 is a disulphide-linked αβ heterodimer, each subunit having a single Ig-like domain. A different less common type which is a CD8 αα homodimer is expressed on some T cells. CD4 is a monomer with four extracellular Ig-like domains. There are two subpopulations of T cells depending on whether TCR associates with CD4 or CD8. These include CD4+ T cells and CD8+ T cells, respectively. Both CD4 and CD8 recognize non-polymorphic regions of MHC molecules. CD4 recognizes the β2 domain of class II MHC, whereas CD8 recognizes the α3 domain of class I MHC molecules (see Chapter 5). *Lck* is a tyrosine kinase which associates with the cytoplasmic tails of CD8 and CD4. It has a role in signal transduction when T cells recognize a specific antigen.

T cells bearing γδ receptors differ from αβ T cells in many ways. A major difference is that some γδ T cells recognize lipids presented by non-polymorphic MHC-like molecules called CD1 molecules. All discussions on T cells throughout the book refer to αβ T cells and not γδ T cells, unless stated.

Just as for B lymphocytes, the repertoire of T lymphocyte specificities is extremely diverse. The following section focuses on the genes coding for TCRs. Since the mechanisms that generate diversity in TCRs are similar to mechanisms that lead to generation of BCR diversity, these are only briefly outlined.

GERMLINE ORGANIZATION OF TCR GENES AND GENERATION OF RECEPTOR DIVERSITY

T cell receptor germline DNA is organized into four loci corresponding to four polypeptide chains, namely, α, β, γ, and δ. Each locus contains multiple gene segments. Their germline organization is essentially the same as the organization of genes that encode Igs. The organization of TCR α and β chain gene segments is depicted in a simplified form in Fig. 8.3.

Some major features of organization of TCR chain genes are outlined in the following text with the main focus on the αβ TCR. These include the following:

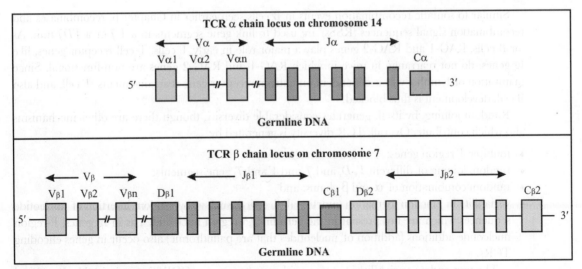

Fig. 8.3 Germline organization of α and β chain loci of αβ TCR. For simplicity, the δ genes are not shown in the α chain locus.

- The TCR α chain locus on chromosome 14, by analogy to the Ig light (L) chain, is composed of a cluster of V segments, a large number of J segments, and a constant gene segment. There are no D segments in the α locus.
- It is interesting that the TCR δ chain genes (which encode the δ chain of the γδ TCR) are embedded inside the TCR α gene region. The δ genes, present between the $V\alpha$ and $J\alpha$ gene clusters, are excised during α chain gene rearrangements.
- The β and γ chains are separate gene regions on chromosome 7.
- The β chain, like the Ig heavy (H) chain, is encoded by $V, D, J,$ and C gene segments. It is noteworthy that there are two sets of $D, J,$ and C genes in the TCR β chain locus. Later in the chapter, we will see that some secreted bacterial proteins called *superantigens* activate many T cells having a particular Vβ sequence, irrespective of antigenic specificity of the TCR.
- While TCR α chain germline DNA has only a single C gene segment, the β chain DNA has two constant region genes—Cβ1 and Cβ2. Their protein products differ by a few amino acids but functional differences are not known to exist. This organization is in sharp contrast to the Ig H chain germline DNA which has multiple C gene segments. These encode products (isotypes) that differ structurally and functionally.

T cell receptor diversity is generated when progenitor cells move into the thymus from the bone marrow. In the thymus, T cells undergo a process of maturation during which germline genes rearrange. The α and β chain genes of the TCR undergo basically the same random rearrangements during T cell development as described earlier for Igs (see Chapter 6). The β chain of the TCR is the first to undergo recombination events. By analogy to Ig H chain DNA, the β chain undergoes two variable region joinings—first $D\beta$ to $J\beta$ followed by $V\beta$ to $D\beta J\beta$. Rearrangement of α chain gene segments, by analogy to Ig L chain DNA, leads to direct $V\alpha$–$J\alpha$ joining. The number of $J\alpha$ gene segments is unusually large due to which receptor diversity increases tremendously. After the rearranged TCR genes are transcribed, the primary transcripts (with the constant domain gene incorporated) are processed to give mRNAs encoding α and β chains of the TCR. Following translation, the α and β chains are expressed on the T cell membrane as disulphide-linked heterodimers. As has been stated earlier, the αβ TCR is more common and is expressed on the majority of T cells.

Similar to somatic recombination events in B cells seen earlier in Chapter 6, recombinases and recombination signal sequences (RSSs) are used to link gene segments in a VJ or a VDJ unit. As for B cells, RAG-1 and RAG-2 genes play a major role in early T cells. T cell receptor genes, like Ig genes, do not rearrange in mice in which RAG-1 and RAG-2 genes are non-functional. Since maturation of lymphocytes is dependent on antigen receptor gene rearrangements, T cell, and also B cell, development is thus blocked.

Random joining, by itself, generates considerable diversity, though there are other mechanisms also which contribute. Overall, TCR diversity is generated by

◆ multiple V region genes;
◆ random joining of different V, D, and J (and V and J) gene segments;
◆ random combination of α and β chains; and
◆ variability in junction formation (junctional diversity), such as by random insertion of nucleotide sequences which are not present in the germline (N-region nucleotide); as in Ig genes, P-region nucleotide additions (addition of nucleotides that are palindromic) also occur in genes encoding TCRs.

The tremendous variability in amino acid sequence seen in CDR3 is maximized by junctional diversity. CDR3 is the hypervariable region of the TCR that makes contact with amino acids in the centre of the peptide associated with an MHC molecule and is most important for antigen recognition by TCR.

Some major differences exist in T and B cell generation of receptor diversity. Since the TCR is bound to the membrane only and does not exist in soluble form like secreted antibody, differential processing of the primary RNA transcript is not required. Although allelic exclusion occurs for the TCR β chain genes, allowing expression of only one β chain, α chain genes do not show allelic exclusion. This allows more than one α chain to be expressed, the reason why some T cells may express two different TCRs on their membrane. Another noteworthy difference is that the high frequency of somatic hypermutation seen among Ig genes, which further magnifies receptor diversity, is not seen in TCR genes. In other words, the sequences generated after initial TCR gene rearrangements during T cell maturation in the thymus show stability, and are same as those present in the mature T cell population at peripheral sites. Thus, affinity maturation seen with antibodies during an ongoing immune response to protein antigens is lacking in the TCR repertoire.

The various mechanisms involved in generation of receptor diversity help to generate a very large repertoire of unique $\alpha\beta$ TCRs equivalent to or even exceeding the number of receptor specificities generated in B cells.

The chapter now progresses to a description of developmental events that lead to the generation of the mature lymphocyte pool that exits the thymus to respond to foreign antigens in the periphery.

SEQUENTIAL EVENTS IN T CELL MATURATION AND SELECTION

Maturation of T cells from bone marrow stem cells occurs in the thymus analogous to the maturation of B cells in the bone marrow (for mammalian cells). The fact that the thymus is of crucial importance for differentiation of immature precursor cells was first recognized in patients suffering from *DiGeorge syndrome* (a congenital immunodeficiency disorder caused by incomplete development of thymus), and also in nude mice which are so called because they lack fur (see Chapter 16). Very low numbers of mature T cells are seen in the circulation and peripheral lymphoid tissues as a result of which T cell-mediated immunity is severely compromised. Removal of the thymus from neonatal mice also leads to failure in T cell maturation.

The various events that occur during T cell maturation are depicted in Fig. 8.4 and are outlined in the following text.

Proliferation of Early T Cells

The early T cells which enter the outer cortex of the thymus do not express TCR, CD3, or the CD4 or CD8 molecules typically found on the surface of T cells. These early T cells called *early thymocytes* show high mitotic activity and proliferate in response to the growth factor IL-7 (and other cytokines) produced by non-lymphoid thymic stromal cells.

Rearrangement of TCR Genes and Co-receptor Expression

The earliest thymocytes called *pro-T cells* contain TCR genes in their germline configuration. RAG-1 and RAG-2 proteins are first expressed at this stage and TCR β chain gene rearrangements occur.

In the *pre-T cell stage*, the newly synthesized β chains are expressed on the cell surface associated with a 33 kDa invariant glycoprotein known as the *pre-T α chain*. In these pre-T cells, pre-T α along with CD3 forms a complex called *pre-T cell receptor (pre-TCR) complex*. It has a role similar to the surrogate L chains in the pre-BCR which is expressed during B cell development. Formation of pre-TCR indicates that a cell has made a productive TCR β chain rearrangement. Further rearrangement of β chain genes is suppressed (allelic exclusion) due to downregulation of RAG proteins that mediate recombination. This ensures that the T cell expresses only one type of β chain.

Maturation proceeds with expression of CD4 and CD8 co-receptors on the surface to form *double-positive (DP)* cells which are found in large numbers in the thymic cortex. It is signalling from the pre-TCR that triggers proliferation in T cells and rearrangement of α chain genes. After a stage of rapid proliferation, pre-Tα is downregulated. TCR α chain gene rearrangements occur after cells have stopped proliferating and RAG proteins are expressed. Following generation of TCRs, DP cells undergo selection processes in the thymus.

Selection of Double-positive Immature Thymocytes

The maturation process in the thymus culminates in the selection of cells that express useful receptors and takes place in two stages: *positive selection* and *negative selection* (Fig. 8.5). Thymic stromal cells, epithelial cells, macrophages, and dendritic cells (DCs) have a major role to play in the selection process.

Positive Selection

This takes place in the thymic cortex and denotes preservation of a thymocyte that can bind to self-MHC. When the TCR on DP thymocytes interacts with MHC molecules expressed on cortical stromal cells (these act as APCs), they receive signals critical for survival and further maturation. This is essential as mature T cells, the key players in activation of immune responses, need to interact with self-MHC molecules associated with foreign peptide.

Those DP cells which fail to make this essential interaction are deprived of survival signals and are permitted to die. Approximately 95 per cent or more of all thymocytes die by apoptosis in the thymus as they fail positive selection. It follows that MHC molecules have a crucial role in selection processes in the thymus. Mice in which genes for class I and class II MHC molecules have been knocked out show lack of mature CD8$^+$ T cells or CD4$^+$ T cells, respectively, as these cells fail to be positively selected.

A salient feature of the positive selection process is that αβ T cells become educated to the MHC molecules on thymic cortical stromal cells. These are self-MHC molecules, whereas all other types of MHC molecules are non-self. This phenomenon is referred to as *self-MHC restriction* and is central to T cell responses. These self-MHC restricted mature T cells will emerge from the thymus and enter the

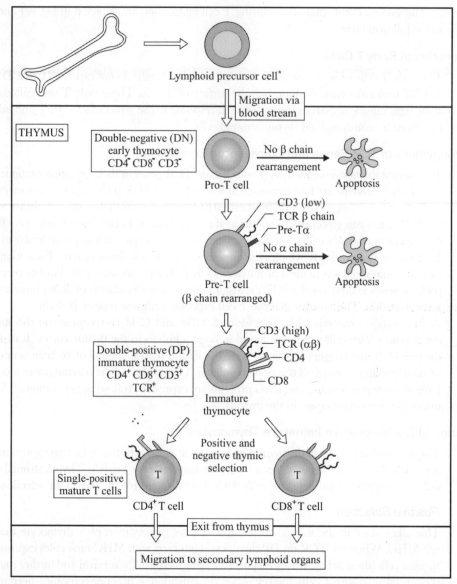

Fig. 8.4 Overview of T cell maturation pathway in the thymus. It should be noted that each stage carries distinct cell surface molecules. Development of CD4$^+$ and CD8$^+$ single-positive mature T cells represents the final stage of the maturation pathway. Failure to express antigen receptors leads to death by apoptosis. The pathway for γδ T cell differentiation separates early from the αβ T cell developmental pathway and has not been shown.
* Common lymphoid precursor that gives rise to both T and B cells.

peripheral lymphoid tissues only after undergoing a second selection process called negative selection, which is discussed in the following text.

Negative Selection

This implies that a thymocyte is eliminated due to some undesirable characteristic that it exhibits. Since gene rearrangements involved in generation of T cell antigen receptors occur in a random manner,

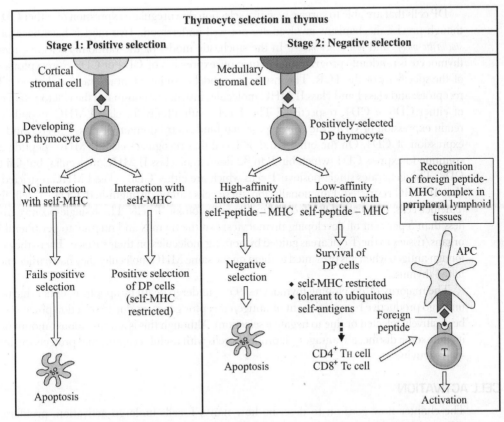

Fig. 8.5   Positive and negative selection of CD4$^+$ CD8$^+$ DP thymocytes in the thymus. Thymocytes undergo selection processes in which they interact with thymic cortical and medullary stromal cells before they leave the thymus as mature single-positive CD4$^+$ or CD8$^+$ T cells.

TCRs specific for both foreign and self-antigens are generated in the thymus. These cells if allowed to escape into the periphery, after surviving positive selection, could lead to undesirable autoimmune reactions. Hence, to avoid this, DP cells undergo another selection process termed *negative selection*. A very high-affinity interaction between the TCR on DP thymocytes and self-peptide-associated MHC molecules on medullary stromal cells delivers signals that lead to deletion of these cells by apoptosis (a low-affinity interaction favours survival). *This is important for development of a state of immunological tolerance due to which immune responses to self are generally avoided* (see Chapter 15).

At this point, it is relevant to mention that in thymus MHC molecules are bound exclusively to peptides derived from degradation of self-proteins. These proteins occur outside the thymus also. A pertinent question that arises here is whether thymus expresses all potential self-antigens that occur outside the thymus. Since all self-antigens are not expressed in thymic tissues, some self-reactive T cells may not be eliminated. To safeguard against this, mechanisms for inducing tolerance exist at peripheral sites also (see Chapter 15).

Overall, the mature T cell repertoire that survives the two-stage selection process and exits the thymus exhibits two significant features:

- Self-MHC restriction
- Tolerance to ubiquitous self-antigens (central tolerance)

DP cells that are able to survive negative selection downregulate expression of either CD4 or CD8, though precise mechanisms involved are not well understood. Two models have been proposed— *stochastic model* and *instructive model*. In the stochastic model or the randomly selective model, a DP thymocyte is randomly programmed to turn off expression of CD4 or CD8 co-receptors, regardless of the specificity of the TCR. The instructive model postulates that interactions between TCRs, co-receptors, and class I and class II MHC molecules instruct or command the cell to retain expression of either CD8 or CD4, respectively. The T cells with affinity for class I MHC–peptide complexes retain expression of CD8 (the co-receptor that binds to α3 domain of class I MHC) and switch off expression of CD4. On the other hand, a T cell that recognizes class II MHC–peptide complexes continue to express CD4 (which binds to β2 domain of class II MHC molecules) but fail to express CD8. This generates single-positive T cells which are either $CD8^+$ class I MHC restricted or $CD4^+$ class II MHC restricted. Functionally, too, these cells can be distinguished: $CD4^+$ T cells function as T helper cells, whereas $CD8^+$ T cells function as cytotoxic T cells. These single-positive mature cells (less than 5 per cent of developing thymocytes) exit the thymus and migrate to peripheral lymphoid organs/tissues to the T cell areas guided by homing molecules on their surface. There they respond to foreign antigen when it is presented to them on the same MHC molecules they had earlier encountered in the thymus.

The majority of developing thymocytes (95%) undergo death by apoptosis, either due to failure to undergo productive rearrangement of antigen receptor genes, or due to selection processes (failure to be positively selected or due to negative selection). Although this is a tremendous amount of wastage, it offers some distinct advantages – it produces cells with useful receptors and protects the host against self-reactivity.

T CELL ACTIVATION

The chapter now goes on to describe how naïve T cells undergo activation, proliferation, and differentiation to effector cells in peripheral lymphoid sites before they participate in adaptive cell-mediated immune responses.

T Cell Activation Occurs in Secondary Lymphoid Organs/Tissues

A naïve T cell's first encounter with an antigen which results in its activation occurs on the surface of an APC, mainly DCs, and also macrophages. This event, called *priming*, occurs in secondary lymphoid sites. In brief, DC progenitors migrate from their site of production (the bone marrow) to peripheral sites (under skin and mucous membranes and in most solid organs) where they are found as immature resting DCs. *Langerhans cells* in the skin are an example of immature DCs. Immature DCs undergo phenotypic and functional changes induced by antigen/pathogen. This transforms them from antigen-capturing cells to efficient APCs which carry foreign peptide–MHC complexes on their surface. These maturational changes occur during their migration from peripheral tissues to the nearest lymph node where they trigger activation of naïve T cells (Fig. 8.6).

An important question that arises here is how rare antigen-specific naïve lymphocytes find their cognate antigen and respond to it. It is the trafficking of naïve T lymphocytes through secondary lymphoid sites, introduced earlier in Chapter 3, that increases the chance that rare T cells will encounter their specific antigen presented by APCs. T cells that do recognize their cognate antigen in T cell areas of lymph nodes (and other secondary sites) are activated to expand and differentiate into effector cells. These cells then migrate via the efferent lymphatics and the circulation to sites of infection. These events are revisited in Chapter 9 (see Fig. 9.4).

The chapter now proceeds to a description of the steps that lead to T cell activation on encounter with a specific antigen.

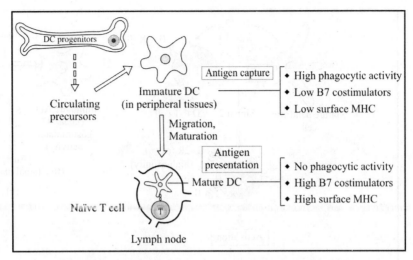

Fig. 8.6   Mature dendritic cells activate naïve T cells in peripheral lymphoid organs. Dendritic cells are important in initiating primary immune responses in peripheral lymphoid tissues.

CD4⁺ T Lymphocyte—APC Interactions

CD4$^+$ T cells interact with APCs which leads to their activation and expansion, followed by their differentiation to effector cells and memory cells. This is depicted in Fig. 8.7 and elaborated in the following text.

Adhesion

Antigen-presenting cells and TH cells initially interact with each other via *cell adhesion molecules (CAMs)* which mediate non-specific transient interaction between the two cell types (see Chapter 2). *Lymphocyte function antigen-1* (LFA-1), an integrin on T cells, binds to *intercellular adhesion molecules (ICAMs)* on APCs. It is reminded here that intercellular adhesion molecules are members of the Ig superfamily (see Chapter 4). In case a T cell encounters its specific antigen, the tightness of binding of LFA-1 with ICAMs increases. This is critical as it allows the TCR to be engaged by antigen long enough to transduce the necessary signals required for T cell proliferation and differentiation. The APC and T cell rapidly dissociate if the T cell fails to recognize a specific peptide–MHC complex. CD2 is an accessory T cell molecule that serves both adhesive and signalling functions. It is a receptor for LFA-3 which is widely distributed on lymphocytes and all APCs.

Specific MHC–Peptide–TCR Interaction (Signal 1)

Recognition of MHC–peptide complexes on the surface of APCs by TCR and CD4 (or CD8 if the interacting cell is a CD8$^+$ T cell) co-receptor constitutes *signal 1*. Signal 1, though essential, is not sufficient to fully activate a T cell. For productive T cell activation, a second costimulatory signal is required.

Costimulation (Signal 2)

Costimulation or *signal 2* required for T cell activation is provided by interaction of costimulatory proteins B7-1(CD80) and B7-2 (CD86) on professional APCs with CD28 on T cells. B7 molecules are members of the Ig superfamily. New B7 and CD28 family members that regulate T cell activation

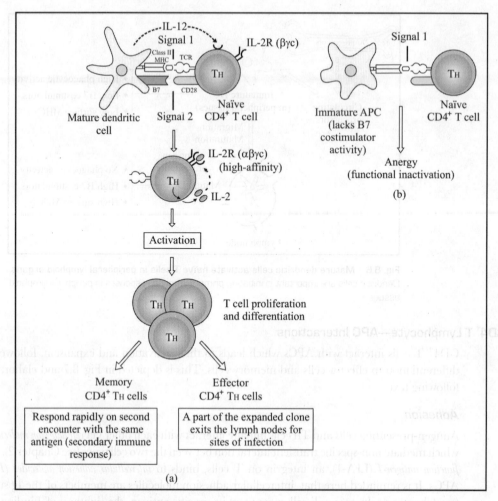

Fig. 8.7 T cells require two signals for productive activation. (a) Both signal 1 and signal 2 combine to trigger T cell responses. Besides direct cellular interactions, cytokines are also important in T cell activation. (b) Delivery of signal 1 alone results in functional inactivation of T cells (anergy).

Note: CD8⁺ T cells are similarly activated by APCs (on recognition of class I MHC—peptide) to memory and effector CD8⁺ cytotoxic T lymphocytes (not shown). Also, IL-12 from activated APCs promotes generation of effector (T$_{H}$1) cells.

have also been identified. Delivery of signal 2 leads to reorganization of signalling proteins in the T cell plasma membrane to the site of contact between the T cell and the APC. This forms an *immunological synapse*, also called *supramolecular activation cluster* or *SMAC* (Fig. 8.8). In SMAC, TCR and associated proteins are concentrated in the centre (*cSMAC*), whereas cell–cell adhesion proteins form a peripheral ring (*pSMAC*). Formation of SMAC enhances intensity and duration of the signalling process activated by signal 1.

A mature DC can simultaneously deliver both signal 1 and 2, and so can activate a T cell to proliferate and differentiate into an effector cell. *It is important that the same cell deliver both the antigen-specific signal and the costimulatory signal.*

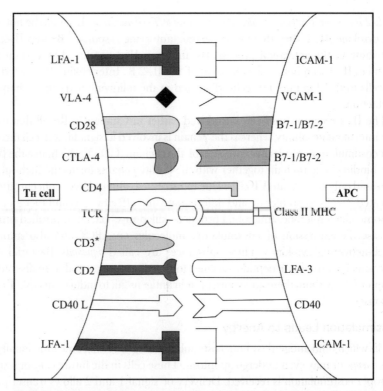

Fig. 8.8   An immunological synapse—the contact region between a T cell and an APC. The figure depicts various cell surface interactions between CD4⁺ Tʜ cells and APCs that lead to the formation of the immunological synapse. The interactions shown trigger T cell activation and cytokine secretion.

* CD3 comprises polypeptide chains which exist as three dimers, namely γε, εδ, and commonly ζζ.

Role of CD40 in T Cell Activation

CD40 ligand (CD40 L) is a key molecule expressed early during T cell activation by an antigen. For sustained expression of CD40 L, costimulatory signals are also needed. Its interaction with CD40 on APCs serves to increase costimulator B7 expression on APCs, and stimulates secretion of T cell-activating cytokines. CD40 L expression on activated T cells, therefore, enhances signals from APCs which further promote T cell proliferation and differentiation. Similar costimulatory signalling through CD40-CD40 L interaction holds significance in promoting activation of B cells (see Chapter 10) and macrophages (see Chapter 9).

T Lymphocyte Response to Antigen and Costimulation

The consequence of signal 2 (and also signal 1) is that genes that were silent in naïve Tʜ cells are now transcribed, leading to increase in synthesis of various proteins. These include

- proteins involved in cell division;
- cytokines, for example, IL-2;
- cytokine receptors, for example, IL-2Rα chain (CD25); and
- anti-apoptotic proteins.

IL-2 is a major T cell growth factor and is central to T cell activation. It should be noted that T cells respond to a cytokine (IL-2) they themselves secrete (autocrine response). Besides IL-2, other cytokines also contribute to the activation process. For instance, IL-1 produced by certain APCs including MØ enhances IL-2 secretion and expression of the IL-2 R. Interleukin-12 secreted by DCs directs naïve TH cells to develop into TH1 cells (discussed in the following text) and enhances interferon (IFN)-γ production.

The IL-2 receptor has been introduced earlier in Chapter 7. Recall that the β chain binds IL-2 with intermediate affinity, whereas the γ chain is involved in signalling. T cell receptor triggering, along with costimulation, results in expression of the α chain (CD25) which, like the β chain, contributes to IL-2 binding. The α chain together with the β and γ chains forms the high-affinity IL-2 R, which is expressed only on activated T cells. Due to increased affinity, lower concentrations of IL-2 can signal activated T cells to proliferate and differentiate into effector cells and memory cells.

Some killed microbes/microbial products (killed mycobacteria; purified protein derivative, PPD) increase the expression of costimulatory molecules on APCs, and also stimulate them to secrete T cell-activating cytokines. These substances are called *adjuvants*. Bacterial antigens are effective adjuvants for protein or peptide vaccines for use in experimental animals (but not in humans) (see Chapter 13). Without these adjuvants, protein antigens fail to induce effective T cell-mediated immune responses.

Lack of Costimulation Leads to Anergy

T cells which bind antigens without costimulation (Fig. 8.7b) become functionally inactivated, referred to as *anergy*, or may even undergo apoptosis. These cells in the future cannot respond to antigens even if proper costimulation is received. Delivery of signal 1 and 2 allows transcription of the IL-2 gene in T cells. It is the second signal which increases the half-life of mRNA specific for IL-2 resulting in IL-2 synthesis. If signal 1 is not accompanied by signal 2, IL-2 mRNA is rapidly degraded and IL-2 is not synthesized. Consequently, T cells fail to proliferate and do not respond to antigens. The importance of anergy in preventing immune responses to self-antigens (called *self-tolerance*) is discussed in Chapter 15.

Activation of CD8⁺ T Cells

The differences in recognition ability of CD4$^+$ and CD8$^+$ T cells have been explained earlier. CD8$^+$ T cells recognize antigenic peptides in association with class I MHC molecules presented on professional APCs. Since these alone have both class I and class II MHC molecules on their surface, they can activate both CD4$^+$T cells (with peptide–class II MHC proteins), as well as CD8$^+$ T cells (with peptide–class I MHC proteins). Naïve CD8$^+$ T cells (cytotoxic T lymphocyte-precursors, CTL-P) that exit the thymus and enter peripheral lymphoid tissues are pre-destined to develop into cytotoxic cells. Recognition of peptide–MHC class I complexes on APCs represents signal 1 for the CD8$^+$ T cell which along with costimulatory signals from APCs results in activation. Cytokines from TH cells also promote the activation process. For this, simultaneous activation of CD4$^+$ T helper cells is essential. This happens when APCs, such as DCs, on ingestion of virally-infected cells may, by a process called *cross-presentation* (see Chapter 5), present cytosolic viral antigens complexed to class I MHC molecules, and vesicular antigens complexed to class II MHC. It should be noted that activation of CD8$^+$ T cells and CD4$^+$ T cells on the same APC enables CD4$^+$ T cell cytokines to provide activating signals to CD8$^+$ T cells. These cells on receiving activation signals clonally expand and differentiate into armed effector cytotoxic cells and memory cells (described in the following text). Although CD4$^+$ T cell–APC interactions have been reasonably well studied, those between CD8$^+$ T cells and APCs are less well understood, though interactions involved are similar.

T Cell Activation by Mitogens and Superantigens

Some substances can induce lymphocyte proliferation, regardless of their antigen specificity (non-specific activation). Such substances are called *mitogens*. A few examples are listed in the following text:

- Phytohaemagglutinin (PHA), a carbohydrate-binding protein (lectin) from red kidney beans (for T cells)
- Concanavalin A (Con A) from castor beans (for T cells)
- Lipopolysaccharide (LPS; for B cells)
- Pokeweed mitogen (PWM; for both T and B cells)

Another group of molecules which can activate T cells non-specifically include the *superantigens*. A large number of secreted bacterial proteins (exotoxins) act as superantigens, including staphylococcal enterotoxins, which are responsible for some types of acute food poisoning. Superantigens differ from conventional antigens. It should be remembered from Chapter 7 that they bind simultaneously to the α chain of class II MHC molecules on APCs and to a particular Vβ domain of the TCR, thereby cross-linking the two (Fig. 8.9). Since the TCR has no specificity for the MHC-associated peptide, many T cells are activated. The consequence of cytokine overproduction due to activation by superantigens of a large number of T cells can be very severe (see Chapter 7).

SIGNAL TRANSDUCTION IN T CELLS

Signal transduction in T cells, as in other cells, begins when a ligand interacts with its receptor. In response, various cellular molecules assemble resulting in the build-up of a signalling cascade or a network. This assembly is dependent on the presence of adaptor or linker proteins which contain certain structural motifs that facilitate interaction. Many linkers are without enzyme activity but some are enzyme linkers, such as cytosolic kinases (enzymes that add phosphate groups—phosphorylation) and phosphatases (enzymes that remove phosphate groups added by kinases—dephosphorylation). Reversible post-translational modifications, such as phosphorylation—dephosphorylation, serve to modulate interactions between various components of the signalling cascade. In the last decade or so, many new effector molecules involved in TCR-linked signal transduction pathways have been identified, making signalling more and more complex. A glance at Fig. 8.10 shows how complex signalling pathways can be.

With this background, some of the very essential features of signalling in T lymphocytes, represented in a simplified form in Fig. 8.11, are discussed in the following text.

Activation of Protein Tyrosine Kinases

Recognition of peptide–MHC complexes by TCR and ligation of costimulatory molecules triggers signalling in T cells. T cell receptors (and also BCRs), just like the receptors involved in cytokine signalling, have no intrinsic tyrosine kinase activity. Instead, cytosolic tyrosine kinases play a key role in the signalling process. These belong to two distinct families which include

- Src family (e.g., Fyn, Lck)
- ZAP-70/Syk family (ZAP70 and Syk for T and B cell activation, respectively).

An early event in T cell activation is induction of protein tyrosine kinase (PTK) activity. The enzyme Lck tyrosine kinase is found non-covalently associated with the intracellular portion of CD4 or CD8 co-receptors, and is inactive in a resting T cell. On TCR triggering, a membrane phosphatase (CD45) catalyzes dephosphorylation of tyrosine residues in Lck, keeping it in an active state. Activated Lck phosphorylates the tyrosine residues in ITAMs in the ζ chains of the TCR complex which

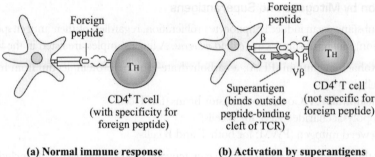

(a) Normal immune response   (b) Activation by superantigens

Fig. 8.9   Stimulation of T cells by superantigens. Superantigens do not undergo processing as other foreign antigens do. They bind directly to class II MHC molecules and a distinct Vβ segment of the TCR.

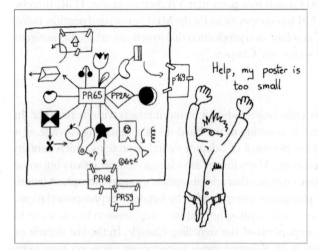

Fig. 8.10   Complexity in signalling pathways.
Source: Reproduced from Zolnierowicz, S. and M. Bollen (2000), 'Protein phosphorylation and protein phosphatases', *EMBO Journal*, 19, pp. 483–488.

provide docking sites for ZAP-70. This event is important in initiation of T cell activation. Lck then phosphorylates ZAP-70 and activates its kinase activity. Activated ZAP-70 phosphorylates adaptor proteins which serve as a platform for recruitment of various molecules including PLCγl to the plasma membrane. Activation of PLCγl by ZAP-70 triggers downstream signalling that leads to activation of the phosphatidylinositol and the Ras/mitogen-activated protein kinase (MAPK) signalling pathways. The phosphatidylinositol pathway is outlined in the following section.

Phosphatidylinositol Signalling Pathway

Activated PLCγl cleaves membrane PIP_2 into inositol 3,4,5-triphosphate (IP_3) and diacylglycerol (DAG). Inositol 3,4,5-triphosphate releases Ca^{2+} from intracellular (endoplasmic reticulum) stores activating calcium-dependent enzymes which, in turn, activate the transcription factor nuclear factor of activated T cells (NF-AT). This translocates to the nucleus and is required for the production of IL-2. Diacylglycerol, along with the increased Ca^{2+}, activates protein kinase C which activates the transcription factor NFκB. This regulates transcription of many genes, including the IL-2 gene and also genes that promote cell-survival.

Thus, coordinated signals from different signalling pathways activate transcription factors required for T cell activation. There is increased transcription of genes including the IL-2 and IL-2R genes, and also the gene for IFN-γ, leading to antigen-specific T cell proliferation and differentiation.

Cyclosporin and FK506, drugs used to prevent graft rejection, interfere in activation of the transcription factor NF-AT and hence IL-2 synthesis. This blocks T cell activation (see Chapter 17).

The activity of tyrosine kinases, such as Lck and ZAP-70, is balanced by tyrosine phosphatases which, thereby, keep the activation process under control. They have a crucial role in control of T cell activation and limiting the ongoing immune response and are referred to again in the concluding part of the chapter.

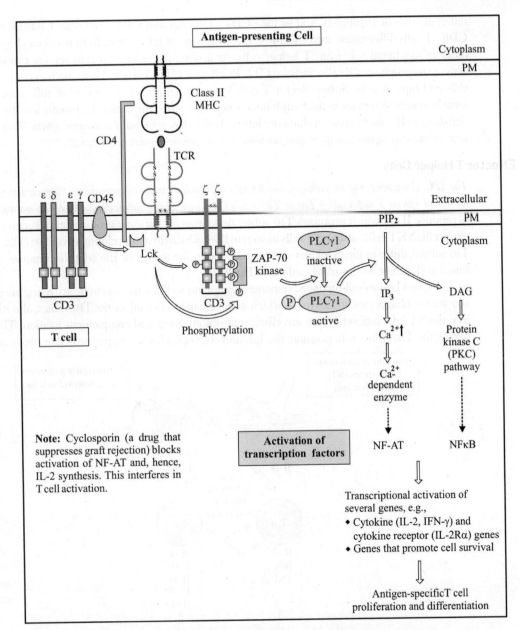

Fig. 8.11 A simplified scheme of signalling in T cells. The RAS/MAPK pathway is not shown. ZAP-70, zeta-associated protein of 70 kDa; NF-AT, nuclear factor of activated T cells; NFκB, nuclear factor kappa B; PLCγ1, phospholipase Cγ1; DAG, diacylglycerol; IP₃, inositol 3,4,5-triphosphate; PIP₂, phosphatidylinositol 4,5-bisphosphate.

T CELL DIFFERENTIATION TO EFFECTOR CELLS AND MEMORY CELLS

Within a day or two after activation, there is increase in number of antigen-specific T lymphocytes referred to as *clonal expansion*. A part of the expanded population of TH cells differentiates into effector cells, whereas some develop into long-lived memory cells. Effector TH cells are specialized to deal with different types of pathogens, and include CD4$^+$ TH1 cells and CD4$^+$ TH2 cells. Clonally expanded CD8$^+$ T cells differentiate into effector CTLs which, as we have learnt from previous chapters also, differ in functional role from T helper cells. As a reminder, while TH cells secrete cytokines that activate macrophages, B cells, and also CTL-Ps, effector CTLs kill target cells, such as virally-infected cells and tumour cells. Some effector T cells leave the lymph nodes for sites of infection, whereas some continue to remain in the lymph node where they stimulate antibody responses to microbes by signalling to B cells, or serve to eliminate infected cells. *Although signal 1 is essential, effector T cells no longer need costimulatory signals to perform their functions, such as cytokine secretion or cytotoxicity.*

Effector T Helper Cells

The APC, characteristics of the pathogen, and the nature of cytokines in the environment are the main determinants of the type of effector T helper cell—TH1 or TH2—which develops. Some intracellular bacteria stimulate DCs to produce IL-12 which promotes TH1 subset development. Parasitic protozoa and worms stimulate mast cells, NKT cells, and also T cells to secrete IL-4, which drives development of TH2 cells. TH1 and TH2 subsets differ in the cytokines they secrete and in the nature of the adaptive immune response stimulated against the invading pathogen (Fig. 8.12).

TH1 subset favours cell-mediated responses against intracellular pathogens by activating microbicidal activities of phagocytes. Interferon-γ, which is the signature cytokine of the TH1 subset, also stimulates secretion of IgG antibodies that are efficient at opsonization and complement fixation. The major role of the TH2 subset is to promote the IgE and eosinophil/mast cell response that protects against

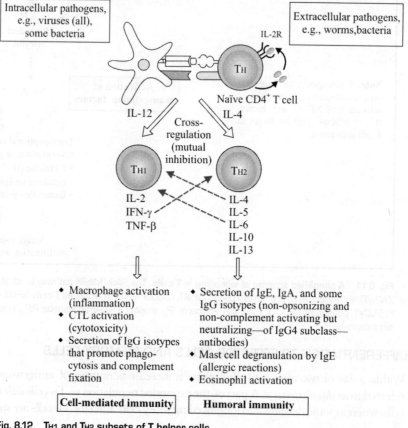

Fig. 8.12   TH1 and TH2 subsets of T helper cells.

helminths. The TH2 subset is also implicated in allergic reactions. It should be noted that the IgG antibodies produced on stimulation of B cells by TH2 cytokines do not enhance phagocytosis or activate complement. The way effector T cells function to protect the host against invading microbes is presented in Chapter 9.

TH1 and TH2 subsets are mutually inhibitory through the cytokines they secrete. Interferon-γ inhibits development of TH2 cells. Interleukin-4 and interleukin-10, produced by the TH2 subset, inhibit development of TH1 cells and, hence, macrophage activation. This is called *cross-regulation*. Cytokines secreted by the two distinct T cell subsets have a major role in isotype switching, details of which are given in Chapter 10.

Effector Cytotoxic T Lymphocytes (CTLs)

Naïve $CD8^+$ T cells entering the peripheral lymphoid organs from the thymus lack the killing machinery and function of armed effector cells. It is only later when they receive the relevant signals that they acquire these properties. Effector CTLs induce target cell killing by two mechanisms, namely, by *perforin/granzyme* and the *Fas/Fas L pathway*. This should be compared with the effector functions of TH cells which act by secreting cytokines. Another significant distinguishing feature is that $CD8^+$ T cells show tremendous ability to clonally expand as compared to $CD4^+$ T cells (see Fig. 9.7). This is not surprising and is essential, considering the large number of cells that may be infected by an invading microbe, and which need to be eliminated. The two mechanisms by which CTLs mediate killing along with effector functions of TH1 and TH2 cells are described in more detail in Chapter 9.

Generation of Memory T Lymphocytes

Some clonally expanded cells develop into long-lived memory T cells (Fig. 8.7). These respond rapidly and more intensely on second encounter with the same microbe, and produce cytokines (memory $CD4^+$ TH cells), or kill target cells (memory $CD8^+$ CTLs). The response generated is called a *secondary response*. Memory T cells, and also effector T cells, do not need costimulators for activation. They re-circulate actively, though their pattern of re-circulation is not the same as that of naïve T cells and effector cells. Other than the circulation, memory T cells are also found in lymphoid tissues and at mucosal sites.

DECLINE OF THE IMMUNE RESPONSE (HOMEOSTASIS)

After the antigen has been eliminated and cytokine levels decline (both are essential survival stimuli for T cells), the expanded pool of antigen-specific T cells decreases and the response subsides. Most of the effector cells die by apoptosis, and only memory cells and some long-lived effector cells survive. *This decrease due to apoptotic cell death is essential as without this the body would soon be filled with expanded clones of lymphocytes.*

The induction of the inhibitory receptor *cytotoxic T lymphocyte antigen-4, CTLA-4*, at the peak of T cell activation holds the activation process in check. It has an important role in termination of the immune response. CTLA-4, too, binds B7 but with higher affinity than CD28. Its cytoplasmic tail carries an *immunoreceptor tyrosine-based inhibition motif (ITIM)* that generates a negative signal in T cells leading to their death by apoptosis. Mice born with a defect in the gene for CTLA-4 suffer from excessive proliferation of lymphocytes. *Immunoreceptor tyrosine-based inhibition motifs* work by recruiting inhibitory tyrosine phosphatases. There are other inhibitory receptors with similar ITIMs such as those expressed on natural killer (NK) cells which when ligated by MHC class I molecules inhibit cytotoxicity (see Chapter 9).

Blocking costimulatory signals (through B7-CD28 and CD40-CD40 L interaction) is a strategy that has practical application. It can be used to prevent undesirable immune responses, such as allograft rejection (see Chapter 17). Various clinical trials to explore this avenue are underway. On the other hand, protective immune responses against tumours can be stimulated by enhancing expression of costimulators (see Chapter 18).

SUMMARY

- Immunity mediated by T lymphocytes (cell-mediated immunity) defends against intracellular microbes.
- There are two types of receptors for antigen on T cells. TCR2 or the $\alpha\beta$ TCR is a commonly found receptor. The second less abundant type is TCR1 or the $\gamma\delta$ TCR which appears earlier than the $\alpha\beta$ TCR during T cell ontogeny.
- The structure of $\alpha\beta$ TCR resembles the Fab fragment of an antibody molecule.
- Associated with the TCR is the CD3 complex. While the TCR functions in antigen recognition, the CD3 complex is involved in signal transduction.
- CD4 and CD8 molecules (co-receptors) are transmembrane glycoproteins that associate with the TCR, and are essential for T cell activation.
- There are two T cell subpopulations depending on whether TCR associates with CD4 or CD8: CD4$^+$ T cells and CD8$^+$ T cells.
- The germline organization of α and β TCR genes is essentially the same as the organization of genes that encode Igs. Mechanisms used to generate a T cell repertoire with diverse TCRs are similar to those that B cells use to generate B cell receptor diversity.
- T cell receptor gene rearrangements occur when progenitor cells enter the thymus from the bone marrow.
- T cell maturation in the thymus involves selection of double-positive thymocytes by two processes. Positive selection preserves thymocytes that bear receptors which can interact with self-MHC molecules (called self-MHC restriction). Negative selection weeds out thymocytes expressing high-affinity receptors that recognize self-MHC molecules bound to self-peptides, and results in self-tolerance.
- Dendritic cells are the major APCs for activating naïve T cells in the peripheral lymphoid organs.
- T cell activation involves interaction between complimentary pairs of molecules on the surface of T cells and APCs. The area of contact between T cells and APCs is the immunological synapse.

- T cells require two signals for activation. Interaction of TCR with peptide–MHC complexes on the APC surface constitutes signal 1, whereas signal 2 is the costimulatory signal provided when B7 costimulators bind to CD28 on T cells. In response to the two signals, activated CD4$^+$ T cells differentiate into effector cells that secrete cytokines which affect phagocytic cells, CD8$^+$ T cells, B cells, and other cells.
- Signal 1 alone without the costimulatory signal results in unresponsiveness (or anergy) in T cells.
- Some bacterial products called superantigens can trigger T cell (having a particular Vβ segment) activation by cross-linking the TCR to MHC class II–peptide complexes on APCs. They do not undergo antigen processing (unlike conventional antigens).
- Different signalling cascades are triggered on T cell activation by antigens. Coordinated signals from these pathways activate transcription factors—NF-AT and NFκB. Critical genes transcribed and translated are those coding for the cytokine IL-2, and the high-affinity IL-2R on the T cell. Binding of IL-2 to the IL-2R leads to antigen-specific T cell proliferation and differentiation.
- Effector T cells require only signal 1 through their TCRs for efficient activation; the costimulatory signal is not required.
- The two subsets of effector CD4$^+$ T cells include TH1 and TH2 cells. They differ in the cytokines they secrete and in function, and are mutually inhibitory.
- CD8$^+$ T cells need to be activated to produce functional CTLs which are equipped with the machinery to kill. Cytokines released by TH cells and APCs are important for their activation. Unlike T helper cells which secrete cytokines, CTLs kill their targets which are virally-infected cells and tumour cells.
- CTLA-4 is an inhibitory receptor which binds to B7 with higher affinity than CD28. It controls the T cell activation process.

REVIEW QUESTIONS

1. Indicate whether the following statements are true or false. If false, explain why.
   (a) IFN-γ suppresses development of the TH2 subset of T cells.
   (b) αβ T cells arise earlier in T cell ontogeny than γδ T cells.
   (c) CD8⁺ cytotoxic T lymphocytes are unable to kill CD4⁺ TH cells.
   (d) The long cytoplasmic domains of the T cell receptor allow interaction with intracellular signalling molecules.
   (e) CD4 binds to the peptide-binding site of class II MHC molecules.
   (f) T lymphocytes fail to proliferate in knockout mice lacking the gene for CTLA-4.

2. Self-assessment questions
   (a) An antigen has breached epithelial barriers and has entered the body. Where is the immune response initiated and how?
   (b) What are the signals required for full T cell activation? How is lymphocyte homeostasis ensured?
   (c) Both antigens and anti-CD3 antibodies stimulate T cells. Do you think there is any difference in stimulation of T cells by the two? Why is it that only antigen-specific T cells clonally expand, whereas those that do not recognize antigen fail to do so?
   (d) What effect do you think knocking out the gene for CD4 or CD8 in mice has on T cell maturation? Explain with reference to the role of CD4 and CD8 molecules in thymocyte interactions with APCs.
   (e) Name two receptor–ligand combinations that function in costimulation. Resting APCs do not express costimulatory molecules. Can you think of any advantage this confers in an individual? In what clinical conditions can costimulatory signals be manipulated for the benefit of patients?

3. For each question, choose the *best* answer.
   (a) Signal transduction in T cells is mediated by
      (i) B7
      (II) TCR
      (iii) CD3
      (iv) MHC
   (b) Presence of which of the following cytokines favours TH1 cell development:
      (i) IL-12
      (ii) IL-4
      (iii) IL-10
      (iv) IL-12 and IL-4
   (c) A T cell receiving signal 1 alone and no costimulatory signal from an APC
      (i) differentiates to a cytotoxic T cell
      (ii) is functionally inactivated
      (iii) proliferates without secreting cytokines
      (iv) differentiates to the TH2 subset
   (d) Effector T cells
      (i) do not require costimulatory signals
      (ii) do not secrete cytokines
      (iii) are not antigen-specific
      (iv) do not migrate

Effector Mechanisms of Cell-mediated Immunity

9

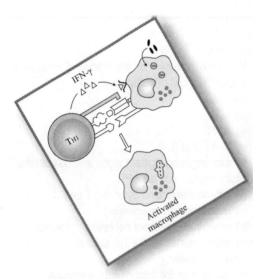

LEARNING OBJECTIVES

Having studied this chapter, you should be able to understand the following:

- The different types of cell-mediated immune responses mediated by effector TH1 cells and CTLs
- How naïve T cells home to lymph nodes and how effector T cells migrate to infected sites
- The signals TH1 cells deliver that activate macrophages to eliminate microbes
- That chronic stimulation of TH1 cells can lead to a DTH response
- Features of DTH reactions and the injury they cause to the host
- The role of TH2 cells in protective immune responses to parasite infections
- Killing mechanisms of target cells by CD8⁺ cytotoxic T cells, and the different ways by which CTLs and NK cells recognize their targets

The immune system functions to protect the body from invading pathogens. This is not an easy task as pathogens are diverse. They gain entry from various sites in the body and grow in different body compartments (Fig. 9.1). Innate defence mechanisms, such as phagocytes, play an important role in their elimination. But when innate mechanisms are unable to deal with the invader, specific adaptive immune responses need to be recruited.

The adaptive immune system employs various effector mechanisms to destroy pathogens—each suiting the type of infecting microbe and the stage of its life cycle. The life cycle of many pathogens involves both extracellular and intracellular phases of infection. Although antibodies can neutralize virus particles circulating in blood, microbes hidden inside the cell's interior are inaccessible to antibodies and also to complement proteins. T cell-mediated immune mechanisms need to be activated to deal with such pathogens efficiently. Obviously, different mechanisms will be suitable at different times.

Cell-mediated immunity (CMI) refers to immunity mediated by T lymphocytes, unlike humoral immunity which is mediated by antibodies and complement. It protects against intracellular microbes, including viruses, many bacteria, fungi, and some protozoa. CMI can be transferred from immunized

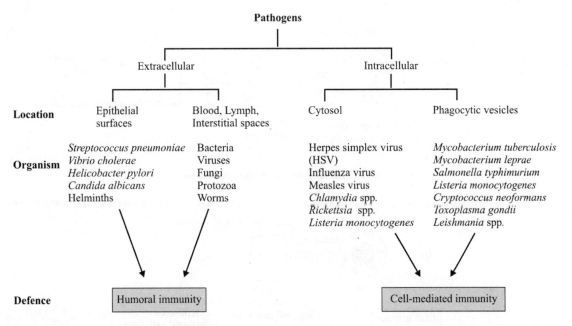

Fig. 9.1 Some infectious agents and body compartments where they grow. The location of the two broad categories of pathogens and the immune response mounted against them are shown.

to non-immunized recipients by T cells, and not by antibodies as for humoral immunity. Also, unlike antibodies, it cannot be transferred to the foetus via the placenta. That cellular immunity is important in the control of intracellular pathogens is well illustrated by the increase in *Mycobacterium tuberculosis* infections linked to the acquired immunodeficiency syndrome (AIDS) epidemic. This is not surprising as human immunodeficiency virus (HIV) infects CD4$^+$ T helper lymphocytes and brings about their depletion in various ways. These cells play a pivotal role in cell-mediated immune responses, which is the reason why HIV infection has devastating effects on the immune system. Infected individuals are prone to various infections including cancer (see Chapter 16). The protective role of CMI in cancer, and its involvement in autoimmunity and in rejection of transplants, will be discussed in subsequent chapters.

The focus of this chapter will be on how effector T lymphocytes exit the lymph nodes for infected sites and on how effector CD4$^+$ and CD8$^+$ T cells help to eradicate the infection. Phagocyte activation which is the principal function of CD4$^+$ T$_{H1}$ cells in CMI is described. Delayed-type hypersensitivity (DTH) responses which result from chronic T cell activation, and which will be revisited in Chapter 14, are discussed. T$_{H2}$ responses are also included in the chapter to bring out the different functional roles of this second subset of T helper cells in immune defence. The mechanisms of CTL-mediated killing of virally-infected cells and the distinct ways these cells and NK cells recognize their targets are emphasized. This chapter concludes with a brief description of some clever strategies microbes deploy to escape CMI and immunopathology due to CMI.

TYPES OF CELL-MEDIATED IMMUNITY

Cell-mediated immune responses dealing with different types of intracellular microbes are of two major types (Fig. 9.2).

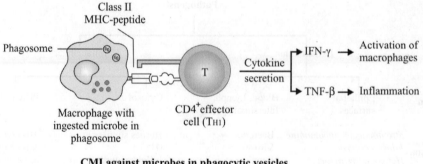

CMI against microbes in phagocytic vesicles

(a)

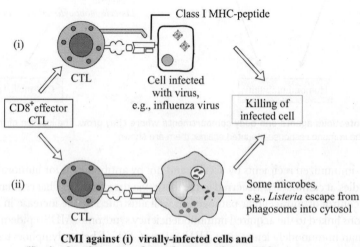

CMI against (i) virally-infected cells and (ii) microbes that escape from phagosome into cytoplasm

(b)

Fig. 9.2   Cell-mediated immunity is of two major types. (a) CMI against microbes in vesicles of phagocytes. TH1 cells activate phagocytes to kill ingested microbes and recruit inflammatory cells. For clarity only signal 1 is shown. (b) CMI against microbes in cytoplasm of infected cells. Specific CD8+ effector CTLs recognize microbial peptide–MHC class I complexes and kill target cells by inducing apoptosis.

TH1-mediated CMI/Delayed-type Hypersensitivity Response

Macrophages ingest microbes into vesicles, process microbial antigens, and display foreign peptide-class II major histocompatibility complexes (MHC) on their surface. Specific CD4+ TH1 effector cells recognize the complexes and are activated to secrete cytokines. These then stimulate the macrophage to kill the microbe and recruit inflammatory cells causing inflammation (Fig. 9.2a).

Sometimes consequences of TH1-mediated CMI can be harmful. The term *delayed-type hypersensitivity (DTH)* is used to refer to such harmful effects, some of which include graft rejection, chronic inflammation seen in tuberculosis infection, and contact dermatitis besides others.

The differentiation of CD4+ T helper lymphocytes into the two major subsets TH1 and TH2 was introduced in Chapter 8 (see Fig. 8.12). Recall that various stimuli present early during the immune response determine the pattern of differentiation. Interleukin-12 (IL-12) produced in innate immune responses to intracellular pathogens by macrophages and dendritic cells (DCs) is the major inducer of

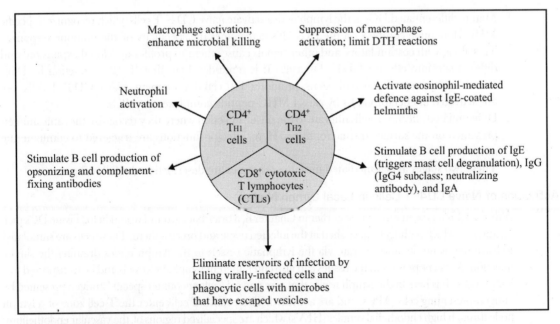

Fig. 9.3 Effector T cell types and their functions.

TH1 cells. This well illustrates the way the early innate immune response guides the development of adaptive immunity. Parasitic protozoa and worms stimulate secretion of IL-4 which is a TH2 inducer. Thus, it is the nature of the pathogen that influences differentiation of naïve T cells into the TH1 or TH2 subset. Importantly, the two subsets differ in functional roles (Fig. 9.3).

Cytotoxic T Lymphocyte Responses

CTLs directly kill infected cells containing microbes/microbial proteins in their cytoplasm, thereby eliminating reservoirs of infection. Viral peptide–class I MHC complexes are displayed on the surface of the infected cell which are recognized by specific effector CTLs. Cytotoxic T lymphocytes then kill their targets by inducing apoptosis. Some ingested microbes escape into the cytoplasm from the phagosome where they are protected from microbicidal activities of phagocytes. The antigenic peptides of these microbes complexed to MHC class I molecules are expressed on the macrophage surface and are recognized by specific CTLs which kill the target cell (Fig. 9.2b).

Involvement of CTLs in anti-tumour immunity is significant. This has motivated development of *adoptive cellular immunotherapy* in which CTLs obtained from a cancer patient are expanded in vitro with IL-2 and then re-infused into the patient. This form of therapy which is aimed at boosting cell-mediated immune responses against the tumour has shown encouraging results (see Chapter 18).

The distinct TH2-mediated response against helminthic parasites needs to be highlighted here. This involves stimulation of immunoglobulin E (IgE) production and eosinophil activation by TH2 cells which together function to eliminate helminthic infections (by extracellular killing).

SEQUENCE OF EVENTS IN CMI/DTH

Broadly speaking, there are two stages in cell-mediated immune responses to protein antigens derived from infecting pathogens:

1. Mature differentiated DCs in the lymph nodes activate naïve CD4$^+$ T cells which recognize a specific MHC II–peptide complex on the DCs (this determines the specificity of the immune response). This along with costimulatory and other signals causes them to proliferate (clonal expansion) and differentiate into effector CD4$^+$ TH1 cells. It is reminded here that IL-12 production by DCs, stimulated by intracellular pathogens, promotes TH1 cell development. Naïve CD8$^+$ T cells too, are activated to effector CTLs by class I MHC-peptide complexes on APCs.

2. Differentiated effector T cells migrate to the site of infection where they recognize the same antigen presented on the surface of macrophages. Here, effector functions are triggered to eliminate the microbe.

These two stages in cell-mediated immune responses are described in the following text.

Activation of Naïve CD4$^+$ T Cells in Local Lymph Nodes

Although this has been introduced earlier in Chapter 8, a brief background would help. Tissue DCs pick up antigens which pathogens have shed in the infected tissue and process them. These cells are stimulated to leave the tissue site and migrate via the lymphatic vessels to the lymph nodes draining the site of infection. Antigens present in the tissues can also enter afferent lymphatic vessels and be transported to a lymph node. It is here in the lymph nodes that rare naïve T cells encounter specific antigen presented by antigen-presenting cells (APCs) and are activated. These naïve T cells enter the T cell zone of a lymph node through high endothelial venules (HEVs) which are specialized regions of the vascular endothelium. L-selectin ligand which is expressed only on HEVs in the lymph nodes directs migration of naïve T cells (which express L-selectin) to these sites from the blood. The mechanism by which selective cell adhesion molecules facilitate the homing/migration process is depicted in Fig. 9.4.

Migration of Effector T Lymphocytes from Lymphoid Organs to Infected Sites

After activation effector T lymphocytes are able to migrate out of the lymph nodes via efferent lymphatic vessels eventually entering the bloodstream through the major lymphatic duct. These cells exit the blood vessels at infected sites where they carry out their effector functions. Differentiation to effector T cells is associated with expression of new adhesion molecules which enable effector cells to migrate to sites of infection. The change in the expression of adhesion molecules expressed on lymphocytes during differentiation from naïve T cells to effector cells is shown in Table 9.1.

The loss of L-selectin which prevents re-entry of effector T cells to the lymph nodes is noteworthy. Tumour necrosis factor-α (TNF-α) and IL-1 (produced by macrophages during innate immune responses to microbes) activate endothelial cells of venules near the infected site to produce selectins, ligands (ICAM-1 and VCAM-1) for integrins, and also IL-8, a chemokine (chemoattractant cytokine) which promotes the migration of lymphocytes to the infected site. When effector TH1 cells recognize the same antigen at infected sites that was presented by DCs in lymph nodes, they secrete cytokines

Table 9.1 Receptor-ligand interactions in T lymphocyte migration.

T cell type	T cell homing receptor	Ligand on endothelial cells	Site of migration
Naïve T cells	L-selectin	L-selectin ligand	To lymph nodes
Activated T cells (T effector cells and memory cells)	E-and P-selectin ligand LFA-1 or VLA-4 (both integrins)	E-or P-selectin (weak adhesion) ICAM-1 or VCAM-1 (stable adhesion)	To peripheral sites of infection

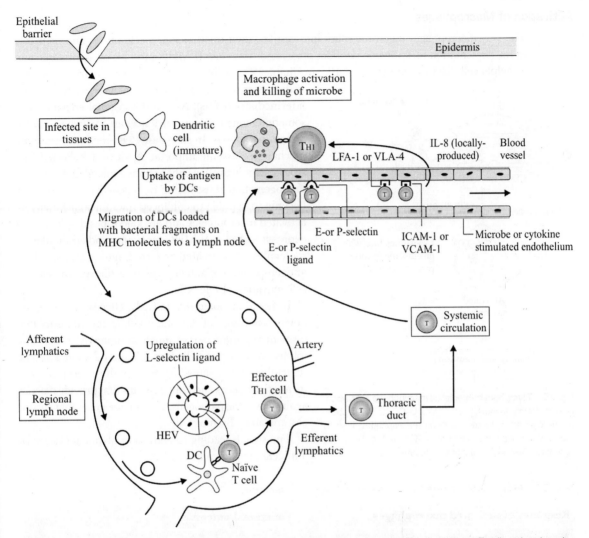

Fig. 9.4 Selective adhesion molecules facilitate homing/migration of lymphocytes. Homing of naïve T cells to lymph nodes where they are activated to effector cells and migration of effector cells from lymph nodes to infected sites in tissues is dependent on presence of selective adhesion molecules.

Note: For convenience and simplicity, molecules involved in cellular interactions have been omitted. Migration of effector CTLs follows a similar pattern.

which activate macrophages to kill ingested microbes. The pattern of migration of effector T cells out of blood vessels is similar to that described earlier for neutrophils (see Fig. 2.14), and monocytes.

EFFECTOR FUNCTIONS OF CD4⁺ Tн1 LYMPHOCYTES

The role of effector Tн1 lymphocytes in enhancing the microbicidal mechanisms of macrophages at infected sites and the way these cells and macrophages are able to stimulate each other to increase the effectiveness of the cell-mediated immune response is elaborated in the following text.

Activation of Macrophages

The way macrophages ingest microbes into vesicles, their microbicidal mechanisms, and their role in the presentation of antigenic peptides associated with class II MHC proteins on their surface to T helper cells have been discussed earlier in Chapter 2. The major microbicidal substances produced in the innate response to microbes include reactive oxygen intermediates (ROIs), NO, and lysosomal enzymes. But sometimes innate immune defences are ineffective against certain pathogens. In such cases, cell-mediated immune mechanisms assume importance, since T cell-mediated macrophage activation enhances their microbicidal activity. Pathogens that resist killing by less active macrophages become susceptible to enhanced microbicidal activity of activated macrophages and are killed. Besides, increased expression of class II MHC molecules and costimulatory molecules on activated macrophages increases their antigen-presenting activity which further promotes TH1 cell activation (Table 9.2).

It should be noted that in CMI, effector TH1 cells are potent activators of the same killing mechanisms that form an important part of innate immune responses. The toll-like receptors (TLRs) from Chapter 2 should also be remembered. It is signalling through these receptors that turns on the genes encoding proteins that provide defence against invading pathogens, and also the genes that encode costimulatory B7 molecules.

The signals leading to activation of macrophages by TH1 cells are shown in Fig. 9.5.

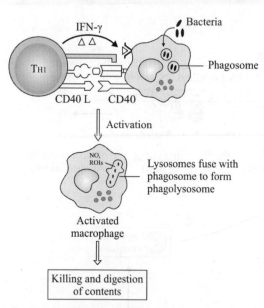

Fig. 9.5   T lymphocyte-mediated macrophage activation. Costimulatory signals from CD40 L–CD40 interaction, and IFN-γ binding to receptors on macrophages, lead to macrophage activation. Effector CTLs, unlike TH1 cells, recognize class I MHC-peptide complexes.

Table 9.2   Response of activated macrophages and functional outcome.

Response of activated macrophages	Functional outcome
Activated macrophages show increased	
◆ fusion of lysosomes with phagosomes	Enhances microbial killing
◆ production of reactive oxygen intermediates (ROIs), NO, and lysosomal enzymes	
◆ secretion of cytokines:	
TNF-α	Increases expression of adhesion molecules on vascular endothelium; recruit inflammatory (neutrophils and monocytes), and effector T cells to the infected site; inflammation
IL-1	
Chemokines (IL-8)	
IL-12	Stimulates differentiation of naïve CD4$^+$ T cells to TH1 subset and IFN-γ production
Platelet-derived growth factor (PDGF)	Aids in tissue repair after infection
◆ expression of MHC and costimulatory (B7) molecules	Enhances T cell responses

Effector T$_{H1}$ cells recognize specific peptide–MHC class II complexes on the macrophage surface and in response express CD40 L that engages CD40 on the macrophages. Besides, T$_{H1}$ cells secrete interferon (IFN)-γ, the defining cytokine of this subset, which binds to receptors on macrophages. The combined signals trigger biochemical signalling pathways which enhance microbicidal functions of macrophages. The costimulatory CD40–CD40 L interaction is important in macrophage activation, which is evident in individuals with an inherited mutation in CD40 L. This is the cause of the immunodeficiency disorder—*X-linked hyper IgM syndrome* (*XHIGM*). Cell-mediated immuntiy to intracellular pathogens is defective in such individuals.

Effector CTLs are also activated on recognition of a specific microbial peptide–MHC class I complex on macrophages. The peptides are derived from microbes in the cytoplasm or from microbes or their proteins that pass through the membrane of the vesicles into the cytoplasm. Effector CTLs directly induce death in target cells, unlike T$_{H1}$ cells which secrete cytokines, thereby eliminating reservoirs of infection.

In summary, macrophages and effector T$_{H1}$ cells that are recruited to peripheral infected sites are able to stimulate each other, increasing the magnitude and effectiveness of the cell-mediated immune response. Cytokines secreted by effector T$_{H1}$ lymphocytes at the site recruit still more monocytes from blood vessels into tissues where they differentiate into macrophages. This amplifies activation of T$_{H1}$ cells. Retention of macrophages at sites of infection is aided by the cytokine *macrophage migration inhibition factor* (*MIF*) secreted by effector cells.

Once the infection has been cleared, the response gradually declines. Macrophages produce other cytokines, for example, platelet-derived growth factor (PDGF), which stimulates the activation of fibroblasts and endothelial cells necessary for repair of tissues.

Tissue Injury due to Chronic T$_{H1}$ Cell-dependent Macrophage Activation—DTH Response

Sometimes tissue injury may accompany normal T$_{H1}$ cell responses to microbes. For instance, in *M. tuberculosis* infection the T cell-mediated immune response becomes chronic as, due to escape mechanisms of the pathogen, the infection is difficult to eradicate (see Chapter 12). Activated T$_{H1}$ cells recruit a large number of macrophages to the site and inflammatory responses are continually activated due to persistence of the pathogen or its products. The resultant inflammation causes injury to normal tissues. Such a response is referred to as a *delayed-type hypersensitivity* (*DTH*) *response* or *type IV hypersensitivity* (see Chapter 14). Infection by *Mycobacteria* is a well-studied example of this type of hypersensitivity. A ball-like mass called a *granuloma* is formed around the persisting microbe (Fig. 9.6).

Granulomas are a hallmark of infection with some intracellular pathogens. Besides macrophages and lymphocytes, multinucleated giant cells (fused macrophages with ingested microbes) and epithelioid cells are also found within a granuloma. There is a central caseous (cheesy) necrosis due to lytic enzymes and ROIs released by activated macrophages. Fibroblasts proliferate under the influence of cytokines secreted by macrophages and synthesize collagen which forms the thick outer layer of the granuloma. Granuloma formation is also seen to occur in tuberculoid leprosy and around schistosome eggs which become trapped in the liver in schistosomiasis.

The tissue injury in DTH reactions caused by overactivity of the immune response frequently accompanies protective cell-mediated immunity. The disease manifestations are due, in large part, to the host's attempt to isolate and restrict the spread of the pathogen.

Skin contact with many small molecules, such as chemicals (nickel in buckle of a watch strap) or plant molecules (uroshiol from poison ivy) can also result in DTH reactions. Interleukin-10, a cytokine of the T$_{H2}$ subset, is a direct inhibitor of macrophages and exerts control over DTH reactions.

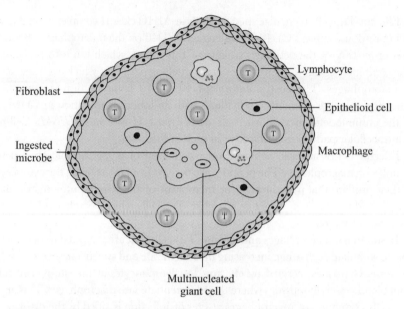

Fig. 9.6   A granuloma. Chronic stimulation of CD4+ TH1 cells by persisting microbes, e.g., mycobacteria, and antigens that are not easily degraded, leads to granuloma formation. Cytokines secreted by various cells contribute to its development.

Apoptosis of T lymphocytes is an important mechanism of immune control and helps to maintain homeostasis in the immune system. *Activation-induced cell death (AICD)* is one way by which T lymphocytes die when they are repeatedly stimulated by antigens (see Fig. 15.3). This helps to control damaging hypersensitivity reactions which occur in response to persisting antigen, allergens, and autoantigens.

TH1 AND TH2 BALANCE IN CMI

To produce an effective and right type of response to a pathogen, it is critical that a CD4+ T cell differentiates into a TH1 or TH2 effector cell. Most pathogens, however, are likely to stimulate both TH1 and TH2 responses; though in many cases one particular type of response predominates. This is exemplified by *Mycobacterium leprae*, a pathogen which survives and replicates in the phagosome of macrophages and causes leprosy (Hansen's disease). Disease progression and clinical outcome vary among individuals as they differ in the pattern of MHC alleles expressed. Such differences may modulate the pattern of immune response to the pathogen.

There are two clinical forms of the disease (Table 9.3). Some infected individuals mount a TH1 response which promotes cellular immunity keeping the number of pathogens low. This form is *tuberculoid leprosy* in which granulomas are formed around nerves. Disease progression is slow as most mycobacteria are killed, and only few survive in tissues.

In contrast, individuals exhibiting defects in TH1 cell activation mount predominantly TH2 responses characterized by high levels of pathogen-specific antibodies. This form is *lepromatous leprosy* in which bacteria multiply unchecked in the macrophages. Due to feeble cell-mediated immune responses, the disease progresses at a fast rate with destructive lesions of nerves, skin, and underlying tissues. *Thus, an immune response can sometimes become so polarized as in M. leprae infection, that the pathogen cannot be eliminated.*

Table 9.3 **T cells and cytokines determine outcome of infection by *M.leprae*.** There are two clinical forms of the disease. Tuberculoid leprosy results when Th1 cells predominate, whereas polarization to Th2 subset leads to lepromatous leprosy. Some patients show a form with intermediate features.

Dominant response mounted by patients	Th1	Th2
Cytokine profile	IL-2, IFN-γ TNF-β	IL-4, IL-5, IL-6 IL-10
Outcome	Tuberculoid leprosy	Lepromatous leprosy
Clinical features	◆ Granuloma formation ◆ Local inflammation ◆ Peripheral sensory nerve defects ◆ Bacterial count low or undetectable ◆ Serum immunoglobulin levels normal	◆ Connective tissue (bone, cartilage) and nerve damage ◆ Uncontrolled growth of bacteria in macrophages ◆ Serum immunoglobulin levels high

ROLE OF Th2 SUBSET IN IMMUNE DEFENCE

Th2 cells represent a second subset of T helper cells. They are the major cells that stimulate B cells to produce certain classes of antibodies, though Th1 cells also contribute to antibody production. Helminthic parasites cannot be easily phagocytosed due to their large size. The Th2 subset mediates protective adaptive immune responses to helminths by stimulating the production of IgE antibodies, and by stimulating eosinophils. Besides, this subset has another important function to perform. It exerts a control over macrophage activation through IL-10, which is important for limiting the DTH response and the injury that it can cause.

Th2 cells on recognition of specific antigen release various cytokines, such as IL-4, IL-5, IL-6, IL-10, and IL-13. Interleukin-4 and interleukin-13 act on B cells to induce class-switching to IgE antibodies specific for helminthic antigens. These bind to high-affinity FcεRs on tissue mast cells and blood basophils. Cross-linking of receptors by parasite antigens causes mast cells to release inflammatory mediators from granules by exocytosis. Interleukin-5 activates eosinophils which on binding to IgE - coated helminths mediate antibody-dependent cell-mediated cytotoxicity (ADCC, see Fig. 11.7). The granule proteins of eosinophils are toxic to the parasite and can destroy even the tough covering of helminths (see Chapter 12). *Worm infections are therefore, characteristically associated with increase in eosinophils (eosinophilia) and serum IgE levels mediated by cytokine secretion by the Th2 subset.* Although IgE has a beneficial role to play in parasite infections, it is also the isotype that is implicated in allergic reactions to environmental antigens (allergens) which are type I/immediate hypersensitivity reactions (see Chapter 14).

The Th2 subset also stimulates production of IgG-neutralizing antibodies of the IgG4 subclass which, unlike other subclasses, do not promote phagocytosis or activate complement efficiently.

EFFECTOR FUNCTIONS OF CD8$^+$ CYTOTOXIC T LYMPHOCYTES

Cytotoxic T lymphocytes are effector cells of CMI which target

◆ cells infected by virus/bacteria,
◆ cancer cells displaying tumour antigens, and
◆ allogeneic grafts.

They function by killing target cells that express specific peptide bound to MHC class I molecules. Since these are expressed by nearly all nucleated cells, these cells when infected can present antigen-derived peptides to effector CTLs and can be killed (Fig. 9.2b).

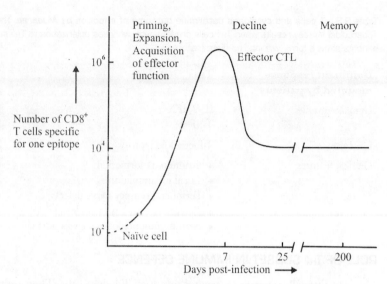

Fig. 9.7 Clonal expansion of CD8+ CTL-Ps on infection of mouse cells with *Listeria*. CTL-Ps which are rare prior to infection, undergo tremendous expansion after infection to generate effector CTLs and long-lived memory cells. After clearance of infection, 90–95% of effector cells die by apoptosis while memory cells are maintained.
Source: Williams, M.A. and M.J. Bevan (2007), 'Effector and memory CTL differentiation', *Annual Review of Immunology,* 25, pp. 171–192.

Naïve CD8+ T cells (CTL-P) cannot kill target cells. In order to do so, they must first undergo activation and clonal proliferation. The massive expansion that CTLs undergo subsequent to infection shown in Fig. 9.7 is amazing. This is followed by differentiation to effector cells in lymphoid organs (see Chapter 8). It is during this process that CTLs acquire the machinery to induce target cell death. Cytotoxic granules are synthesized de novo when the cell receives signals to activate and proliferate, and several proteins including *perforins*, *granzymes*, and *granulysin* are stored in them. Besides acquiring granules, there is expression of *Fas ligand* (*Fas L*), and also cytokines including IFN-γ and TNF-β through which CTLs regulate immune responses.

Steps Involved in Target Cell Killing by CTLs

The initial event in CTL-mediated killing of target cells involves binding to the target cell. The sequence of events that follow leading to apoptotic target cell death is outlined in the text that follows.

- Recognition of specific peptide–MHC class I complex on the surface of infected cells and other target cells
- Conjugate formation due to tight binding of adhesion molecules on CTL surface to ligands on target cell (an initial transient interaction becomes stable)
- Clustering of antigen receptors (TCRs) and co-receptors (CD8) on CTL at the contact site
- Polarization of granules to contact site
- Granule exocytosis triggered by signals from TCR
- Delivery of the lethal hit
- Detachment of CTL after target cell killing
- Killing of other target cells

Two distinct pathways, both triggered in response to signals from the TCR, are involved in death of infected cells by effector CTLs (Fig. 9.8). Natural killer cells have granules similar to those in CTLs. The pathways they use to induce apoptosis in their target cells are similar too.

Granule Exocytosis Pathway

This is dependent on perforin which, in the presence of Ca^{2+}, polymerizes to form a transmembrane channel in the plasma membrane of the target cell. This is similar to the pore-forming membrane

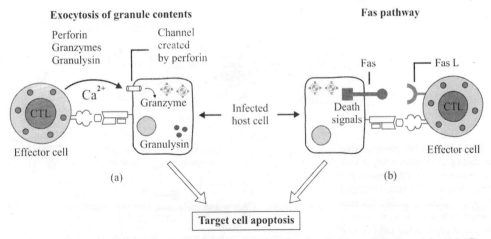

Fig. 9.8 CTL induction of cell death in virally-infected cells. The granule exocytosis pathway (a) and the Fas pathway (b), both of which induce apoptosis in a target cell, are shown. Pathways used by NK cells are similar.

attack complex (MAC) whose formation is initiated on complement activation by microbes or antibodies bound to their target (see Chapter 11). Granzymes are a collection of serine proteases which pass into the target cell through transmembrane channels created by perforin. Once inside the target cell, they cleave and activate enzymes called caspases. Caspases cleave proteins at aspartic acid residues and function in induction of apoptosis (see Chapter 15). Granulysin, an antimicrobial peptide, results in pathogen killing. The granule exocytosis pathway described in the preceding text is in sharp contrast to phagocytosis where killing mechanisms are restricted to phagosomes and phagolysosomes.

A CTL detaches after killing its target and goes on to kill another target cell. Since contents of the granules are re-synthesized, a single CTL can sequentially kill many target cells. The close intercellular contact between the CTL and the target cell minimizes risk of damage to normal host cells. Cytotoxic T lymphocytes do not destroy themselves when they kill their target, as there are mechanisms which contribute to resistance of CTLs to the perforin released.

Fas Pathway

Interaction of Fas L expressed on the surface of mature activated $CD8^+$ T cells with Fas (CD95) on target cells results in aggregation of Fas. Fas, expressed on many cell types and a member of the TNF receptor family, is a death-inducing receptor having a death domain in its cytoplasmic tail. Fas–Fas L interactions trigger intracellular signalling events that lead to Ca^{2+}-dependent target cell apoptosis. This pathway, also, involves activation of caspases but does not trigger granule exocytosis.

Apoptotic cells are rapidly cleared by phagocytosis (see Box 2.1).

CTLs and NK Cells Recognize Their Targets in Different Ways

Natural killer cells have a major role to play in innate responses. Like CTLs, they too target virally-infected cells, tumour cells, and allogeneic grafts. Although killing mechanisms of NK cells are similar to those used by CTLs, the two cell types use different mechanisms to recognize their targets (Fig. 9.9). Recall the 'missing-self' hypothesis described in Chapter 2 (see Fig. 2.7).

In brief, NK cells recognize target cells that fail to express class I MHC molecules on their surface. Some viruses, such as herpes virus, downregulate MHC class I molecule expression on the surface of host cells. Although the cell is no longer a target for CTLs, it is now a target for NK cell killing. Natural killer cells have inhibitory receptors which on recognition of class I MHC molecules

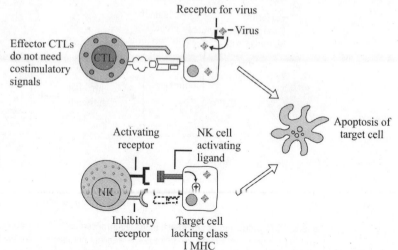

Fig. 9.9 CTL and NK cell-mediated cytotoxicity. CTLs with the help of their TCRs recognize class I MHC-associated peptide complexes presented on target cells and mediate apoptosis. NK cells kill target cells, such as some tumour cells and virally-infected cells lacking class I MHC molecules as these fail to deliver the inhibitory signal.

expressed on all nucleated cells deliver signals that inhibit cytotoxicity. This explains why healthy host cells are not killed by NK cells. Being relevant to the context, it needs mentioning here that NK cell inhibitory receptors carry the same inhibitory *immunoreceptor tyrosine-based inhibition motifs* (*ITIMs*) in their cytoplasmic tails which are also present in the inhibitory receptor CTLA-4 (cytotoxic T lymphocyte antigen-4) on activated T cells (see Chapter 8) and in the inhibitory FcγRIIB (CD32) present in the B cell membrane (see Chapter 10). These inhibitory receptors have an important role to play in the contraction phase of an immune response. On the other hand, NK cell activating receptors carry activating motifs called *immunoreceptor tyrosine-based activation motifs* (*ITAMs*) which are also present in signalling molecules of T and B lymphocyte receptors.

Interestingly, both perforin and MAC, which is formed from terminal complement components, act similarly to produce pores in the target cell membrane. However, the killing mechanisms induced by perforin and MAC differ markedly. Cytotoxic T lymphocytes and also NK cells activate apoptosis in which the target cell is induced to self-destruct or to commit suicide. A calcium-dependent nuclease is activated which leads to fragmentation of DNA. Although MAC produces nuclear changes following pore formation other changes that are the hallmark of apoptosis (see Box 3.1) are not seen.

EVASION OF CMI BY MICROBES AND IMMUNOPATHOLOGY

Microbes have evolved various ways to evade host cell-mediated immune defences and survive. A balance between the efficacy of host defences mounted, and resistance offered by pathogens to host defence is important in determining the outcome of the infection. Some ways by which pathogens evade CMI and cause immunopathology are briefly outlined here. Both aspects are described more fully in Chapter 12.

Listeria monocytogenes secretes a protein called *listeriolysin* which creates pores in the phagosome membrane through which it can escape into the cytoplasm. Here, it is protected from microbicidal mechanisms of phagocytes. *M. tuberculosis* inhibits fusion of lysosomes with the phagosome, and is thus able to survive and replicate in phagocytes. Viruses, also, have evolved an amazing variety of clever strategies to escape immune defences (see Figure 12.6). Since the surface expression of class I MHC molecules is very essential in antiviral defence, many viruses, to their favour, downregulate

MHC class I molecule expression on the surface of host cells they infect. For instance, HIV proteins prevent cell surface expression of class I MHC molecules. Herpes simplex virus (HSV) expresses a protein that interacts with transporter associated with antigen processing (TAP, see Chapter 5) and blocks transport of antigenic peptides from cytosol to the endoplasmic reticulum (ER). When not loaded with peptides, class I MHC molecules are unstable and not expressed on the cell surface. Such cells are not recognized by $CD8^+$ T lymphocytes as they are class I MHC restricted. There are other ways too by which viruses evade the immune system.

Activated macrophages release many toxic substances during cell-mediated immune responses which cause some injury to normal tissues at the site of infection or antigen persistence. Although this normally resolves once the microbe is eliminated, microbial infections persist sometimes or antigens cannot be degraded. In such cases, as discussed in the preceding text, chronic stimulation of T cells and macrophages leads to DTH reactions in which there is continual production of cytokines and other factors. The resultant granulomatous inflammation is associated with necrosis and fibrosis. Replacement of normal tissue by connective tissue leads to functional impairment of the tissue/organ at the affected site. Some examples of damage due to DTH reactions are cited here:

♦ Granuloma formation around eggs of *Schistosoma mansoni* which deposit in the liver results in fibrosis. Due to obstruction to venous blood flow and cirrhosis, liver functioning is impaired.

♦ Much of the breathing difficulty seen in patients suffering from *M.tuberculosis* infection is due to the fibrosis that occurs in the lung.

♦ Some autoimmune disorders show DTH responses similar to those seen in persistent infections. Destruction of pancreatic β islet cells seen in IDDM (type I diabetes) is mediated by cytokines released during the DTH response. T_{H1} cells are implicated in chronic inflammation of the joints seen in rheumatoid arthritis (see Chapter 15).

In the examples cited above, an overactive immune response against the antigen/pathogen causes damage and functional impairment of the affected site. Hence, the term *hypersensitivity* is used for such reactions.

SUMMARY

♦ Cell-mediated immunity (CMI) is the branch of adaptive immunity that functions to defend against microbes that survive in phagocytes or infect non-phagocytic cells.

♦ Cell-mediated immunity is due to the action of T cells. Two distinct effector T cell subpopulations implicated include $CD4^+$ T helper cells (T_{H1}) and $CD8^+$ CTLs. CMI can be transferred to other animals of the same inbred strain by T cells, unlike humoral immunity that is transferred by antibodies.

♦ There are two main types of $CD4^+$ effector T_H cells which are defined by the cytokines they produce. These include the T_{H1} and the T_{H2} subsets. The nature of the pathogen determines into which subset the $CD4^+$ T cell differentiates into. The two subsets have different functional roles to perform.

♦ $CD4^+$ T_{H1} cells mediate activation of macrophages

that have phagocytosed microbes and enhance their killing ability. T_{H2}-mediated responses target helminthic parasites. $CD8^+$ CTLs kill infected cells directly, thereby eliminating reservoirs of infection. To carry out their function, T cells need to interact directly with cells they are going to help/kill. Specific recognition molecules are involved.

♦ Naïve T lymphocytes are activated in peripheral lymphoid organs by DCs which are the principal APCs involved in activation of naïve T cells.

♦ Effector T cells that are generated migrate to sites of infection, where, on recognition of a specific antigen, they are activated to release cytokines. Adhesion molecules have an important role to play in homing and migration of lymphocytes.

♦ At infected sites, effector T_{H1} cells are stimulated to express CD40 L and produce high levels of

IFN-γ which together are involved in activation of macrophages.

♦ Activated macrophages show enhanced production of ROIs, NO, and lysosomal enzymes that kill the ingested microbe. They upregulate surface molecules that enhance T cell responses. The cytokines they release induce inflammation and also fibrosis and tissue repair.

♦ Effector TH1 cells promote generation of CTLs and certain classes of antibodies.

♦ The TH1/TH2 balance is important in determining the outcome of an infection.

♦ TH2 effector cells are mainly involved in protection against helminthic parasites by stimulating IgE production and eosinophil activation. Besides, they

stimulate production of some antibody classes and inhibit activation of macrophages.

♦ The two pathways involved in killing of target cells by CTLs include the granule exocytosis pathway and the Fas pathway. Both these pathways induce target cell apoptosis.

♦ Cytotoxic T lymphocytes and NK cells recognize their targets in different ways, though their killing mechanisms are similar.

♦ Many pathogenic microbes resist cell-mediated immunity.

♦ DTH reactions occur due to persistent microbes/ antigens which cause chronic activation of T cells. Such reactions can lead to immunopathology.

REVIEW QUESTIONS

1. Indicate whether the following statements are true or false. If false, explain why.
   (a) TH2 subset limits activation of macrophages.
   (b) CTLs participate in ADCC.
   (c) IL-4 inhibits development of the TH2 response.
   (d) CD40 L is expressed on activated macrophages.
   (e) Unlike CTLs, NK cell activity does not require priming.
   (f) ADCC is an important mechanism for killing intracellular microbes.

2. Self-assessment questions
   (a) How is it that naïve T cells home to lymph nodes, whereas effector T cells migrate preferentially to infected sites in tissues? Can you explain the significance of homing/migration in the life of a T cell?
   (b) What is a delayed-type hypersensitivity response and what are its consequences? Which principal cell types participate in such reactions?
   (c) Do you think that development of the TH2 subset would have a favourable effect on cell-mediated immunity? Why or why not? Explain how clinical outcome varies in individuals infected with Mycobacterium leprae.
   (d) What are the two pathways used by cytotoxic T cells to kill their targets? Are the same pathways used by NK cells to kill target cells?

   (e) What are the signals needed for activation of macrophages in CMI? Illustrate with an example of an inherited mutation how defective signalling can lead to deficiency in killing intracellular pathogens.

3. For each question, choose the best answer.
   (a) CD8+ cytotoxic T lymphocytes
      (i) recognize antigens associated with class II MHC molecules
      (ii) can phagocytose virus
      (iii) recognize and kill virus-infected cells
      (iv) do not produce IFN-γ
   (b) Cell-mediated immune responses are
      (i) activated by histamine
      (ii) normal in a DiGeorge patient
      (iii) not dependent on macrophages
      (iv) activated by T cells
   (c) What is not true about NK cells?
      (i) Release perforin on target cells.
      (ii) Express TCR as do T cells.
      (iii) Lyse tumour cells and virally-infected cells.
      (iv) Bear Fc receptors.
   (d) A defining cytokine of TH2 cells is
      (i) IFN-γ
      (ii) IL-4
      (iii) IL-12
      (iv) IL-2

Activation of B Lymphocytes

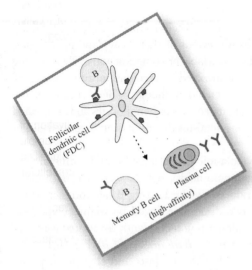

LEARNING OBJECTIVES

Having studied this chapter, you should be able to understand the following:

♦ The structural and functional features of the B cell receptor and associated proteins

♦ That antigens to which B cells respond are of different types depending on whether T cell help is needed or not

♦ Salient features of signalling in B cells and how complement enhances B cell responses

♦ How antigen stimulation of B lymphocytes leads to their differentiation to antibody-secreting plasma cells

♦ Role of T helper cells and cytokines in humoral immune responses to protein antigens

♦ The late events in germinal centres that increase antibody affinity and generate memory cells

♦ The factors that enable B cells to switch the class of antibody they make and how the B cell response is terminated

On activation by antigens, B lymphocytes produce antibodies which represent a major defence mechanism against extracellular microbes and their toxins. Immunity mediated by antibodies, and also complement proteins, is referred to as humoral immunity. This is in contrast to cell-mediated immunity which involves T cell-mediated immune responses. Membrane-bound immunoglobulin (Ig), the antigen receptor on B lymphocytes, recognizes intact unprocessed antigens, such as proteins, carbohydrates, lipids, other non-protein antigens, and also small chemicals. T cells, on the other hand, generally recognize and respond only to protein antigens, and so are ineffective in providing protection against many microbes with polysaccharide-rich capsules.

B cell developmental processes in the bone marrow leading to their maturation have been outlined earlier in Chapter 6. Mature naïve B cells (IgM$^+$ IgD$^+$) exit the bone marrow and circulate in blood and lymph from where they are carried to peripheral lymphoid organs, such as lymph nodes and spleen. Their activation, proliferation, and differentiation to plasma/memory cells in peripheral lymphoid organs are dependent on the presence of antigens. B cells have a short life-span, and in absence of antigen-induced activation, they die by apoptosis.

The chapter commences with a description of the structural features of the B lymphocyte receptor and the different types of antigens to which B cells respond. The role of antigens in initiation of humoral responses, activation of signalling pathways leading to expression of specific genes, and how complement enhances B cell activation are discussed. The humoral response to protein antigens, T helper cell interactions with B cells in lymphoid tissues, and late events in germinal centres which enhance the protective functions of antibodies are explained. The chapter concludes with the concept behind the mechanism of antibody feedback.

The diverse effector functions of antibodies produced during humoral immune responses and the way they afford protection against microbes and their products are the purview of Chapter 11.

B CELL ANTIGEN RECEPTOR–CO-RECEPTOR COMPLEX

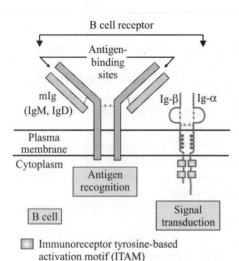

▢ Immunoreceptor tyrosine-based activation motif (ITAM)

Fig. 10.1 The B cell receptor (BCR). The BCR comprises membrane-bound Ig (IgM/IgD) associated with a disulphide-linked Ig-α and Ig-β heterodimer. While mIg recognizes antigen, phosphorylation of tyrosine residues in ITAMs in cytoplasmic tails of Ig-α and Ig-β initiates signal transduction.

Antigen receptors of naïve B cells include membrane IgM and IgD. The variable (V) regions of their heavy and light chains, particularly the hypervariable or complimentarity determining regions (CDRs), are involved in recognition and binding of antigens, just as for secreted antibodies. The V regions of the receptor differ in different clones of lymphocytes and are created by unique genetic mechanisms that have been described earlier in Chapter 6.

As the intracytoplasmic tails of membrane Ig (mIg) are too short (have three amino acids), signals generated on antigen binding are transduced by the Ig-α/Ig-β heterodimer which is comprised of two disulphide-linked invariant polypeptide chains. The heterodimer is non-covalently associated with mIg and together they form the *B cell receptor (BCR)* (Fig. 10.1).

The cytoplasmic domains of Ig-α and Ig-β polypeptides contain *immunoreceptor tyrosine-based activation motifs (ITAMs)* which are also found in CD3 proteins of the T cell receptor (TCR) complex. Cross-linking of mIg brings several ITAMs close together, triggering signalling events that lead to activation of transcription factors and expression of various genes. The function of Ig-α/Ig-β polypeptide chains in B cells is comparable to that of CD3 proteins in T lymphocytes.

The BCR is associated with at least three cell membrane molecules which include

- CR2 (complement receptor type 2; CD21)—a receptor for C3d, a degradation product of complement component C3b, which coats pathogens;
- CD19; and
- TAPA-1 (target of antiproliferative antibody; CD81).

Together, these three proteins comprise the *BCR co-receptor complex* (Fig. 10.2). It provides costimulation for efficient B cell activation in which CD19 plays a predominant role.

On BCR stimulation, the kinases that are associated with the BCR phosphorylate tyrosine residues in ITAM motifs present in the cytoplasmic tail of CD19. This creates docking sites for several proteins. How activating signals are transduced is described in a later section of this chapter. As signalling cascades are triggered by both the BCR and the co-receptor complex, B cell immune responses are

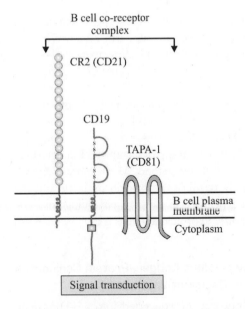

B cell co-receptor complex

CR2 (CD21)

CD19

TAPA-1 (CD81)

B cell plasma membrane

Cytoplasm

Signal transduction

Fig. 10.2   B cell co-receptor complex. The co-receptor complex serves to enhance signals from the BCR.

greatly enhanced. It should be recalled that co-receptors for TCR include CD4 and CD8 molecules (see Chapter 8).

The B cell antigen receptor performs an additional role besides its role in initiating the process of B cell activation. Antigen binding to mIg leads to internalization of the complex into an endosome. Processing/presentation pathways lead to display of peptides bound to class II MHC molecules on the B cell surface for recognition by TH cells. The specialized role of B cells as APCs was introduced earlier in Chapter 3 (see Fig. 3.16).

B CELL RESPONSE TO THYMUS-DEPENDENT (TD) AND THYMUS-INDEPENDENT (TI) ANTIGENS

As protein antigens (or protein conjugates) stimulate weak B cell responses by themselves, B cells require help from T cells for maximal antibody production. These antigens are referred to as *thymus-dependent (TD)* antigens. It should be remembered that MHC molecules can only bind peptides derived from protein antigens, and generally, it is only these peptide–MHC complexes that are recognized by T cells. This is unlike *thymus-independent (TI) antigens* which generally, on their own, provide a strong activating stimulus to B cells without requiring help from T cells. Thymus-independent antigens which include *TI type 1 (TI-1)* and *TI type 2 (TI-2)* antigens are briefly described in the following text.

Thymus-independent type 1 antigens include mostly bacterial cell wall components, such as lipopolysaccharide (LPS). They deliver mitogenic signals at high concentrations which activates many B cells in a non-specific manner (polyclonal activation), producing antibodies of many different specificities (Fig. 10.3).

Thymus-independent type 2 antigens include molecules containing multiple identical epitopes, such as pneumococcal polysaccharide and polymeric protein antigens, such as bacterial flagellin (Fig. 10.4). Thymus-independent type 2 antigens cause clustering and cross-linking of several mIg receptors on specific B1-B cells. This delivers a strong activating stimulus to the B cell. These atypical cells, which represent a minority of the B cell population, respond well to carbohydrate antigens and poorly to protein antigens (see Chapter 6).

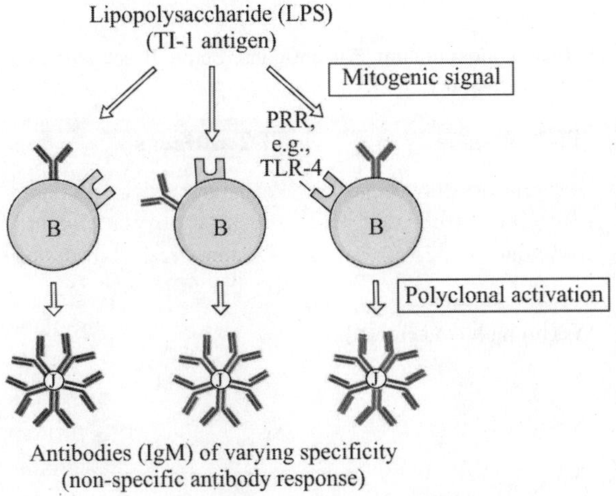

The B cell response to TI antigens described in the preceding text does not require T cell help though the response to TI-2 antigens may be partly dependent on TH cell cytokines. The TI response, thus, differs markedly from the response to TD antigens which is depicted in Fig. 10.9.

Both types of TI antigens generate mostly low-affinity IgM antibodies. This is because germinal centre events, which are T cell-dependent, do

Lipopolysaccharide (LPS) (TI-1 antigen)

Mitogenic signal

PRR, e.g., TLR-4

B   B   B

Polyclonal activation

Antibodies (IgM) of varying specificity (non-specific antibody response)

Fig. 10.3   Thymus-independent type 1 (TI-1) antigens.

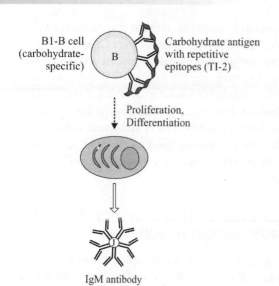

B1-B cell
(carbohydrate-
specific)

B

Carbohydrate antigen
with repetitive
epitopes (TI-2)

Proliferation,
Differentiation

IgM antibody
(e.g., anti-blood group A and
anti-blood group B antibodies)

Fig. 10.4   Thymus-independent type 2 (TI-2) antigens.
Note: Exposure to bacterial carbohydrates triggers formation of antibodies. Some cross-react with blood group A and B antigens (cross-reactivity).

not occur. There is little, if any, isotype switching, with no (or poor) generation of long-term memory B cells. The secondary response to TI antigens resembles the primary response. For TD antigens, on the other hand, the secondary response is more intense with IgG antibodies predominating. These important facts should not be forgotten at any stage. Table 10.1 summarizes some key features of TD and TI antigens.

The way antibody responses against TI antigens are induced is not well understood. Much more is known about antibody responses to protein antigens and the key role that T helper cells play in their stimulation. The immune response to protein antigens is discussed later in this chapter.

Thymus-independent Antigen–Protein Conjugates are Useful in Design of Vaccines

A carbohydrate can be converted into a TD antigen by covalently linking it to a protein. The complex is internalized by a B cell specific for the carbohydrate, and peptides derived from the protein are presented to T helper cells. These, in turn, provide signals to the B cell to secrete antibodies specific for the carbohydrate (see Fig. 13.4). This has important implications in the design of vaccines. A polysaccharide vaccine against *Streptococcus pneumoniae* elicits a poor response in children below 2 years of age. The problem has been overcome by linking it to a protein carrier (conjugate vaccines). Another example is the Hib vaccine which is linked to tetanus toxoid and is used to prevent meningitis in children (see Chapter 13).

T cell–B cell collaboration also explains the ability of protein carriers to help in antibody responses to haptens (see Fig. 4.1). While B cells recognize the hapten, T cells recognize the carrier.

The following section describes how antigen recognition and receptor-induced signalling initiates activation of naïve B lymphocytes.

Table 10.1   Major features of thymus-dependent (TD) and thymus-independent (TI) antigens. Some TI antigens (e.g., polysaccharides) on second exposure may stimulate a response typical of memory.

Feature	TD antigens	TI-1 antigens	TI-2 antigens
Chemical nature	Proteins, e.g., tetanus and diphtheria toxin, haemagglutinin (influenza virus)	Bacterial lipopolysaccharide (LPS) and other cell wall components	Polymeric antigens, e.g., capsular polysaccharide (*Pneumococci*), bacterial flagellin (*Salmonella*)
Polyclonal activation	No	Yes (in high concentration)	No
Isotype switching	Yes	No	No or limited
Affinity maturation	Yes	No	No
Memory generation	Yes	No	No or poor

INITIATION OF B CELL RESPONSE BY ANTIGENS AND B CELL SIGNALLING PATHWAYS

Microbial or other antigens from tissues or circulation are transported to B cell-rich follicles (primary follicles) in peripheral lymphoid organs. Recognition and binding of native antigen by specific Ig receptors induces cross-linking of two or more B cell receptors. Thymus-independent antigens which contain many identical epitopes cross-link several mIg receptors on a B cell, and generally provide a strong activating stimulus (signal 1; described in the following text). Soluble protein antigens, however, are unable to cross-link adjacent membrane receptors as they lack repetitive epitopes. As they stimulate feeble responses on their own, humoral responses to such antigens, as has been mentioned earlier, are T cell dependent (Fig. 10.9).

Although recognition of antigens by B and T cells differs significantly, intracellular signalling in the two cell types bears similarity. As membrane receptors of naïve B cells have cytoplasmic tails that are too short, signals are transduced by the Ig-α/Ig-β heterodimer (Fig. 10.1). Their cytoplasmic domains contain ITAM motifs which are crucial for signal transduction. Figure 10.5 depicts a very simplified scheme of intracellular signalling triggered in B cells.

The salient features of the way receptor-induced signalling in B cells leads to their activation are outlined in the following text.

1. Cross-linking of surface Ig by antigen activates protein tyrosine kinases (PTKs) of the *Src family* which are *Blk*, *Fyn*, and *Lyn* in B cells.
2. Activated kinases phosphorylate tyrosine residues in ITAM domains of the B cell receptor creating docking sites for the downstream adaptor protein *Syk* that has an affinity for phosphorylated proteins. Phosphorylation of protein tyrosine residues is an important feature in both B and T cell activation.
3. Syk, a cytoplasmic tyrosine kinase which is analogous to ZAP-70 in T cells (see Fig. 8.11), binds to phosphorylated ITAMs, and is itself phosphorylated and activated by Src kinases.
4. Activated Syk, as was seen for ZAP-70 in T cells, stimulates *PLCγ2* activity.

    This acts on membrane *phosphatidylinositol 4,5-bisphosphate (PIP₂)* to generate *inositol 3,4,5-triphosphate (IP₃)* which increases intracellular Ca^{2+}, and also *diacylglycerol (DAG)*. As a consequence, Ca^{2+}-dependent enzymes and *protein kinase C (PKC)*, respectively, are activated.
5. Another pathway that is activated is the Ras/MAPK pathway.

In summary, antigen-induced B cell signalling leads to activation of transcription factors—*NFκB*, *NF-AT*, and *AP-1*. These promote expression of specific genes whose protein products lead to B cell division and differentiation (described in the following text).

Serious consequences can arise if signal transduction is defective in B cells. For instance, there is a block in B cell activation due to a mutation in *B cell-specific tyrosine kinase (Btk)*, which also is activated by Syk and has a crucial role in the B cell signalling network. In pre-B cells, Btk is associated with the pre-BCR. When Btk is mutated, pre-B cells fail to mature leading to the immunodeficiency disorder *X-linked agammaglobulinemia (X-LA)*. Mature B cells are lacking or reduced in patients, and antibodies of most isotypes are absent (see Chapter 16).

Role of B Cell Co-receptor Complex and Complement in B Cell Activation

The B cell co-receptor, which as seen earlier is comprised of at least three proteins, provides costimulation that leads to efficient B cell activation (Fig. 10.6).

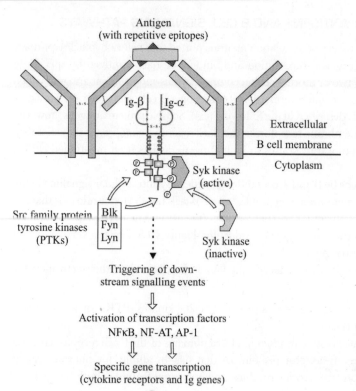

Fig. 10.5 B cell activation. The scheme is an oversimplification. Activation of Syk kinase triggers diverse signalling pathways in B cells, the net result of which is the transcription of genes, such as those for Igs and cytokine receptors.
Note: Only one Ig-α/Ig-β heterodimer is shown here.

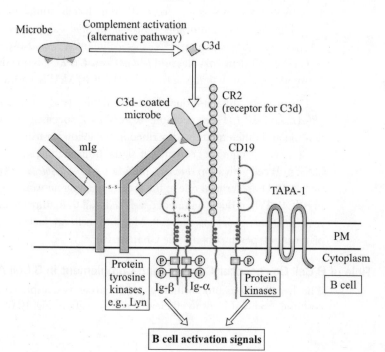

Fig. 10.6 Role of B cell co-receptor complex and complement in enhancing B cell activation. Simultaneous binding of C3d to CR2 and of the antigen to mIg on the same B cell delivers activation signals which enhance B cell activation.

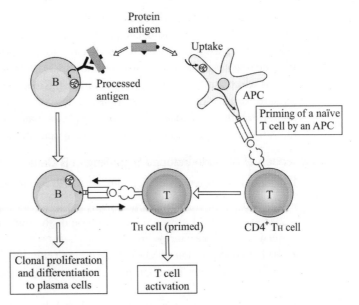

Fig. 10.7 B cell response to a protein antigen depends on a primed TH cell. Only the MHC–peptide–TCR interaction has been shown in the figure. There are other interactions also which, for B cells and TH cells, are depicted in Fig. 10.9. *Note:* B and T cells recognize different epitopes on the same antigen making the response antigen-specific.

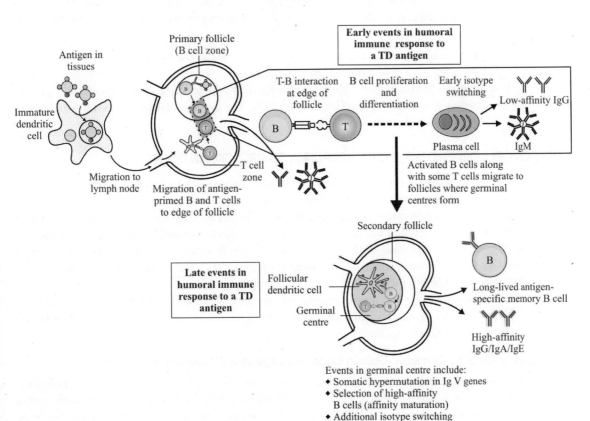

Fig. 10.8 T helper cell-dependent antibody response to a thymus-dependent (TD) antigen. Interaction of antigen-primed B cells and T cells at the edge of the follicle and the early and late cellular events to a protein antigen are shown here.

Simultaneous binding of C3d (a complement split product which deposits on the pathogen surface) to CD21 (CR2), and of antigenic determinants on the pathogen surface to mIg on the same B cell, brings kinases associated with the BCR close to the co-receptor. This leads to phosphorylation of tyrosine residues in the long cytoplasmic tail of CD19. Docking sites are thus created for several protein kinases which are activated on antigen binding. Kinases on association with the co-receptor complex serve to enhance signals from the BCR, underscoring the importance of the complement system in humoral immunity. Antigen–Antibody complexes coated with C3d, generated via the classical pathway of complement activation, can deliver similar activation signals.

Consequences of Antigen-induced Signalling in B Cells

Functional consequences of signalling in B cells include the following.

- Entry into cell cycle and clonal expansion
- Secretion of IgM during the early phase of the humoral immune response (this response is best seen with polysaccharide antigens)
- Increased expression of class II MHC molecules, B7 (B7-1 and B7-2) costimulatory molecules, and receptors for T cell-derived cytokines (this is unlike T cells in which cytokine genes are expressed)
- Change in expression of receptors on B cells for chemokines produced in lymphoid follicles (this facilitates migration of B cells to edges of lymphoid follicles to T cell-enriched sites where B cell–T cell interaction occurs)

Induction of costimulatory B7 molecules enables the B cell to function as an antigen-presenting cell and interact with an appropriate T helper cell if the antigen is a protein (TD) antigen.

With the preceding background, the chapter proceeds to a discussion of the B cell response to protein antigens and the crucial role played by T helper cells. The key interactions between B lymphocytes and T helper cells are described.

T HELPER CELL-DEPENDENT B CELL RESPONSE TO PROTEIN ANTIGENS

The B cell response to a protein antigen is a two-way process in which B and T cells interact with each other and are mutually activated. For antigen-specific B cells to differentiate into plasma cells, they must be helped by primed CD4$^+$ TH cells. As has been explained earlier in Chapter 3, a primed CD4$^+$ TH cell is a cell that has seen the same antigen, also recognized by the B cell, presented on an APC surface as a peptide–MHC complex. B cells present antigens to primed T cells, which then signal to B cells to clonally expand and differentiate (Fig. 10.7). Referring to Figs 3.11 and 3.16 at this stage would be helpful.

Before proceeding to the signals required for complete B cell activation, priming of TH cells by dendritic cells (DCs), and their subsequent migration to sites of interaction with B cells is briefly outlined in the following section.

Priming of TH Cells by Dendritic Cells in Lymphoid Organs and Migration

Although TH cell priming by DCs has been focused on earlier in Chapter 8, some salient points are reiterated here. It is lymphocyte re-circulation that allows T cells and B cells to migrate into the lymph nodes to which antigen-loaded DCs/antigens also migrate. Stimulation of a humoral response by a protein antigen requires initial activation of naïve T cells in T cell zones by DCs. These antigen-primed T cells migrate to the edges of the lymphoid follicles to which B lymphocytes which have been activated by the same antigen (in the lymphoid follicles) also migrate (Fig. 10.8).

This migration is facilitated by a change in expression of certain chemokine receptors on activated lymphocytes, and production of chemokines in follicles and T cell areas of the lymph node. This ensures that naïve B and T cells, which initially are segregated in lymphoid organs, come close together only when required, that is, after activation. Antigen-primed B and T cells interact at the interface of the primary follicle and the T cell-rich zone, where B cells present processed antigens to T helper cells that have already recognized the same antigen/pathogen and are, in turn, activated by them. It is important to remember that B cells and T helper cells that cooperate must be specific for the same protein antigen, though generally the two cell types respond to different epitopes on that antigen. Interaction with TH cells leads to B cell proliferation and differentiation up to plasma cells which secrete predominantly IgM, though some early isotype switching to IgG (low-affinity) antibodies also occurs (early events). Activated B cells along with some T cells also migrate into follicles where they rapidly proliferate. Subsequent events (late events) occur in the *germinal centres* (GCs). These are regions formed within lymphoid follicles during T cell-dependent B cell responses to protein antigens. They are the sites of affinity maturation, an event described in a later section of this chapter.

B Cell–TH Cell Interactions

B cell activation involves two stages which are described in the following text (Fig. 10.9).

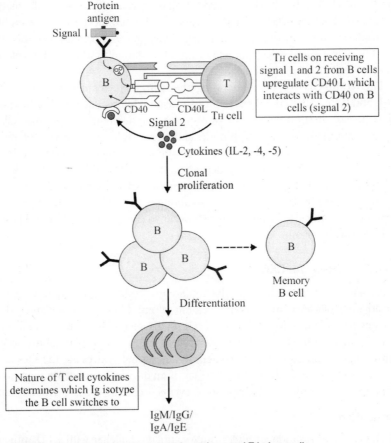

Fig. 10.9   B cell activation by a protein antigen and T helper cells.
Note: The above TD response should be compared to a TI response in which there is no memory generation, and no (or limited) class-switching from IgM isotype.

B Cells as Antigen-presenting Cells in T Helper Cell Activation

As has been described in Chapter 8, TH cells need two signals for activation:

Signal 1 A protein antigen bound to mIg on B cells is endocytosed and then processed via the endocytic pathway into peptide fragments. These associate with class II MHC molecules for presentation to *primed* CD4$^+$ TH cells (this makes the response antigen specific). Recognition of the peptide–MHC complex by the T cell receptor provides *signal 1* to the TH cell.

Signal 2 This is delivered when *B cell costimulatory molecules (B7-1* and *B7-2)* interact with *CD28* on the TH cell.

T Helper Cell Activation of B Lymphocytes

Just as for T cells, two signals are required for complete B cell activation:

Signal 1 This is delivered when antigen in its native form interacts with Ig receptors on B cells. It should be kept in mind that as protein antigens deliver a weak stimulus, an additional costimulatory stimulus is needed.

Signal 2 This is the costimulatory signal from a TH cell. These cells on receiving signal 1 and 2 from B cells transiently express *CD40 L*. This interacts with B cell *CD40* molecule and delivers signal 2 to the B cell. If a B cell receives signal 1 alone, it is usually functionally inactivated (anergized) or eliminated. T helper cell-mediated activation of B lymphocytes bears resemblance to activation of macrophages in cell-mediated immunity (see Chapter 9). It should be remembered from Chapter 8 that TH2 cells favour the development of humoral immunity, whereas TH1 cells favour predominantly cell-mediated immune responses.

The CD40–CD40 L interaction, together with the cytokines secreted by TH cells (mainly IL-2, IL-4, and IL-5), signals the B cell to proliferate and differentiate into antibody-secreting effector cells (plasma cells). In a primary immune response, the differentiated plasma cells move to the *medulla*, the innermost layer of the lymph node, and secrete IgM. Some early isotype switching to IgG also occurs. Specific antibodies enter the circulation and mucosal secretions, but plasma cells do not circulate actively. Most of them undergo apoptotic cell death within 2 weeks and do not contribute to long-term antibody production. Cells from the expanded B cell clone, besides differentiating into IgM-secreting plasma cells, may undergo additional events which characterize the humoral immune response to a protein antigen and which occur in the germinal centres. These events are described in the following section.

EVENTS IN THE GERMINAL CENTRE

To provide long-term antibody production, some members of the expanded B cell population migrate into adjacent follicles in the lymph nodes (or in spleen). These follicles enlarge to form secondary follicles with germinal centres. Many germinal centres are seen to form after initial contact of B cells with a protein antigen. TH cells which activated B cells migrate along with them and surround the germinal centres. Besides intensive B cell proliferation, germinal centres are the sites of various events which are significant as they increase the efficiency of an ongoing immune response to protein antigens. The chapter now proceeds to a description of events occurring in the germinal centres.

Affinity Maturation

The IgG antibodies produced after primary antigen challenge with a TD antigen are generally of low average affinity. However, during the course of a humoral response, the affinity of antibodies increases (*affinity maturation*). This process, shown in Fig. 10.10, is described in the following text.

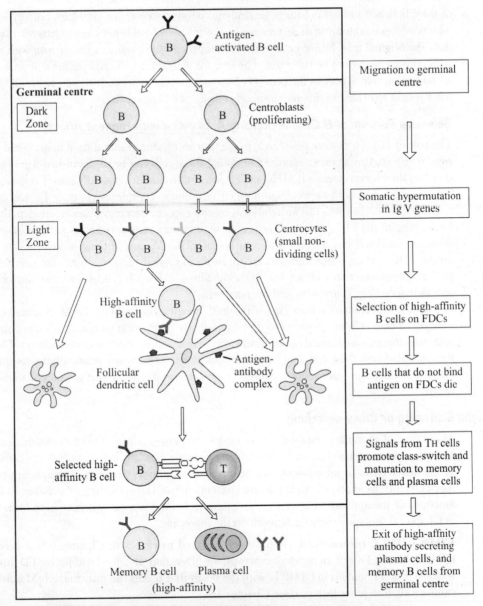

Fig. 10.10 Events in the germinal centre. Germinal centre events involve interaction between B cells, FDCs, and TH cells. B cells with very high-affinity mIg receptors are selected by FDCs presenting antigens on their surface. These cells are rescued from undergoing apoptosis by interacting with TH cells. High-affinity activated B cells undergo isotype switching and mature into plasma cells/memory B cells which exit the GC.
Note: Affinity maturation occurs in response to T helper cell-induced B cell activation and is seen only with TD antigens.

Somatic Hypermutation in Ig Heavy and Light Chain Variable Genes

Activated B cells (*centroblasts*) entering the germinal centres proliferate rapidly. Germinal centres include a *dark zone*, where centroblasts undergo rapid cell division, and an adjacent *light zone* which is rich in follicular dendritic cells (FDCs). During proliferation of activated B cells in the dark zone, the V regions of their Ig heavy and light chain genes undergo point mutation at a very high rate (hypermutation). This produces mutated mIg molecules, some of which may be able to bind antigens with higher affinity than the original mIg. However, adverse consequences due to generation of mIg with reactivity to self-components cannot be ruled out. The enzyme activation-induced cytidine deaminase (AID) has an important role to play in the process of somatic hypermutation. It should be recalled that it also has a role in switching to different antibody classes (see Chapter 6).

Selective Survival of B Cells Producing Antibodies with Highest Affinity

The role of *follicular dendritic cells* (*FDCs*) in the process of affinity maturation in germinal centre light zone is crucial. It is again emphasized here that these cells can be distinguished from other DCs in that they do not express class II MHC molecules, and so cannot act as APCs for T cells (see Fig. 3.15). They capture and hold unprocessed antigen in immune complexes via their Fc and complement receptors. As B cells (*centrocytes*) with different receptor specificities encounter an antigen, they compete for binding to the FDC surface. B cells with high-affinity receptors for an antigen have a selective advantage and will stay longer on the surface of FDCs. As just binding of centrocytes to antigens on the FDC surface is not sufficient for survival, additional survival stimuli are needed which are provided by interaction with a CD4$^+$ TH cell. These selected B cells differentiate into high-affinity antibody-secreting plasma cells and memory cells.

Somatic hypermutation leaves many B cells that express low-affinity receptors and so cannot bind antigens. These cells are destined to die. As antibody production increases in an ongoing immune response, antigens are cleared rapidly and are available only in very low concentration. This accounts for survival of only those cells that bear high-affinity receptors, whereas low-affinity receptor-bearing cells die by apoptosis (survival of the fittest). Germinal centres, therefore, are sites of tremendous cell death.

Isotype Switching or Class-switching

Maturation of a primary response to a secondary response is closely linked to switching of antibody isotypes, a phenomenon known as *class-switching* or *isotype switching*. In this process, the constant region of the heavy chain of an antibody can be changed without a change in its unique antigen-binding specificity (i.e., its idiotype). An important consequence of class-switching is a change in the effector functions of the antibody. The genetic mechanisms behind isotype switching have been focused on in Chapter 6. Isotype switching depends on the following:

CD40–CD40 L interaction It has been referred to earlier in Chapter 9 that a mutation in CD40 L blocks TH cell–dependent macrophage activation. B cell activation by TD antigens, too, is blocked by a mutation in CD40 L, with the result that B cells can only make IgM antibodies and cannot switch to other isotypes (see Chapter 16).

Cytokines secreted by TH cells Cytokines, too, have a key role to play in isotype switching (Fig. 10.11).

TH2 cells secrete IL-4 and IL-13 which induce isotype switching to IgE, the antibody class that plays a key role in defence against helminths. This function of IgE is mediated by eosinophils which are activated by IL-5, another key cytokine of the TH2 subset. Increase in eosinophils is a characteristic of parasitic diseases. In addition, eosinophils mediate allergic reactions (immediate hypersensitivity). The site of the immune response also determines the antibody class produced. In mucosal tissues, B cells switch to IgA which is very efficiently transported through epithelia into mucosal secretions. This class-switch to IgA is stimulated by IL-5, and transforming growth factor-beta (TGF-β) produced by many cell types in mucosal and other tissues.

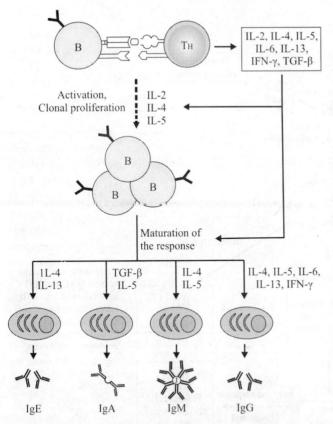

Fig. 10.11   Role of T$_H$ cell cytokines in class-switching. Class-switching to isotypes other than IgM occurs during the humoral response to a TD antigen. T cell-derived cytokines play an important role. The CD40–CD40 L interaction is also crucial for class-switching in response to TD antigens.

The major role of T$_{H1}$ cells in promoting cellular immunity has been described in earlier chapters. Although these cells do not initiate antibody formation, they can induce class-switching to certain isotypes. For instance, many bacteria and viruses stimulate the T$_{H1}$ subset to release interferon-gamma (IFN-γ) which stimulates production of opsonizing and complement-fixing IgG (IgG1, IgG2, and IgG3) antibodies.

Overall, T$_H$ cells secrete different cytokines in response to various types of microbes. The cytokines released stimulate production of antibodies of different classes/subclasses capable of performing distinct effector functions. Isotype switching enables the host to mount antibody responses that are best at fighting the microbe.

Differentiation of Germinal Centre B Cells into Plasma Cells and Memory Cells

B cells that survive selection in the germinal centres and receive survival signals from T$_H$ cells differentiate into plasma cells and long-lived memory cells.

Plasma Cells

These are end-stage B cells that do not express mIg and do not respond to antigens or divide. They exit germinal centres and migrate to the extrafollicular regions of peripheral lymphoid organs (such as to medulla in lymph nodes), and the bone marrow, and do not circulate actively. Bone marrow plasma cells continue to produce high levels of antibodies for months or years (after antigen elimination) providing quick protection against re-infection. Only secreted antibodies enter the circulation.

Memory Cells

Some progeny of germinal centre B cells become memory cells which differentiate rapidly into high-affinity antibody secretors on second contact with antigens (secondary response). Memory cells localize mainly in germinal centres in secondary lymphoid organs. Others, after exiting the germinal centres, reside in mucosal tissues and re-circulate in blood. They often express membrane IgG, IgA, or IgE in contrast to naïve mature B cells which express IgM and IgD. Also, they express higher levels of adhesion molecules compared to naïve cells. This promotes migration of memory cells to sites of infection anywhere in the body.

The germinal centre events discussed in the preceding text are highly significant as they enhance the protective functions of antibodies. An overview of the sequential steps from recognition of a protein antigen by mIg on specific B cells to generation of plasma cells and memory cells, and activation of memory B cells in a secondary immune response, is depicted in Fig. 10.12.

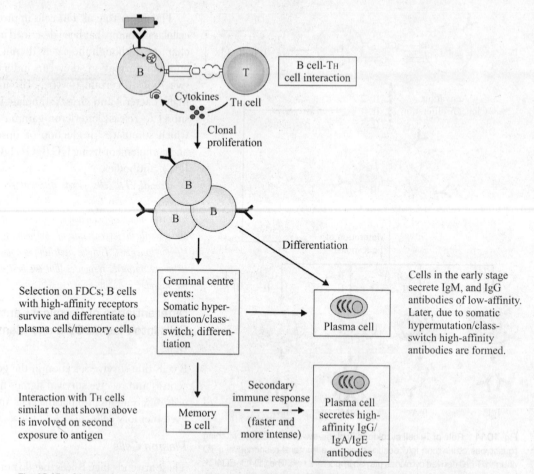

Fig. 10.12 An overview of the humoral immune response to a protein antigen. The figure depicts B cell activation, proliferation, and differentiation triggered on recognition of a protein antigen by mIg (see main text for details). For simplicity, some interactions between B cells and Tн cells have been omitted. Figure 10.9 should be referred where additional interactions between the two cell types are shown.

Formation of memory cells is important and has been exploited in vaccine development. An effective vaccine is one that can induce a good memory response to the antigen(s) in the vaccine. On subsequent re-exposure to the original antigen/pathogen, a faster and more intense immune response is mounted (secondary response) which helps to eliminate the pathogen. Interactions with Tн cells, similar to those in a primary response, are involved in secondary immune responses.

REGULATION OF THE B CELL RESPONSE

Humoral immune responses are downregulated when enough antibodies have been produced and antigen–antibody complexes are present. For instance, an antigen coated with an antibody can bind simultaneously to mIg and to the FcγR (Fc receptor for IgG; FcγRIIB or CD32) inducing clustering of the two. As seen in Fig. 10.13, an inhibitory signalling cascade is activated through the cytoplasmic tail of the Fc receptor terminating B cell activation (antibody feedback). Another B cell surface molecule, CD22, also negatively regulates B cell signalling. Both CD32 and CD22 are inhibitory receptors

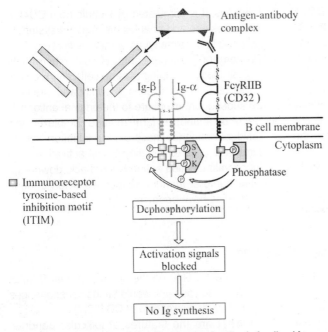

Ig-β Ig-α FcγRIIB (CD32)

B cell membrane

Cytoplasm

☐ Immunoreceptor tyrosine-based inhibition motif (ITIM)

Antigen-antibody complex

Phosphatase

| Dephosphorylation |
| ⇩ |
| Activation signals blocked |
| ⇩ |
| No Ig synthesis |

Fig. 10.13   Termination of B cell activation (antibody feedback).

which carry *immunoreceptor tyrosine-based inhibition motifs* (*ITIMs*) in their cytoplasmic tails. Immunoglobulin-G binding to CD32 leads to tyrosine phosphorylation in the ITIM motif. An inhibitory phosphatase is recruited to the phosphorylated ITIM motif in the intracellular region of CD32 bringing the two in close association with each other. The phosphatase by dephosphorylating phosphotyrosine residues in kinases, such as Syk, and in cytoplasmic domains of Ig-α/Ig-β polypeptides (signalling molecules) delivers a switch-off signal to B cells. B cell-activation signals are thereby blocked. Thus, both phosphorylation and dephosphorylation events play an important role in B cell (and also T cell) signalling.

Another mechanism for control of B cell responses proposed by Neils Jerne and described as the *network hypothesis* is briefly explained. Its central principle is that B lymphocytes, besides recognizing foreign antigens, also recognize the binding regions of antibodies evoked by that antigen. In other words, the antibodies induced in an individual by an antigen entering the body are immunogenic in the same individual and will, in turn, evoke an immune response (anti-idiotypic response) forming a network. The immune response triggered against the idiotype would block B cells producing the antibody with that idiotype resulting in decline of the immune response to the antigen. The concept is bewildering, yet interesting. Reciprocal idiotypic–anti-idiotypic interactions may in part be responsible for maintaining homeostasis by anergizing lymphocytes to self-antigens. However, actual involvement of such interactions in regulation of physiological immune responses is as yet unclear.

SUMMARY

- On activation by antigens in peripheral lymphoid organs, B lymphocytes secrete antibodies which provide defence against extracellular microbes and their toxins.
- B cells recognize antigens through membrane Ig (IgM/IgD) which along with Ig-α/Ig-β heterodimer constitutes the B cell receptor (BCR).
- B cell co-receptor complex, which consists of at least three proteins including CD19, CD21, and CD81, enhances signals from the BCR.
- Antigens to which B cells respond are of two types: thymus-independent (TI) and thymus-dependent (TD). Thymus-independent antigens activate B cells without requiring help from T cells and are of two types—type 1(TI-1) and type 2 (TI-2).
- TI antigens, on their own generally, provide strong

activating signals to B cells. Thymus-dependent antigens require help from CD4+ TH cells to activate B cells to produce antibodies.
- B cell responses to protein antigens require initial activation of naïve T cells by DCs in the T cell zones of lymphoid organs. T cells then receive activating signals from B cells at the edges of the follicles.
- Protein antigens bind to specific mIg receptors and are taken up inside the B cell. They are processed and presented on the surface complexed to class II MHC molecules to specific TH cells. This constitutes signal 1, whereas costimulatory B7-1/B7-2 molecules provide the second signal. TH cells on activation by signal 1 and 2 express CD40 L and secrete cytokines.
- While antigen binding to mIg constitutes signal 1

for the B cell, the costimulatory CD40–CD40 L interaction constitutes signal 2. It parallels the B7 costimulatory signal required for T cell activation.

♦ Cytokines from CD4⁺ TH cells are important for B cell proliferation and differentiation.

♦ Germinal centres are sites where late events in T cell-dependent antibody responses, such as affinity maturation, isotype switching, and memory B cell formation occur. Affinity maturation increases the affinity of antibodies for protein antigens. It is due to mutation in Ig genes followed by selection of high-affinity clones.

♦ Isotype switching in B cells leads to production of various Ig classes which mediate diverse effector functions. It is stimulated by signals from CD40 L and cytokines and enables the immune system to respond to different types of microbes.

♦ Progeny of germinal centre B cells differentiate into antibody-secreting plasma cells and memory cells. Memory cells respond swiftly and intensely on subsequent exposure to the original antigen.

♦ Secreted antibodies form immune complexes with residual antigens. These bind to inhibitory receptors on B cells terminating B cell activation. This mechanism, called antibody feedback, downregulates humoral immune responses when enough antibodies have been secreted.

REVIEW QUESTIONS

1. Indicate whether the following statements are true or false. If false, explain why.
   (a) Centrocytes are rapidly dividing B cells which are found primarily in the light zone of germinal centres.
   (b) Immune response to a hapten in a hapten–protein carrier conjugate involves recognition of the hapten by a specific T cell.
   (c) The cytoplasmic region of membrane-bound IgM consists of only three amino acid residues.
   (d) The progeny after a class-switch has specificity identical to the parent B cell.
   (e) IL-5 in combination with TGF-β stimulates IgA production.
   (f) Plasma cells express surface immunoglobulin having specificity identical to that of the B cell receptor.

2. Self-assessment questions
   (a) Mice depleted of C3 (the major complement protein) were immunized with antigen A. Do you think this would have any affect on development of the humoral immune response? Why or why not?
   (b) Describe salient features of TI-1, TI-2, and TD antigens. What accounts for differences in the humoral immune response triggered by them?
   (c) What signals are essential for activation of B lymphocytes by T helper cells? Compare with T cell-mediated macrophage activation in cell-mediated immunity.
   (d) Knockout mice were generated that failed to express CD40 on the surface of their B cells. What do you think would be the consequences of lack of expression of CD40?
   (e) What are the features of follicular dendritic cells that set them apart from other dendritic cells? In your opinion, is there any advantage of their long-term presentation of antigen on development of the immune response?

3. For each question, choose the *best* answer.
   (a) Which of the following cell types secretes IgE?
       (i) Plasma cells
       (ii) B lymphocytes
       (iii) Mast cells
       (iv) Basophils
   (b) Plasma cells within a lymph node are found primarily in
       (i) medulla
       (ii) cortex
       (iii) paracortex
       (iv) primary follicles
   (c) Follicular dendritic cells
       (i) express class II MHC molecules
       (ii) are efficient at processing antigens
       (iii) are found in the medulla
       (iv) are found in germinal centres
   (d) Which event does not occur in the germinal centre?
       (i) Somatic hypermutation
       (ii) B cell proliferation
       (iii) Rearrangement of immunoglobulin genes
       (iv) Apoptosis

Effector Mechanisms of
Humoral Immunity

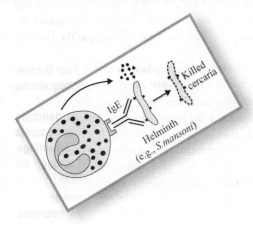

LEARNING OBJECTIVES

Having studied this chapter, you should be able to understand the following:

◆ The different ways in which antibodies produced in a humoral response protect against infectious agents and their toxins, and that Fab and Fc regions of antibodies have different functional roles
◆ The importance of neutralization, agglutination, precipitation (Fab functions), and opsonization and ADCC (Fc functions) in protection
◆ The importance of Fc receptors in mediating effector functions of antibodies
◆ The different pathways by which the complement system is activated and the various roles of complement proteins in host defence
◆ How antibodies protect at mucosal surfaces and how they confer protection on the foetus and newborn
◆ How some pathogens are able to evade humoral immunity

Specific immunity mediated by antibodies is referred to as *humoral immunity*. It is that effector arm of adaptive immunity that provides defence against extracellular microbes and their toxins. The complement system is another important element of humoral immunity which is activated when an antibody reacts with its specific antigen/pathogen, or directly by microbial components (innate). Antibodies cannot reach microbes (such as viruses) that live inside host cells. To combat intracellular microbes, the host has to activate cell-mediated immune mechanisms involving T cells (see Chapter 9). Humoral immunity, however, is important for extracellular phases of such microbes as antibodies prevent them from gaining entry into host cells.

The importance of humoral immunity in defence is reflected in patients suffering from a congenital immunodeficiency disorder called *X-linked agammaglobulinemia* (*X-LA*; see Chapter 16). Such patients show defects in antibody production and are prone to infections by many bacteria, viruses, and parasites. Lack of antibodies in the patient's serum can be revealed by a technique called immunoelectrophoresis (see Fig. A.22).

To recapitulate some salient points which have been discussed in earlier chapters, B cells use antibodies bound to the cell membrane as antigen receptors. Binding of antigens triggers activation and allows the B cell to present antigens effectively to T helper lymphocytes. Signals from antigen-primed T cells lead to differentiation of B cells into antibody-secreting plasma cells and memory cells. Plasma cells do not express membrane-bound antibodies. They are actively engaged in antibody synthesis and can release several thousand antibody molecules per second. In peripheral lymphoid organs, such as lymph nodes and spleen, B lymphocytes, on stimulation by antigen (protein), produce antibodies of different heavy chain classes (isotypes) which can function at any distant site of infection in the body. Antibodies are also present in mucosal secretions where they prevent entry of microbes through epithelia. Each immunoglobulin (Ig) class and subclass has a distinct set of effector functions to perform (though some functions may overlap) due to differences in the Fc region of various antibody classes/subclasses. For instance, recognition of antigens by IgM, and also IgG, can trigger complement activation, whereas IgE recognition leads to inflammatory responses due to mast cell degranulation, and anaphylaxis. Most antibodies, however, possess several protective capabilities. An antibody such as IgG that agglutinates bacteria may also opsonize the bacteria and lyse the bacteria by complement fixation.

The chapter deals with the various effector mechanisms used by antibodies to combat different types of pathogens and their toxins. The way antibodies defend against microbes entering via the respiratory and gastrointestinal tracts (mucosal immunity) and how they protect the foetus and newborn from infections are also covered. The components of the complement system, its activation pathways, and biological role are described. Interestingly, pathogens have devised some ingenious ways to evade humoral responses. Some of these strategies are also explained. Antibodies are essentially protective, but they are also a cause of damage to our own tissues. Such undesirable reactions that lead to immunopathology are also included in the concluding part of this chapter.

ANTIBODY-MEDIATED EFFECTOR MECHANISMS

It should be recalled from Chapter 4 that antibodies are bifunctional, and their *two* essential functions shown in Fig. 11.1 are structurally separated.

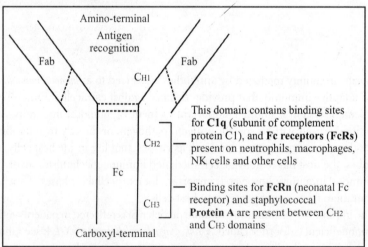

Fig. 11.1 The bifunctional role of antibodies. The Fab portions of antibodies recognize antigens, whereas the Fc tails trigger various effector functions when they interact with Fc receptors (FcRs) and complement. Their binding sites and also sites for binding of FcRn and Protein A (see Chapter 12) are indicated.

The two major ways in which antibodies function in immune defence include:

Recognition   The Fab region of antibodies recognizes and binds specifically to anything foreign, such as antigenic components on the surface of microbes.

Activation of diverse effector mechanisms   These are mediated by the Fc region after an antibody recognizes and binds to the foreign cell surface. The effector functions of antibodies result from interactions between the heavy chain constant regions with components of the innate immune system, such as the complement protein C1q, or with cell membrane receptors such as Fc receptors (FcRs) on phagocytes.

Fab-mediated Functions

Following are some of the Fab-mediated functions.

Neutralization

The pathological effect of many bacteria, seen especially in diseases such as tetanus, diphtheria, and botulism (a severe kind of food poisoning), is due to the toxins (proteins/enzymes) they secrete (exotoxins). Many toxins have two polypeptide chains: the receptor-binding domain is on one chain, whereas the toxic function, such as inhibition of protein synthesis, is carried out by the second chain. Antibodies (antitoxins) binding to the receptor-binding site on the toxin can prevent the toxin from binding to the cell, thereby protecting the cell from toxic attack. This is called *neutralization*. Toxin–antitoxin complexes are removed by phagocytosis, digested intracellularly, and exocytosed (Fig. 11.2). Immunoglobulin-G is efficient as a neutralizing antibody.

Inactivated exotoxins which no longer exert harmful effects are called *toxoids*. These have a very important practical application. Toxoid vaccination is used to prevent diphtheria and tetanus caused by *Corynebacterium diphtheriae* and *Clostridium tetani*, respectively (see Chapter 13).

Besides toxins, antibodies can also neutralize bacteria and viruses, blocking pathogen attachment to host cells. For instance, secretory IgA (sIgA) prevents colonization and infection by pathogenic microbes, such as *Vibrio cholerae* at mucosal sites. Also, by binding to viral surface molecules, through which viruses gain entry into host cells, sIgA prevents viruses from establishing infection at these sites

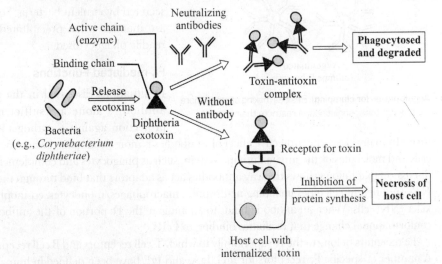

Fig. 11.2   Neutralization of toxins. Toxins neutralized by antibodies are unable to interact with cell surface receptors, whereas free toxin causes host cell necrosis.

(Fig. 11.9). Antibody-coated pathogens/antigens can finally be expelled from the body by a variety of mechanisms, such as entrapment in mucus and expulsion by peristalsis in the gut.

Some insect and snake venoms are extremely toxic and can even be fatal. Passive immunization with neutralizing antibodies can be used to counteract their adverse effects. Such antibodies can be generated in animal species, usually horses. Horse antitetanus toxin can be administered passively to patients to protect against tetanus toxin. However, an adverse response called *serum sickness* may develop (see Chapter 14).

Agglutination

This is antibody-induced clumping of *particulate antigens*, such as whole bacteria (Fig. 11.3).

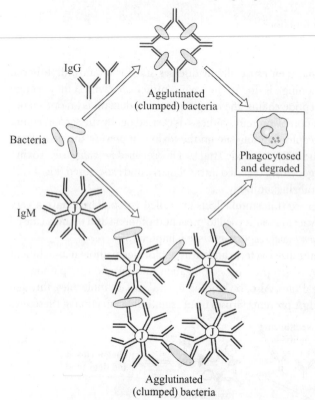

IgG

Agglutinated (clumped) bacteria

Bacteria

Phagocytosed and degraded

IgM

Agglutinated (clumped) bacteria

Fig. 11.3 Agglutination (or clumping). Besides making bacteria more susceptible to phagocytosis, agglutination restricts their spread.

Each antibody attaches to identical antigenic determinants (epitopes) on separate antigen particles to form a network of clumped cells. Besides preventing the spread of the infectious agent in the body, the large number of agglutinated bacteria can be engulfed together by a single phagocyte. Otherwise, a much larger number of phagocytes would be required to engulf the same number of unclumped bacteria. As IgM has many more antigen-binding sites than IgG (see Fig. 4.21), it is much more efficient at cross-linking particulate antigens and agglutinating them.

It should be noted that agglutination is an important in vitro technique which has various applications such as in disease diagnosis (see Appendix 1).

Precipitation

Precipitation occurs when an antibody combines with *soluble antigens*, such as extracellular enzymes secreted by virulent bacteria. Soluble molecules are inactive when precipitated and are more readily phagocytosed.

Fc-mediated Functions

In situations discussed in the preceding text, antibodies alone are sufficient in affording protection against a pathogenic microbe or a toxin. In many cases, the protective effect of antibodies is more pronounced when they are assisted by cells and molecules of the innate immune system, such as phagocytes and complement proteins. The discussion that follows shows the way antibodies act as adaptors that bind through their Fc regions to *FcRs* on different cell types including neutrophils, macrophages/monocytes, eosinophils, and natural killer (NK) cells. When an antibody binds to an antigen, the Fc portion of the antibody undergoes a conformational change that facilitates binding to FcRs.

Fc receptors belong to the Ig superfamily to which T cell receptors and B cell receptors also belong. A number of specific Fc receptors for IgG, IgA, and IgE have been defined in humans that differ in cellular distribution, specificity for Ig classes and subclasses, and also in signalling mechanisms and function. Fc receptors play an active role in triggering various activities and do not simply bind the antigen–antibody complex. Cross-linking of receptors on binding to antigen–antibody complexes activates effector functions such as phagocytosis, antibody-dependent cell-mediated cytotoxicity (ADCC), and release of cytokines and inflammatory mediators. Some receptors deliver inhibitory signals. Immunoreceptor tyrosine-based activation motifs (ITAMs) or immunoreceptor tyrosine-based inhibition motifs (ITIMs), which are activating and inhibitory motifs, respectively, are present in the intracellular regions of the receptors. Some selected FcRs are represented diagrammatically in Fig. 11.4 with their characteristics shown in Table 11.1.

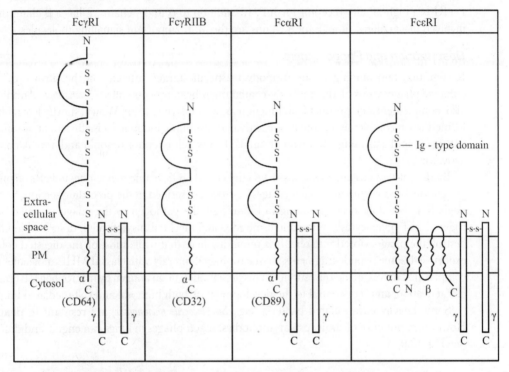

Fig. 11.4 Schematic diagram of human Fc receptors. Some selected FcRs for IgG, IgA, and IgE are shown. FcγRIIB differs from the other receptors. The cytoplasmic tail of its α chain delivers inhibitory signals.

Table 11.1 Specific human leukocyte Fc receptors. Expression of FcαRI is inducible rather than constitutive.

FcR	Cellular distribution	Antibody class/subclass bound	Function
FcγRI	Macrophages, neutrophils, eosinophils	IgG1, IgG3 (high-affinity)	Activation of phagocytosis and killing
FcγRIIB	B lymphocytes	IgG1, IgG3 in an immune complex/bound to microbes	Blocks B cell activation by delivering inhibitory signals
FcαRI	Neutrophils, monocytes/macrophages, eosinophils	IgA1, IgA2	Phagocytosis, release of inflammatory mediators, and ADCC
FcεRI	Mast cells, basophils, eosinophils	IgE (high-affinity)	Degranulation on cross-linking of IgE (bound to FcεRI) by antigens

While the α polypeptide chain of FcRs is involved in Fc binding, additional polypeptide chain(s) are involved in transducing signals. These are the β and/or γ polypeptide chain (s). Immunoglobulin-G and its subclasses bind to FcγRs, which are of several types. FcγRI and FcγRIIB are two such receptors. FcγRI consists of an α chain which is the binding chain and two identical disulphide-linked γ chains that have a role in transducing activating signals. FcγRIIB, found only on B cells, has two Ig-like domains in the α chain. As it is not associated with other chains, signalling is mediated by the cytoplasmic region of the α chain itself. The receptor differs in the fact that its intracellular region delivers an inhibitory signal which is important in regulating B cell responses (see Fig. 10.13). FcαRI binds IgA1 and IgA2. FcεRI is a high-affinity receptor for IgE. In addition to α and γ chains, it has a β chain that is also involved in signalling, though the γ chains are the more important signalling molecules.

Opsonization and Phagocytosis

Recognition and binding of an antibody to specific target antigens on the surface of microbes enhance phagocytosis of the antibody-coated microbe, a process called *opsonization*. Antibodies and, also, complement split product C3b function as opsonins (Fig. 11.5). We will shortly learn how C3b is formed when complement proteins are activated. Immunogloubulin-G is efficient at opsonization of pathogens and activating complement, unlike IgA which is a poor opsonin and a weak complement activator.

Binding of the constant Fc regions of IgG (IgG1 and IgG3) bound to microbes to FcRs on professional phagocytes (neutrophils and macrophages) has been described in the preceding section. Several such Fc–FcR interactions occur resulting in binding of the pathogen to the phagocyte membrane and triggering of phagocytosis. Subsequent microbicidal mechanisms activated, described in Chapter 2, destroy the phagocytosed microbe. It is reminded here that while most of the digested contents are exocytosed, some peptide fragments, in macrophages, interact with class II MHC molecules to form a complex that moves up the cell's surface. This presentation of an antigen by macrophages is critical to TH cell activation, an event central to the development of both humoral and cell-mediated immunity.

Some heavily encapsulated bacteria (e.g., *Streptococcus pneumoniae*) are resistant to phagocytosis. However in presence of anticapsular antibodies, macrophages in lungs can engulf and destroy them (see Fig. 12.9).

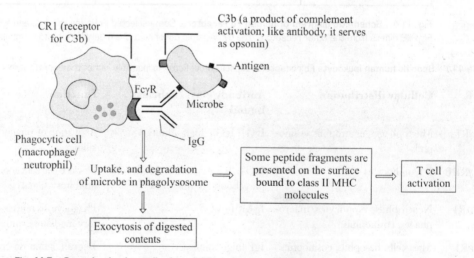

Fig. 11.5 **Opsonization by antibody and C3b enhances phagocytosis.**

C3b synergizes with antibodies in triggering phagocytosis. It attaches to the pathogen surface and interacts with *C3b receptors (CR1)* on phagocytes. This is not the only way by which complement proteins function. There are other important roles also. Red blood cells (RBCs) which also express receptors (CR1) for C3b can bind cells or complexes to which C3b has adhered. This allows RBCs to deliver these complexes to the liver or spleen where macrophages remove them without destroying the red blood cells (see Fig. 12.18).

Antibody-dependent Cell-mediated Cytotoxicity

Antibody-dependent cell-mediated cytotoxicity, a specific (adaptive) immune response mounted against the antibody-coated target cell, involves killing of the target cell by cytotoxic effector cells, such as NK cells, eosinophils, macrophages, and neutrophils. Natural killer cells play an important role in ADCC (Fig. 11.6). When Fc receptors on NK cells (FcγRIII; CD16) bind to the Fc regions of an array of IgG antibodies bound to the target cell surface, signals are transduced that activate the NK cells to discharge the contents of their granules (perforin and granzymes) on the target cell resulting in its death by apoptosis. A large number of perforin molecules inserted in the target cell membrane can also induce cell death by lysis.

Host cells infected with viruses and bacteria can also be killed by ADCC mediated by macrophages and neutrophils. Eosinophils, which are weakly phagocytic, can also mediate ADCC. As depicted in Fig. 11.7, eosinophil-mediated ADCC involves extracellular killing of pathogens. The difference with phagocytosis, which involves intracellular killing of the ingested microbe, should be noted. Eosinophils express many molecules of high-affinity *FcεRI* on their surface. These receptors bind to the Fc region of IgE antibodies that coat helminthic parasites, such as schistosomes, which, due to their large size, are not easily engulfed. The signals, thus, transduced cause eosinophils to degranulate and release their toxic contents directly onto the target (exocytosis). While helminths are somewhat resistant to the toxic substances released by macrophages and also neutrophils, they are killed by major basic protein (MBP) and other toxic substances present in eosinophil granules.

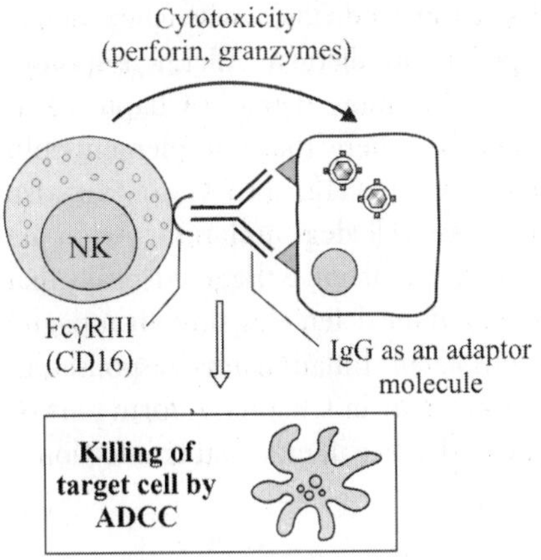

Cytotoxicity
(perforin, granzymes)

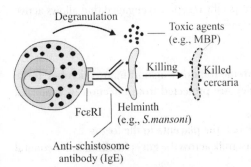

FcγRIII
(CD16)

IgG as an adaptor
molecule

**Killing of
target cell by
ADCC**

Fig. 11.6 Antibody-dependent cell-mediated cytotoxicity (ADCC). A target cell tagged with antibodies is marked as foreign and destroyed by cytotoxic NK cells via binding to FcRs and release of granule contents.

Degranulation

Toxic agents
(e.g., MBP)

Killing

Killed
cercaria

FcεRI

Helminth
(e.g., *S.mansoni*)

Anti-schistosome
antibody (IgE)

Fig. 11.7 Eosinophil-mediated ADCC.

However, the importance of ADCC in immune defence in vivo is not very clear. Although this mechanism is normally protective, extracellular release of granule contents by neutrophils may cause injury to host tissues as is exemplified by the pathogenesis in immune complex (IC) disease (type III hypersensitivity reaction; see Chapter 14).

A salient feature of the humoral immune response to helminths is the dominance of IgE antibodies. B cells respond to helminths by switching to IgE, whereas the response to most bacteria and viruses involves switching to IgG antibodies. B cells have unique mechanisms by which they can change the heavy chain constant region of the antibody from μ (IgM) and δ (IgD) to γ (IgG), α (IgA), or ε (IgE) keeping the same heavy and light chain variable region (V_H and V_L). This changes the class of the antibody, though specificity is not altered (see Chapter 6). *This pattern of isotype switching which is determined by the type of cytokines produced by T helper cells in response to different types of microbes is highly significant as it ensures optimal host defence.* Besides isotype switching, *affinity maturation* is another change that occurs which results in antibodies having higher affinity for antigens. This further enhances the protective functions of antibodies (see Chapter 10).

Mast Cell/Basophil Activation by IgE

Another use of Fc receptors is in mast cell activation by IgE (Fig. 11.8). The Fc portion of IgE binds to high-affinity FcεRI present on tissue mast cells and blood basophils. Mast cells are located throughout the body including skin, submucosal tissues, and lungs. Binding of a specific antigen (entering the body for the second time) to IgE results in cross-linking of FcεRI which triggers activation and degranulation of the mast cell/basophil. There is release of mediators such as histamine and chemotactic factors that help to recruit various effector cells to the site.

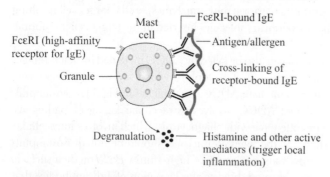

Fig. 11.8 IgE-mediated mast cell activation. A mast cell with an antigen/allergen cross-linking FcεRI-bound IgE on its surface is shown here. Signalling through the receptor triggers degranulation of the mast cell with release of inflammatory mediators.

Unfortunately, this can lead to undesirable allergic symptoms for certain antigens called allergens (type I or immediate hypersensitivity). For instance, symptoms of hay fever can develop in some individuals when they contact grass pollen, an allergen. Allergic responses are covered in more detail in Chapter 14. It is emphasized here that complement-split products (C3a, C4a, and C5a) can also induce mast cell degranulation. An acute inflammatory reaction is triggered locally that helps in immune defence against an antigen/infectious agent. Inflammatory responses, as described earlier in Chapter 2, form part of the body's defence in eradicating infection.

FUNCTION OF ANTIBODIES AT SPECIFIC ANATOMIC SITES

Antibodies which are produced in peripheral lymphoid organs are secreted into the bloodstream from where they can access various sites of infection. But, for transport across epithelia, specialized mechanisms exist which are dependent on the Fc tails of antibodies. This allows antibodies to be delivered to places, such as foetal circulation by transplacental passage from the mother (IgG), and to mucus secretions, milk, and tears (IgA). In both cases, a specific receptor is engaged that allows active transport through cells to the above sites.

Immunity in the Newborn (Neonatal Immunity)

Newborn mammals are unable to mount effective immune responses against many microbes as the immune system is not fully developed or mature. They are protected from infection by maternal antibodies which are acquired through two routes:

+ By active transport of IgG (except subclass IgG2) across the placenta to the foetus
+ By transport of IgA and IgG isotypes present in breast milk across the gut epithelium into neonatal blood

The routes by which the foetus and neonates acquire maternal antibodies depend on a special Fc receptor called the *neonatal Fc receptor (FcRn)*. This differs from other leukocyte Fc receptors in that it shows structural resemblance to MHC class I molecules. However, it differs in that a peptide-binding groove is not involved in IgG/IgA binding. The FcRn–IgG interaction involves residues located at the C_{H2}–C_{H3} domain interface in the Fc tail of IgG (Fig. 11.1).

The ability of maternal antibodies to be transported across the placenta to the foetus, and those present in milk to pass through neonatal gut into blood, is because FcRn can bind and traffic IgG within and across cells. Newborns are thus able to acquire protective antibodies to various infectious microbes to which mothers have been exposed/vaccinated. *Maternal antibodies are important as they provide protection to the newborn, an excellent example of passive immunity.* Owing to low proteolytic activity in the gastrointestinal tract (GIT) of newborns and presence of colostral trypsin inhibitors, degradation of Igs in the early first few days of life is prevented.

Immunity at Mucosal Sites

Mucosal epithelial surfaces lining the gastrointestinal and respiratory tracts are the major entry sites for many pathogens. Defence at these surfaces is provided largely by secretory IgA which is very efficient at neutralizing microbes that have been ingested or inhaled. This prevents bacterial colonization and viral infection of cells.

B lymphocytes underlying mucosal areas internalize antigen that is recognized by their surface Ig. The internalized antigen is processed and presented to primed $CD4^+$ T helper cells which provide signals to B cells to class-switch to IgA (see Chapter 10). Dimeric IgA produced in the lamina propria, which underlies epithelium at mucosal sites has to be transported to the lumen. This, and also the transport of antibody to breast milk, requires movement of the antibody across epithelial layers, a process known as *transcytosis* (Fig. 11.9).

A special Fc receptor called the *poly-Ig receptor (p-IgR)* which also is a member of the Ig superfamily, is involved in transport. On binding to p-IgR, expressed on the basal surface of epithelial cells, IgA is endocytosed into vesicles and transported across the cytoplasm to the apical surface of the cell. The vesicles fuse with the plasma membrane and the receptor is cleaved by a protease. Immunoglobulin-A is released into the lumen still carrying a part of the bound p-IgR called *secretory component (SC)*. Besides its role in the transport of dimeric IgA, the SC serves to protect IgA from proteolysis in the lumen. It masks sites present in IgA susceptible to proteolytic cleavage. This protection enables IgA to exist longer in a protease-rich environment, such as the lumen. Immunoglobulin-M is also present in mucosal secretions, though in much lesser amounts than IgA.

Mucosal immunity serves to protect against many viruses such as polio and influenza virus, and also against bacteria including *V. cholerae*, *Salmonella*, and *Neisseria gonnorhoeae*. Antibodies bound to the surface of microbes can be eliminated by peristaltic movements in the gut.

Some vaccines stimulate humoral immunity and production of neutralizing IgA antibodies at mucosal surfaces. A good example is the attenuated oral polio vaccine (OPV) of Sabin which induces protective secretory IgA (sIgA) antibodies against polio virus infection (the vaccine stimulates cell-mediated immunity as well).

THE COMPLEMENT SYSTEM

The complement system is a major effector system of both innate and antibody-mediated acquired immunity. It is composed of more than 30 proteins in plasma and on cell surfaces. The complement proteins on cell membranes are receptors for activated complement proteins or proteins that regulate complement activity. The complement proteins are synthesized mainly by liver hepatocytes, and also by

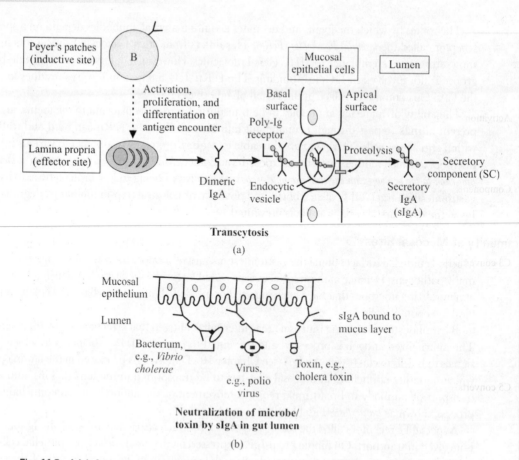

Fig. 11.9 (a) IgA transport across the mucosal epithelium (transcytosis). Dimeric IgA is transported into the intestinal lumen with the help of the poly-Ig receptor. It is released as sIgA with the SC attached to it. **(b) Neutralization of microbes/toxins by sIgA.** Secretory IgA (SC not shown) affords protection against viruses, bacteria, and toxins at mucosal surfaces.

blood monocytes and tissue macrophages. In plasma, complement proteins are normally in an inactive form (zymogens). They are activated sequentially by proteolysis under particular conditions, such as infection to generate products that mediate the effector functions of complement. The system, like the blood coagulation system, works as a cascade and results in tremendous amplification. Although complement proteins perform various critical roles, the system also has the potential to cause damage to host tissues when overactivated.

The following section describes the pathways that lead to complement activation. The effector functions performed by the system and some regulatory mechanisms which prevent uncontrolled complement activation are also discussed.

Complement Activation Pathways

There are three pathways of complement activation that are shown in schematic form in Fig. 11.10.

The *classical pathway*, the first to be worked out, is activated mainly by binding of antibodies to surface of microbes. The two remaining pathways, which include the *mannose-binding lectin (MBL)* and the *alternative pathways*, are antibody-independent routes of complement activation. *The central event*

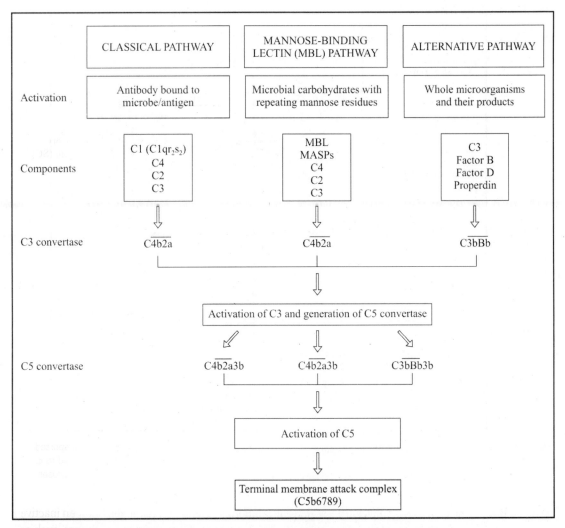

Fig. 11.10   Pathways of complement activation. The complement system can be activated via three pathways, of which the classical pathway is dependent on antibody (adaptive), unlike the lectin and alternative pathways (innate). The generation of C3 and C5 convertases which lead to formation of the terminal membrane attack complex (MAC) is shown.

in all the three pathways is the generation of a C3 convertase which converts C3 to C3b. With the subsequent generation of *C5 convertase*, the three pathways converge on a common terminal pathway that leads to formation of the *membrane attack complex (MAC)* which results in microbial lysis. The sequence of reactions in the three pathways is outlined in Fig. 11.11.

The Classical Pathway

The classical pathway is initiated mainly by the binding of antibody (IgM, IgG1, IgG2, and IgG3) to an antigen on a target surface such as bacterial cells or by a soluble antigen–antibody complex. C1, the first enzyme complex in the cascade, is found in the circulation as a pentamer $C1qr_2s_2$ in which C1q is the recognition subunit (Fig. 11.12). Activated C1r and C1s are serine proteases that cleave the complement proteins C4 and C2 (described in the following text).

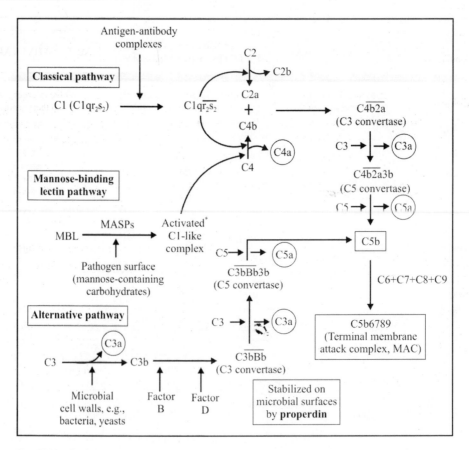

Fig. 11.11 Activation of complement. The complement split products encircled are inflammatory mediators, designated anaphylatoxins.
*C2 is also cleaved by the complex, as is C4, but is not shown here.

Binding of C1q to two adjacent Fc regions of antibodies bound to a pathogen/antigen results in activation of the associated C1r and C1s dimers. This leads to cleavage of C4 to give a large fragment C4b which attaches covalently near C1 on the pathogen surface. C2 (which binds to C4b) is then cleaved by C1s to give a large fragment C2a which remains associated with C4b. The complex $\overline{C4b2a}$ is the C3 convertase which generates C3a and C3b from C3. Some of the C3b generated binds to $\overline{C4b2a}$. The resultant $\overline{C4b2a}$3b complex is a C5 convertase, generation of which marks the end of the classical pathway. *A part of C3b generated by C3 convertase, instead of associating with $\overline{C4b2a}$, diffuses and coats ICs and particulate antigens, and functions as an opsonin. It is recognized by receptors for C3b on phagocytes and is phagocytosed.*

The Mannose-binding Lectin Pathway

The lectin pathway, like the alternative pathway, represents an important innate defence mechanism as it can be activated in absence of a complexed antibody. It is initiated by the binding of a plasma protein *MBL*, a protein of the innate immune system, to mannose residues on microbial surfaces. Mannose-binding lectin was introduced earlier in Chapter 2 as a pattern-recognition protein whose synthesis is induced in liver as part of the acute-phase response. Mannose-binding lectin circulates as

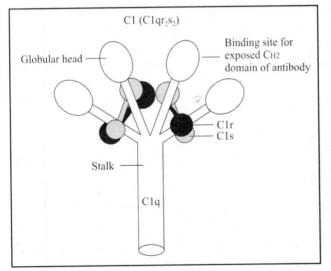

Fig. 11.12 Structure of C1 – the first component of the classical pathway. C1q can bind to IgM and IgG complexed to pathogen/antigen and trigger complement activation.

a complex with a group of protease zymogens known as *MBL-associated serine proteases (MASPs)*. Interestingly, MASPs are structurally and functionally similar to the proteases C1r and C1s, whereas MBL is structurally similar to C1q.

Binding of MBL/MASP complexes to specific microbial carbohydrates leads to autocatalytic activation of MASPs. Activated MASPs which mimic activities of C1r and C1s cleave C4 and C2 to generate first the classical pathway C3 convertase ($\overline{C4b2a}$), and then the C5 convertase ($\overline{C4b2a3b}$). Further activation leads to final assembly of the MAC. Overall, the mechanism of the lectin pathway is more like that of the classical pathway.

The Alternative Pathway

This pathway is activated by cell wall consti-tuents in both Gram-positive (e.g., teichoic acid) and Gram-negative (e.g., LPS) bacteria. Low-level C3 hydrolysis occurs spontaneously in plasma with formation of C3b. Although most of the C3b is inactivated by hydrolysis, some C3b attaches covalently to the surface of pathogens. C3b is prevented from binding stably to normal host cells by several regulatory proteins that are present on host cells but are absent from microbes. The binding of factor B to C3b and its cleavage by factor D generates Bb which remains associated with C3b forming the C3 convertase ($\overline{C3bBb}$) of the alternative pathway. This can activate C3 molecules by cleaving them to C3a and C3b. C3b can be fed back into the pathway to create more C3 convertase forming a positive feedback amplification loop. On certain microbial surfaces, $\overline{C3bBb}$ is stabilized by binding of a serum factor *properdin*. Subsequent binding of C3b molecules creates the alternative pathway C5 convertase ($\overline{C3bBb}3b$) which is analogous to the ($\overline{C4b2a}3b$) complex of the classical pathway. Thus, the alternative pathway is initiated through spontaneous hydrolysis of C3b, the rate of which increases considerably by activating surfaces such as microbial cell walls.

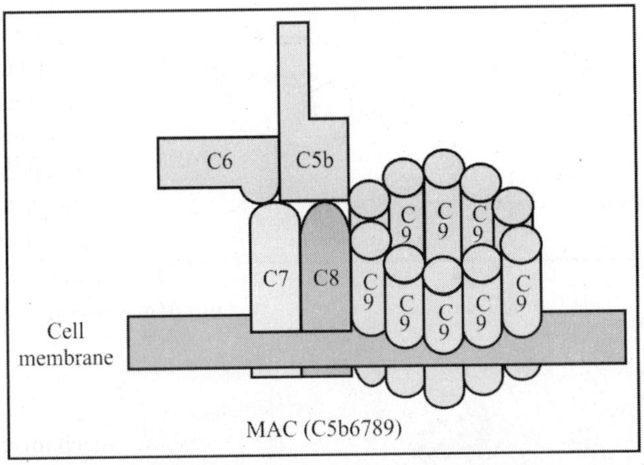

The Membrane Attack Pathway

The non-enzymatic C3b component of the C5 convertase of the classical and lectin pathway ($\overline{C4b2a}3b$), and of the alternative pathway ($\overline{C3bBb}3b$) binds to C5 which is cleaved to generate a small fragment C5a and a larger fragment C5b. C5a is a very potent mediator of inflammation, whereas C5b binds to antigenic surfaces and initiates formation of MAC (Fig. 11.13). It first binds C6 and then C7 from the plasma to form a trimolecular complex C5b67

Fig. 11.13 The terminal membrane attack complex (MAC). MAC, formed from terminal complement components, creates a transmembrane channel in the membrane that disrupts membrane integrity leading to cell lysis.

which is able to insert into the lipid bilayer of a target cell. Further binding of C8 and C9 occurs with the latter polymerizing to form the complete MAC creating a pore in the cell membrane. This destroys membrane integrity. There is osmotic lysis due to influx of water and loss of electrolytes which can diffuse freely through the central channel of MAC. It is noteworthy that C9 is structurally homologous to *perforin*, a pore-forming protein found in granules of CTLs and NK cells. The pores created by polymerized C9 are similar to the pores that perforin forms in the target cell membrane, though killing mechanisms induced are different (see Chapter 9).

Biological Role of Complement Components

Some of the major physiologic activities of the complement system which have been depicted earlier in Fig. 2.3 are summarized in Fig. 11.14 and are discussed in the following text.

Opsonization

After antibodies bind and coat the surface of an infectious agent, C1q binds to the antibodies and initiates the complement cascade. C3b functions as opsonin and is recognized by receptors (CR1) on the surface of phagocytes. This, along with binding of antibodies to Fc receptors on phagocytes, stimulates phagocytosis (Fig. 11.5).

Chemotaxis and Activation of Leukocytes

Inflammatory responses, as was described in Chapter 2, form part of the body's defence in eliminating an infectious agent. The small fragments generated by cleavage of complement proteins, namely, C3a, C4a, and C5a, bind to receptors on mast cells and basophils causing them to degranulate. Histamine and other pharmacologically active mediators are released which induce an inflammatory response. C5a is also an important chemotactic agent. It is able to induce monocytes and neutrophils to adhere to vascular endothelial cells, extravasate, and migrate towards the site of complement activation in tissues. Besides, it enhances phagocytosis.

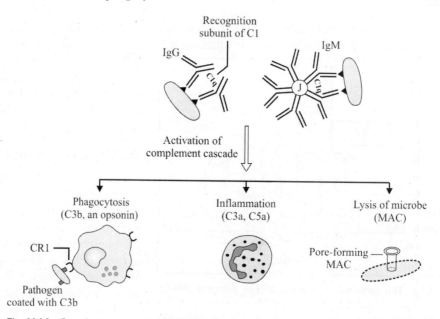

Fig. 11.14 Complement proteins and their role.

Overproduction of these small complement fragments induces a generalized inflammatory collapse leading to a shock-like syndrome, features of which are similar to that seen in IgE-mediated allergic reactions. The term *anaphylactic shock* is used for such a reaction, and the small peptides C3a, C4a, and C5a are designated *anaphylatoxins*.

Lysis of Bacteria and Cells

The terminal MAC of the complement pathway provides major defence against most gram-negative bacteria, particularly *Neisseria* species. Individuals deficient in MAC components are prone to a form of bacterial meningitis.

Enhancing B Cell Responses to Antigens

C3d, the main fragment of covalently bound C3b, is a ligand for *complement receptor type 2 (CR2)* on the B cell surface. When C3d coupled to antigen cross-links surface IgM and CR2 activating signals to the B cell are amplified enhancing B cell response to the antigen (see Fig. 10.6).

Clearance of Immune Complexes

Immune complexes containing microbial antigens or antigens from dying host cells are formed continuously both in health and disease. Complement plays an important role in handling these ICs. Complement fragments, such as C3b bound within ICs provide ligands for clearance by phagocytic cells via complement receptors. This is beneficial as it prevents ICs from being deposited in tissues. Immune complexes can also bind to CR1 on erythrocytes which carry the complexes to sites of disposal such as liver and spleen (see Fig. 12.18). Deficiency in early components of the classical pathway (e.g., C1, C2, or C4) results in inefficient clearance of ICs and leads to increase in the incidence of IC disease resembling systemic lupus erythematosus (SLE) (see Chapter 15).

Regulation of Complement Activation

The complement pathway is potentially dangerous for host cells as it can lead to inflammatory and destructive effects. Control proteins, present in the plasma and host cell membranes, which act on complement components at several key points in the activation sequence, prevent activation of complement on surfaces of host cells. Their lack in microbes allows complement activation to proceed only on foreign surfaces.

Activation of C1, the first step in the classical pathway of complement activation, is controlled by *C1 inhibitor (C1INH)*, a plasma protease. Its deficiency leads to the disease *hereditary angioedema (HAE)* in which there is abnormal C1 activation. The serum protein *factor H* has important regulatory functions in the alternative pathway. First, it competes with factor B for binding to C3b on host cell surfaces which thus, stay protected. Factor H can also displace Bb from the convertase already formed, forming C3bH. This prevents further activation of the complement cascade. Once factor H binds to C3b, the latter becomes susceptible to cleavage by serum *Factor I*. The inactive derivative iC3b formed is further degraded to C3d which has important functions to perform. *Decay accelerating factor (DAF)*, a cell surface molecule, besides competing with factor B (as does factor H) for binding to C3b on cell surfaces, dissociates the convertase complex as well. Similar control mechanisms exist for the classical pathway C3 convertase. Regulatory mechanisms that prevent MAC insertion into host cell membranes also exist. *CD59* (also called *protectin*) prevents insertion of MAC into the membrane.

EVASION OF HUMORAL IMMUNITY BY MICROBES AND IMMUNOPATHOLOGY

Many wily pathogens have very cleverly evolved strategies which help them to evade our humoral defences. Some of the strategies deployed are cited in the following text:

1. Certain microbes mutate surface molecules that are the targets of neutralizing antibodies *Escherichia coli* escapes recognition by varying antigens contained in its pili, structures which help in its attachment and entry into host cells. African trypanosomes *(Trypanosoma brucei)* are flagellated protozoans which cause sleeping sickness in humans. They too can evade antibody mediated defences by expressing new surface glycoproteins (see Fig. 12.15). Viruses also, particularly influenza virus and human immunodeficiency virus (HIV), mutate their surface antigens, and so are at a selective advantage.
2. Vaccinia virus, Epstein–Barr virus (EBV), and some other microbes contain proteins that mimic complement regulatory proteins.
3. Herpes simplex virus (HSV) produces glycoproteins which bind to FcγRs on immune cells. This blocks action of antiviral antibodies.
4. Interestingly, *Staphylococcus aureus* makes Protein A which binds to the Fc region at sites which are critical for binding to FcRs on various immune cells (Fig. 11.1).
5. Some membrane proteins, in resistant strains of *Neisseria*, prevent MAC from inserting into the cell membrane.
6. Certain bacteria, for example, *Pseudomonas aeruginosa* possess an elastase that inactivates the anaphylatoxins C3a and C5a thereby preventing an inflammatory response.

Binding of antibody to a pathogen/antigen is essentially protective. But action of antibodies can, in some instances, cause damage to the host (immunopathology).

1. Small antigen–antibody complexes that escape phagocytosis are deposited at certain sites where they activate the complement cascade causing inflammatory damage. For example, kidney glomeruli are destroyed by immune complexes in the disorder glomerulonephritis (type III hypersensitivity).
2. Antibodies can also react with our body's own cells and can be critically implicated in the pathogenesis of autoimmune disease. Such antibodies called *autoantibodies* are seen in both systemic and organ-specific autoimmune disease. They contribute to the disease in two ways: by effector mechanisms discussed in the preceding text or through formation of immune complexes formed by reacting with autoantigens. A good example is SLE where autoantibodies bind to DNA and form immune complexes that cause glomerulo nephritis and vascular injury (see Chapter 15).
3. Cross-linking of IgE bound to mast cells and basophils by some antigens (allergens) can initiate an allergic response. This produces severe undesirable reactions of type I or immediate hypersensitivity. It should be borne in mind that the same reactions which afford protection against worm infections (Fig. 12.14) can, inappropriately, cause adverse reactions as well.

SUMMARY

◆ Humoral immunity is that arm of adaptive immunity that is mediated by antibodies produced by plasma cells, and also complement proteins. It represents a major defence mechanism against extracellular microbes and their toxins.

◆ Production of antibodies usually requires help from

T cells (TH) specific for a foreign peptide derived from a protein antigen that is also recognized by the B cell.

◆ In an antibody molecule, the antigen recognition and binding portion (Fab) is spatially segregated from the effector (Fc) region. Fab region is involved in neutralization of microbes and toxins. Antigen binding by the Fab region activates effector functions of antibodies.

♦ The different biologic functions of each class of antibodies are due to differences in the Fc regions of the heavy chains. Isotype switching is directed by cytokines produced by T$_H$ cells. Antibodies of various isotypes produced are distributed to various body compartments. Due to affinity maturation, and isotype switching, protective functions of antibodies are enhanced.

♦ Antibodies prevent microbes from gaining entry into host cells, and toxins from exerting harmful effects. Many vaccines that are being used currently work by stimulating production of neutralizing antibodies.

♦ Effector cells recognize antibody-coated pathogens through Fc receptors (FcRs) that bind to Fc tails of antibodies. Binding transduces signals that stimulate phagocytosis, microbicidal activities of phagocytes, and pathogen destruction.

♦ Some parasites are too large to be engulfed. Eosinophils which express high-affinity receptors for IgE, and also FcRs specific for the constant region of IgG, play a key role in their destruction. Mechanism of killing involves release of toxic substances onto the parasite surface (exocytosis).

♦ Antibodies can also initiate destruction of pathogens by activating the complement system. This system which includes many circulating and cell surface proteins plays an important role in host defence.

♦ There are three pathways leading to complement activation. The classical pathway is activated after the binding of an antibody to an antigen and is an essential component of adaptive immunity. The alternative pathway is activated by microbial surfaces in absence of antibodies and is a component of innate immunity. In a third pathway, called the lectin-MBL pathway, the plasma protein MBL interacts with mannose residues on the surface of microbes triggering complement activation.

♦ The late steps of complement activation via the three pathways are common and lead to the formation of the membrane attack complex (MAC)–a protein complex which leads to lysis of the pathogen.

♦ Products of complement activation include C3b which functions as opsonin and C3a/C5a which induce inflammation. Fc receptors and complement receptors synergize in enhancing uptake and destruction of pathogens and immune complexes.

♦ Cell surface and circulating regulatory proteins in mammals exert a control over inappropriate complement activation on host cells which would otherwise cause considerable damage to the host.

♦ FcRn, a neonatal Fc receptor, transports maternal antibodies to the newborn.

♦ A poly-Ig receptor (poly-IgR) transports sIgA into the gut lumen.

♦ Many microbes evade humoral immunity. Some strategies include antigenic variation, resistance to phagocytosis, and inhibition of complement activation. Antibodies, in some instances, can be a cause of immunopathology.

REVIEW QUESTIONS

1. Indicate whether the following statements are true or false. If false, explain why.
   (a) Antibodies bound to microbial surfaces trigger the alternative pathway of complement activation.
   (b) C3b is an anaphylatoxin.
   (c) Protective antibodies against infectious agents are often neutralizing antibodies.
   (d) Properdin participates in the alternative pathway of complement activation.
   (e) Transport of IgM across the placenta is important for immunity in neonates.
   (f) IgG is more efficient at agglutinating particles than IgM.

2. Self-assessment questions.
   (a) IgG is subjected to proteolytic digestion by pepsin. Would antigen-binding and effector functions be retained in the fragments obtained on digestion?
   (b) What are the major biological activities of the complement system? Freshly prepared antiserum is generally decomplemented before being put to practical use. Can you explain why this step is necessary?

(c) Explain the term antibody-dependent cell-mediated cytotoxicity (ADCC). What is the importance of ADCC by eosinophils in host defence?

(d) How do Fc receptors expressed on B cells differ from Fc receptors expressed on neutrophils/macrophages? Give examples of two non-leukocyte Fc receptors and their functional importance.

(e) Outline the late cell surface events that lead to formation of MAC. Do you think there is any similarity between lysis induced by MAC and that induced by porforin roloasod from CTLs and NK cells?

3. For each question, choose the *best* answer.

(a) Which complement component promotes neutrophil chemotaxis?
   (i) C3b
   (ii) C6
   (iii) C5a
   (iv) C5b

(b) All are complement inhibitory proteins except
   (i) DAF
   (ii) CD59
   (iii) C1 inhibitor
   (iv) LFA-1

(c) What is not true about IgG?
   (i) It is cleaved by papain to yield two Fab fragments.
   (ii) It is not a complement-activating antibody.
   (iii) Its half-life is approximately 23 days.
   (iv) It is present in serum in highest concentration.

(d) Humoral immune response to helminths is dominated by
   (i) IgM
   (ii) IgG
   (iii) IgE
   (iv) IgA

Immune Response against Microbes

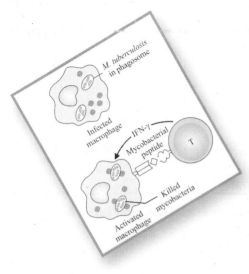

LEARNING OBJECTIVES

Having studied this chapter, you should be able to understand the following:

♦ The different types of immune responses activated by various classes of microbes

♦ That microbes have devised various strategies to evade elimination by the immune system

♦ How continual change in surface proteins of microbes poses a big problem for vaccine development

♦ The obstacles in the way of malarial vaccine development and some targets for vaccination

♦ That infection by pathogens may be a cause of severe immunopathology and that chronic persistence of microbial antigens can induce a DTH response

♦ How superantigens produce symptoms of septic shock by inducing excessive production of cytokines

The major physiological role of the immune system is to defend the host against various infectious microbes. Both natural and acquired immune responses function as an integrated system to ward off pathogens. An infectious disease is likely to occur if immune responses mounted by the host are unable to deal with the intruder. These diseases can have disastrous effects on the host and can often be fatal. They are the leading cause of mortality worldwide, and according to WHO estimates (2002), account for over 14 million deaths a year. Most deaths—almost 90 per cent—are caused by six infectious diseases, namely, pneumonia, AIDS, diarrhoeal diseases, tuberculosis (TB), malaria, and measles (Fig. 12.1). Developing countries of the world are the most affected, with children under the age of 5 years being the most vulnerable.

There are many other problems to be faced in addition to the burden due to infectious diseases. These include newly emerging infections such as H5N1 and H1N1 influenza, and severe acute respiratory syndrome (SARS) which is caused by a corona virus (Box 12.1). Besides, there are some infections that have re-emerged, such as dengue and TB. Another major problem and a cause of serious concern is the multi-drug resistance that is seen with diseases such as malaria and TB.

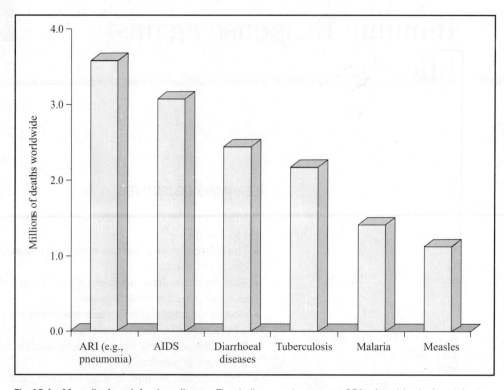

Fig. 12.1   Mortality from infectious disease. The six diseases shown cause 90% of total deaths from infectious disease worldwide (over 14 million).
ARI, acute respiratory infections

Whether an infection occurs or not depends on the effectiveness of the immune response to the infectious agent. This, in turn, is dependent on many factors:

+ Nature of the infectious microbe
+ Extent of infection
+ Host factors such as
    □ presence of an immunodeficiency disorder;
    □ use of immunosuppressive therapy; and
    □ infection with viruses, such as human immunodeficiency virus (HIV) that causes immuno-deficiency.
+ Genetic factors, such as major histocompatibility complex (MHC) haplotypes (see Chapter 5)

The immune status of the host is a major factor that determines susceptibility to disease. Immunodeficient patients are particularly prone to infections with certain types of microbes depending on the immunodeficient component (see Chapter 16).

The main focus of this chapter is on how mammalian hosts protect themselves against a diverse range of pathogenic microbes which include viruses, bacteria, parasites, and fungi. The chapter describes the main features of immunity to the four broad categories of infectious agents. Some of the ingenious strategies deployed by microbes to escape host defence mechanisms are discussed. Parasite vaccines with special focus on malarial vaccines and the damaging consequences of infection by pathogens are considered in the later part of the chapter.

Box 12.1   Severe acute respiratory syndrome (SARS): Emergence of a new disease

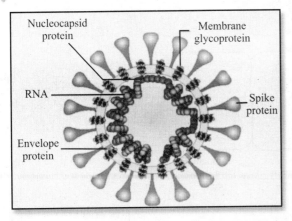

Nucleocapsid protein

Membrane glycoprotein

RNA

Spike protein

Envelope protein

Fig. 12.2   SARS-CoV—the cause of severe acute respiratory syndrome. Surface spike proteins are characteristic of the virus. *Source:* https:/.../kristopher-ulrich--sars-specialist, accessed on 10 July 2010.

Severe acute respiratory syndrome (SARS), a new viral disease, emerged in China in November 2002 in the Guangdong Province. It spread rapidly to many countries due to international mobility, and within weeks the disease had affected over 8,000 people spread over many countries with 774 deaths reported by WHO. The causative agent is a novel coronavirus (CoV)–*SARS-CoV*–having surface spike proteins (S proteins) which give the virus a crown-like appearance (Fig. 12.2); hence, the name. The protein associated with a cellular receptor *angiotensin converting enzyme 2 (ACE2)*, localized mainly in the lung, small intestine, liver, and kidney allowing the virus to gain entry into cells.

The mechanism used by SARS-CoV to gain entry involves membrane fusion similar to that used by human immunodeficiency virus (HIV) envelope glycoproteins and influenza virus haemagglutinin. Although the viral receptor is present on many cell types, the disease caused by the virus is limited to the lungs. Most of our understanding regarding the pathology of SARS has been based on the outbreak in 2002–2003. It presents with an atypical pneumonia characterized by fever, dyspnea, and lymphopenia.

Innate immune mechanisms with natural killer (NK) cells dominating have an important protective role. The virus, however, has the ability to block induction of the antiviral interferon (IFN) response which may be a mechanism of immune evasion by the virus.

It is believed that the disease may have been transmitted to humans from the wet markets which are common in South China. These wet markets, which house many different animals, flourish as the restaurant trade relies on them for supply of various unusual varieties of meat.

In 2005, there was an important finding that a virus from Chinese bats closely resembled SARS-CoV. It was suggested that bats in the wild may be a reservoir from which the virus infected civet cats. Studies have shown that mutations in two amino acids of the civet virus (which does not bind to the human receptor ACE2) converted it to a virulent form that bound to the human receptor with very high affinity. This explains the transmission of the virus to humans from wet markets where civet cats were found to be infected with SARS-CoV.

In preceding chapters, different components that comprise the immune system and the way immune responses are generated have been adequately dealt with. Presumably, by now the reader is well-familiarized with the basic concepts that underlie innate and adaptive immune defences. The chapter commences with immunity to viral infections.

IMMUNITY TO VIRUSES

Viruses are intracellular pathogens that can infect a wide variety of cell populations by using normal cell surface molecules as receptors to gain entry. Epstein–Barr virus (EBV) infects B cells by binding to the complement receptor CR2 on the B cell surface. Human immunodeficiency virus-1 uses the CD4 molecule and chemokine receptors (CCR5/CXCR4) to gain entry into macrophages/T helper cells. Defence mechanisms against viruses are briefly discussed in the following section.

Early Innate Defence Mechanisms against Viruses

The early antiviral innate defences are highly coordinated events and are shown in Fig. 12.3.

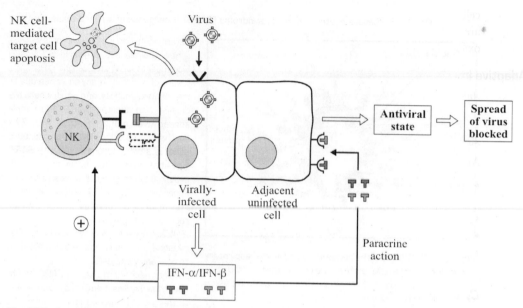

Fig. 12.3 **Innate immune response against virus.** Interferons induce an antiviral state in nearby uninfected cells.

Cytotoxicity of natural killer (NK) cells is enhanced by interferons (IFN), and interleukin-12 (IL-12) released by activated macrophages in response to infection.

Type I Interferons

Interferon-α/interferon-β are antiviral proteins produced by infected cells in response to viral infection. They induce an antiviral state in nearby uninfected cells making them resistant to infection. Many

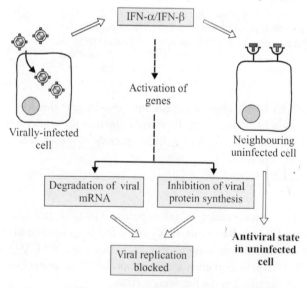

Fig. 12.4 **Activation of intracellular antiviral defences by IFN-α/ IFN-β.** Type I interferons activate genes whose products degrade viral RNA and block viral protein synthesis.

genes are activated which have direct antiviral activity (Fig. 12.4). As IFNs lack specificity, their synthesis in response to one type of viral infection will also protect against other viruses. Interferon-α is in clinical use as an antiviral agent in some forms of viral hepatitis.

Natural Killer Cells

These come into play about 2 days following a viral infection. Natural killer cell-mediated killing of infected cells makes use of the *perforin/ granzyme* mechanism similar to that used by cytotoxic T lymphocytes (CTLs). Natural killer cells differ from CTLs in some important ways which have been referred to in earlier chapters (see Chapters 2 and 9).

By secreting IFN-γ, NK cells activate macrophages which form part of the initial defence against many pathogens. Macrophages have the ability to phagocytose viruses and virus-infected cells and kill them. Potent killing mechanisms, both oxygen-dependent and oxygen-independent, that are detrimental to viruses exist in the phagolysosomes. Tumour necrosis factor-alpha (TNF-α), nitric oxide (NO), and IFN-α are some of the very potent antiviral molecules produced by macrophages.

Adaptive Immune Response to Viral Infection

Antibodies and *CTLs* are important components of the specific antiviral adaptive immune response (Fig. 12.5).

Antibodies

Antibodies exert their antiviral effect in various ways. They

- neutralize free viral particles and so, block their entry into host cells; secretory IgA provides defence at mucosal surfaces by preventing infection of epithelial cells;
- opsonize viruses or infected cells for phagocytosis;
- mediate lysis of virus-infected cells by complement (classical pathway); and
- mediate antibody-dependent cell-mediated cytotoxicity (ADCC) by non-specific immune cells, such as NK cells, macrophages, and neutrophils.

Cytotoxic T Lymphocytes

Once viruses have gained entry into host cells and have established themselves comfortably, a cellular adaptive immune response is needed to cope with the infection. CD8$^+$CTLs are the principal effector cells that operate against virally-infected cells. As they are class I MHC restricted, they can recognize and kill host cells displaying viral peptides in context of class I MHC molecules.

CD4$^+$ T Helper Lymphocytes

T$_H$ cells function in antiviral immunity by

- recruiting macrophages to infected sites and activating them;
- releasing IL-2 which facilitates proliferation and differentiation of B cells, and CTL-precursors (CTL-Ps) to effector cells, and recruiting them to sites of virus infection; and
- facilitating affinity maturation and isotype switching for an optimal antibody response.

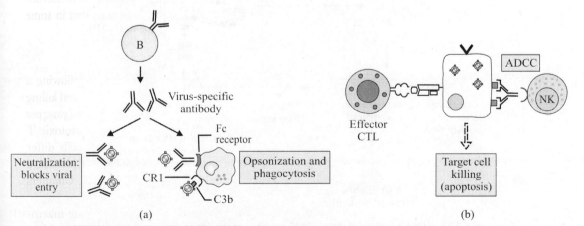

Fig. 12.5 Adaptive immune response against virus. (a) Antibodies prevent viral entry into host cells and opsonize virus (as does complement product C3b) enhancing phagocytosis. (b) Cytotoxic T lymphocytes and NK cells target infected cells.

Evasion of Immune Responses by Viruses

Viruses have evolved many interesting mechanisms by which they escape our immune defences. Some of these are listed in the following text along with illustrative examples.

Antigenic Variation

Human immunodeficiency virus, rhinovirus (the cause of the common cold), and influenza virus change their surface antigens very rapidly due to mutation. Effective immunological memory fails to develop. Antigenic variation in the influenza virus is described in the following section.

Sequestration

Human immunodeficiency virus integrates into host T cell DNA as a provirus and stays hidden from the immune system. It may stay dormant for up to 10–15 years. Some herpes simplex viruses (HSVs) establish themselves in sensory neurons.

Inhibition of Antigen Processing

Herpes simplex virus expresses a protein which binds to the peptide-binding site of transporter associated with antigen processing (TAP). This blocks delivery of peptides to class I MHC molecules in HSV-infected cells. Owing to lack of presentation of viral antigens, CD8$^+$ cytotoxic T cells do not receive activation signals. There are other viruses also which act in different ways (Fig. 12.6).

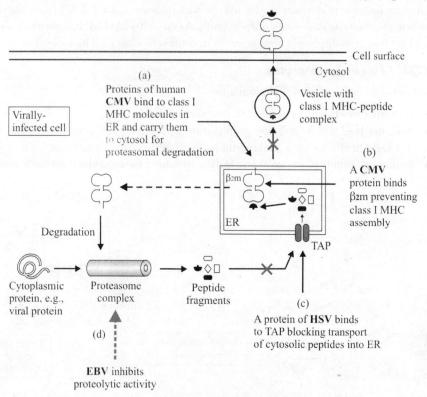

Fig. 12.6   Virus inhibition of class I MHC antigen processing and presentation pathway.
The strategies depicted in the figure help viruses to evade immune responses.
CMV, cytomegalovirus; HSV, herpes simplex virus; EBV, Epstein–Barr virus

Downregulation of Class I MHC Expression

Adenoviruses, shortly after infection, produce a protein that suppresses transcription of class I MHC genes.

Immunosuppression

Epstein–Barr virus which infects B cells produces a protein viral IL-10 (vIL-10) that is homologous to IL-10, a macrophage-suppressive cytokine. The protein suppresses cytokine production by TH1 subset resulting in decreased levels of IL-2, TNF-β, and IFN-γ. Macrophage function and cell-mediated immunity (CMI) are inhibited.

The various evasive strategies described in the preceding text are summarized in Table 12.1.

Table 12.1   Evasion of immune responses by viruses.

Mechanism of evasion	Examples/Comments
Antigenic variation	HIV, rhinovirus, influenza virus
Sequestration	Herpes simplex virus (in sensory neurons), HIV (integrates into host cell DNA)
Inhibition of antigen processing ◆ by blocking peptide-binding site of TAP ◆ by inhibiting proteolytic activity of proteasome	 Herpes simplex virus Epstein–Barr virus
Downregulation of class I MHC expression	Adenovirus
Immunosuppression	Epstein–Barr virus (secretes viral IL-10)

Influenza Virus Continually Varies the Structure of Its Surface Proteins

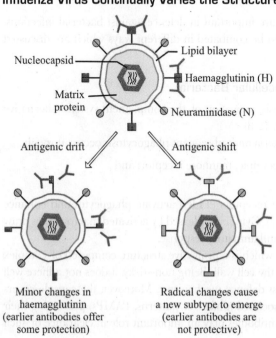

Nucleocapsid — Lipid bilayer

Matrix protein — Haemagglutinin (H)

Neuraminidase (N)

Antigenic drift   Antigenic shift

Minor changes in haemagglutinin (earlier antibodies offer some protection)

Radical changes cause a new subtype to emerge (earlier antibodies are not protective)

Influenza virus, which affects the respiratory system, has three types: A, B, and C. Of these, influenza type A is the most common. It contains two major surface glycoproteins in its outer lipid envelope: *haemagglutinin* (*H*) and *neuraminidase* (*N*). Haemagglutinin enables the virus to attach to cells and is important for inducing protective neutralizing antibodies. The name neuraminidase derives from the fact that it can cleave *N*-acetylneuraminic acid—sialic acid—present in host cell glycoproteins. This facilitates release of newly formed virus from infected cells. Unlike haemagglutinin, neuraminidase does not induce effective humoral immunity.

Fig. 12.7   Antigenic drift and shift in the influenza virus. Antibodies to haemagglutinin are protective. When antigenic drift occurs, antibodies to previous strains may afford some protection. However, in antigenic shift, these earlier antibodies fail to protect causing a pandemic to break out.

Subtypes of type A influenza virus are distinguished by variations in the two surface proteins. The official nomenclature is based on assigning an H number and an N number depending on the type of haemagglutinin and neuraminidase the subtype contains, for example, H1N1, H2N2, H3N2, and so on.

Influenza virus which changes its surface antigens rapidly does so by two processes: *antigenic drift* and *antigenic shift* (Fig. 12.7).

Antigenic drift, a perpetual process, occurs due to minor variations in haemagglutinin caused by point mutations in the viral genome. These minor variations may cause mild disease. Radical changes in haemagglutinin due to exchange of large segments of two different viral genomes is called antigenic shift. These larger changes, which occur occasionally, cause a new subtype to emerge and may occur when, for instance, human and bird influenza viruses infect the same cell, for example, pig cells.

Antigenic shifts cause widespread viral epidemics (pandemics) to break out because earlier antibodies fail to offer protection. Many influenza pandemics due to antigenic shifts in the influenza A virus have been documented, with the 1918 pandemic killing millions of people.

Due to tremendous antigenic variation by influenza virus, it has not been possible to produce an effective vaccine. So, prophylactic vaccination (a preventive strategy) against influenza virus is not possible. Human immunodeficiency virus also shows antigenic variation, even more so than the influenza virus. In such cases, targets of immunization would be the invariant proteins of the virus. Since the emergence of the avian influenza virus (H5N1), which infected humans in Hong Kong in 1997, many other avian influenza viruses such as H9N2 and H793 have emerged. These have crossed the species barrier and are spreading to humans. A new strain of influenza A virus (H1N1) of swine origin, which emerged in Mexico in March/April 2009 and was responsible for the flu pandemic commonly called 'swine flu', is also a cause of grave concern.

IMMUNITY TO BACTERIA

Both innate and adaptive immune responses are important in defence against bacterial infections. Intracellular and extracellular bacteria need to be combated in different ways which are discussed in the following text.

Early Innate Defence Mechanisms against Extracellular Bacteria

Early defence mechanisms include phagocytosis, activation of the complement system (alternative pathway), and the inflammatory response (Fig. 12.8).

Binding of phagocytes to extracellular bacteria and subsequent phagocytosis occurs through

- pattern-recognition receptors (PRRs), for example, mannose receptor; and
- complement receptor for C3b (an opsonin)

It is relevant to mention here that toll-like receptors (TLRs) activate phagocytes and enhance microbicidal killing mechanisms (see Chapter 2). Cytokines released by activated macrophages draw leukocytes to sites of infection amplifying the inflammatory response.

Many bacteria synthesize an outer capsule which is a protective structure composed of complex polysaccharides in a loose gel that lies outside the cell wall. Being non-sticky, it does not adhere well to the phagocyte surface and interferes in host defence mechanisms. Moreover, the capsule covers surface carbohydrate molecules (pathogen-associated molecular patterns, PAMPs) preventing their recognition by phagocyte receptors (PRRs). Antibodies play an important role in clearance of such

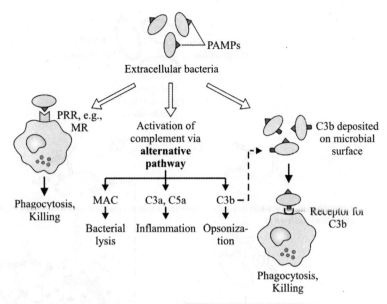

Fig. 12.8 Innate immune response to extracellular bacteria.

encapsulated bacteria (Fig. 12.9). Presence of the capsule often prevents insertion of lytic C5b-9 membrane attack complex (MAC) into bacterial cell membranes.

Cell surface properties of bacteria are important determinants of the type of immune response triggered. Gram-positive and Gram-negative bacteria, which differ in cell wall and membrane composition, respond differently to complement (Fig. 12.10). The thick peptidoglycan layer of Gram-positive organisms prevents insertion of lytic C5b-9 MAC into cell membranes, whereas Gram-negative organisms are lysed by MAC. It should be recalled from Chapter 2 that lipopolysaccharide (LPS) of Gram-negative bacteria is recognized by TLR-4 on antigen-presenting cells (APCs) and represents a danger signal that alerts the immune system.

Adaptive Immune Response to Extracellular Bacteria

In adaptive immunity, antibodies represent the major defence mechanism against extracellular bacteria and their toxins. Antibody-mediated defence mechanisms are summarized in the following text:

- Neutralization of bacteria and their toxins
- Opsonization and enhancement of phagocytosis
- Complement activation (via classical pathway)

Besides antibodies, TH cells have a key role to play. They are activated by protein antigens to release cytokines that help B cells to produce antibodies, activate macrophages, and stimulate inflammatory responses (Fig. 12.11).

Intracellular Bacteria

Although *innate defences* such as phagocytes, both neutrophils and macrophages, and NK cells have a role in controlling infection by intracellular bacteria, elimination of infection requires *adaptive cell-mediated immune responses* in which TH cells have a key role. Acquired immunodeficiency syndrome (AIDS) patients show increased susceptibility to infection by intracellular bacteria as due to depletion of T helper cells, CMI is compromised is such patients.

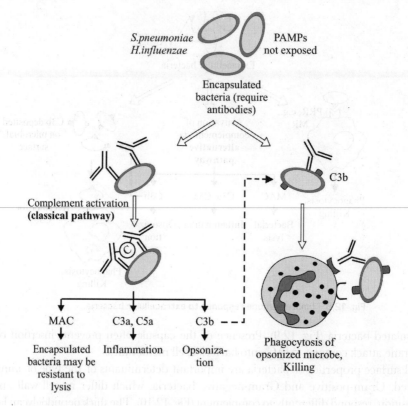

Fig. 12.9 Adaptive immune response to extracellular (encapsulated) bacteria.

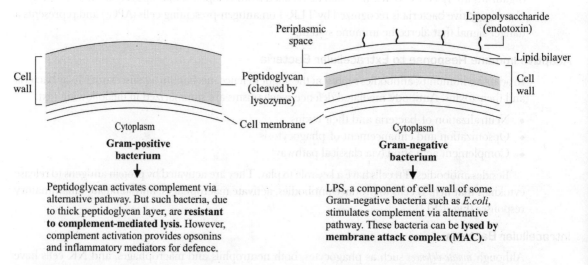

Fig. 12.10 Gram-positive and Gram-negative bacteria respond differently to complement-mediated lysis. The cell wall of *E. coli*, a Gram-negative bacterium, contains LPS which is a potent stimulator of innate immunity.

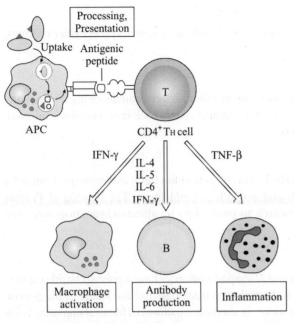

Fig. 12.11 Activation of CD4⁺ T cells by extracellular bacteria.

The major types of cell-mediated immune reactions which have been described earlier in Chapter 9 include

- activation of macrophages by TH1 cells to kill phagocytosed microbes and
- cytotoxic T lymphocyte-mediated killing of infected cells.

It is once again emphasized here that the TH2 subset responds to helminths which are not easily engulfed.

Both CD4⁺ and CD8⁺ T cells cooperate with each other in protecting against intracellular pathogens such as *Listeria monocytogenes* (a food-borne intracellular microbe and the cause of one type of meningitis), a bacterium that survives in macrophages (Fig. 12.12). Cell-mediated immune responses are also important in defence against *Mycobacterium tuberculosis*. This is discussed in a section that follows along with other key features of TB infection.

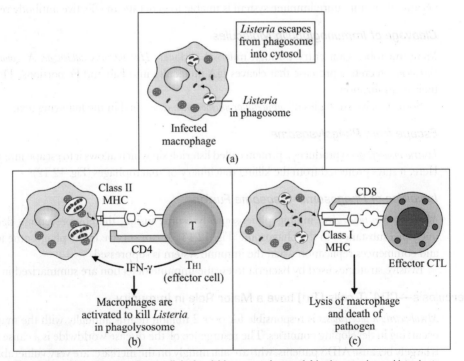

Fig. 12.12 *Listeria* grows intracellularly within macrophages. (a) In the cytoplasm, *Listeria* stays protected from bactericidal activity of macrophages. (b) and (c) Elimination of infection by *Listeria* requires participation of both TH cells and CTLs.

Evasion of Immune Responses by Bacteria

Some evasive strategies of *extracellular bacteria*, which have briefly been introduced in earlier chapters, are listed in the following section.

Antigenic Variation

Escherichia coli and *Neisseria gonorrhoeae* vary the structure of outer surface proteins giving rise to many different strains. As a 'new' antigen is presented to the immune system each time a person is infected, only primary immune responses are mounted.

Fc Binding

Protein A from some staphylococci binds to the Fc tails of antibodies (IgG) and prevents them from binding to Fc receptors on phagocytic cells and activating complement. The binding of Protein A to IgG is exploited in immunological research to purify IgG by affinity chromatography (see Appendix 1).

Encapsulation

Many bacteria such as *Streptococcus pneumoniae* and *Haemophilus influenzae* have a polysaccharide capsule that has anti-phagocytic properties. It protects the pathogen from ingestion and killing by phagocytic cells and also interferes with complement activation (via alternative pathway). Humoral immunity is the major defence against such bacteria. Antibodies can promote phagocytosis directly through Fc receptors or indirectly by activating complement. Infants are very prone to infection with encapsulated bacteria because their immature immune system is unable to generate an effective antibody response.

Cleavage of Immunoglobulin Molecules

Many microbes gain entry through mucosal surfaces. *Haemophilus influenzae*, *N. gonorrhoeae*, and *S. pneumoniae* secrete a protease that cleaves IgA molecules into Fab and Fc portions. This interferes in their neutralization.

Some evasive strategies of *intracellular microbes* are described in the following text:

Escape from Phagolysosome

Listeria monocytogenes produces a protein called listeriolysin which allows it to escape into the cytoplasm. Here, it stays protected from the killing machinery of macrophages (Fig. 12.12).

Inhibition of Phagosome–Lysosome Fusion

Mycobacterium tuberculosis inhibits phagosome–lysosome fusion, thereby preventing delivery of anti-microbial substances to the phagosome (Fig. 12.13). It can survive in the phagosome for many years and commences replication when the immune system is suppressed.

Evasive strategies used by bacteria to escape immune detection are summarized in Table 12.2.

Tuberculosis—CD4⁺ T cells (TH1) have a Major Role in Immunity

Mycobacterium tuberculosis is responsible for over 2 million deaths annually with the majority of cases occurring in developing countries. The resurgence of the disease worldwide is a cause of concern. It is largely because AIDS patients, who are alarmingly on the increase, are very vulnerable to infection. This is seen especially in areas where number of HIV-infected people is large, such as South Africa. Here, co-infection with *M. tuberculosis* and HIV is very common. Another cause is the emergence of drug-resistant strains.

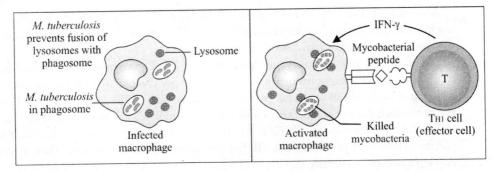

Fig. 12.13   CMI against intracellular infection by mycobacteria. Inter £ron-gamma released by activated TH1 cells activates macrophages to release reactive oxygen intermediates (ROIs) and nitric oxide that kill the mycobacteria, though they are not completely eliminated.

Table 12.2   Evasion of immune responses by bacteria.

Mechanism of evasion	Examples/comments
Extracellular Antigenic variation	*Escherichia coli* *Neisseria gonorrhoeae*
Fc binding	*Staphylococci* (protein A inhibits binding of antibody to Fc receptors, and complement activation)
Encapsulation	*Streptococcus pneumoniae* *Haemophilus influenzae* (resist phagocytosis)
Cleavage of Ig molecules	*Neisseria gonorrhoeae*
Intracellular Escape from phagolysosome into cytoplasm Inhibition of phagosome–lysosome fusion	*Listeria monocytogenes* *Mycobacterium tuberculosis*

Infection by *M. tuberculosis* occurs by the respiratory route. Alveolar macrophages phagocytose the inhaled bacilli, but as the bacteria inhibit phagolysosome formation, they survive and multiply intracellularly. However, TH1 cells , on recognition of mycobacterial peptides complexed to class II MHC molecules on the macrophage surface, deliver signals that induce lysosomal fusion and activate killing mechanisms (Fig. 12.13).

As the pathogen is not completely eliminated, there is chronic stimulation of macrophages by T helper cells and granuloma formation occurs. Granulomas, which have been described earlier in Chapter 9, are a collection of activated lymphocytes and macrophages with fibrosis and tissue necrosis around the microbe (see Fig. 9.6). Infection by *M. tuberculosis* does not usually lead to active disease and only approximately 10 per cent of infected individuals develop clinical symptoms (chronic pulmonary tuberculosis). This is because within a granuloma, T cells activate macrophages to kill the mycobacteria, or suppress proliferation so that infection is contained, though the pathogen is dormant and is not eliminated. The chronic granulomatous inflammation that occurs is a type IV hypersensitivity reaction (see Chapter 14) and is the cause of immunopathology seen in the disease. Re-activation of viable organisms inside granulomas may cause them to rupture and spread infection to other tissues severely impairing their functioning. Some factors that allow re-activation of dormant bacilli include infection with HIV as in AIDS patients, and immunosuppressive therapy.

Activation of TH1 cells and recruitment of macrophages forms the basis of a recall or memory test in which purified protein derivative (PPD) from *M. tuberculosis* is injected into the skin. The test is used to assess immunity to *M. tuberculosis* (see Chapter 14).

Cell wall *of M. tuberculosis* is rich in lipids. Some γδ T cells recognize mycobacterial lipid antigens which associate with non-polymorphic CD1 molecules (see Chapter 5). This is unlike the conventional recognition by T cells of antigenic peptides associated with MHC molecules on cell surfaces. The extent to which these cells function in protective immunity to TB is not well understood.

Bacillus Calmette-Guerin (BCG) is an attenuated strain of *Mycobacterium bovis* that is used as a vaccine to immunize people against TB. But as it shows varied effectiveness, efforts are underway to develop a new more effective vaccine.

IMMUNITY TO PROTOZOA AND WORMS

Parasitic infections, which include the single-celled protozoa and multicellular worms, pose a major threat to health in tropical countries, particularly in the developing world. Malaria is a widespread disease and infection by intestinal worms affects billions of people. Worm infections in children result in stunted growth, anaemia, and slowing down of mental development. Malnutrition exacerbates disease severity. Some major parasites are listed in Table 12.3.

Table 12.3　Some parasites and the diseases they cause.

Parasite	Disease
Protozoan	
Trypanosoma brucei	African sleeping sickness (trypanosomiasis)
Entamoeba histolytica	Amoebic dysentery
Trypanosoma cruzi	Chagas disease
Plasmodium spp.	Malaria
Toxoplasma gondii	Toxoplasmosis
Leishmania donovani	Kala azar
Leishmania braziliensis	Leishmaniasis
Roundworm	
Wuchereria bancrofti	Filariasis
Trichinella spiralis	Trichinosis
Flatworm	
Schistosoma mansoni	Schistosomiasis

The immune response stimulated by parasites depends on the individual parasite, its location, and on the developmental stage. Both innate and adaptive mechanisms are activated. But as innate immunity is weak and parasites have devised various ways of evading adaptive immune responses, infections are generally chronic.

Innate Immune Response

The major innate defence mechanism against protozoan parasites is phagocytosis. Trypanosomes stimulate the alternative pathway of complement, and are phagocytosed by neutrophils and macrophages. However, some parasites resist killing mechanisms and are able to survive and even replicate within the interior of phagocytes.

Adaptive Immune Response

Parasites in blood (amoeba and trypanosomes) stimulate antibody production, whereas those residing inside cells (*Toxoplasma* and *Leishmania)* activate a cell-mediated immune response. By secreting IFN-γ, TH1 cells activate macrophages to kill parasites that have been phagocytosed.

Helminthic infections are dominated by a TH2 response which is characterized by generation of *IgE antibodies* and *eosinophilia*. As seen in earlier chapters, major cytokines involved in a TH2 response include IL-4, IL-5, IL-6, IL-10, and IL-13. Interleukin-4 provides help to B cells and stimulates production of IgE, whereas IL-5 is an activator of eosinophils. Immunoglobulin-E has a major protective role in infection by helminths. Serum levels are found to be elevated enormously from a normal value of about 50 ng ml^{-1} to 10,000 ng ml^{-1}.

Immunoglobulin-E has the unique ability of binding to high-affinity FcεRs expressed on mast cells and basophils. Immunoglobulin-E bound to cells can be retained on the surface for long periods of time. Cross-linking of IgE by worm antigens activates mast cells to degranulate and release the contents of their granules. Histamine is a major mediator which increases vascular permeability causing serum components such as IgG to leak out from the blood vessels. Eosinophils also are drawn to the site of worm infestation due to chemotactic effects of *eosinophil chemotactic factor-A (ECF-A)* released by mast cells. Eosinophils are stimulated to degranulate on binding to IgE/IgG-coated worms by their Fc receptors or by complement products generated due to triggering of alternative pathway by helminths. The main toxic proteins released from granules are *major basic protein (MBP)* and *eosinophil cationic protein (ECP)*. These, along with other toxic constituents, cause considerable damage to the worm. Extracellular killing is thus important in worm infections (Fig. 12.14).

Expulsion of helminthic worms from the intestine is facilitated by

- mast cell-mediated increase in intestinal motility and diarrhoea and
- secretion of mucus by cytokine-activated goblet cells.

Unfortunately, the reactions described in the preceding text which evolved to defend against worm infections can also produce very severe adverse reactions of type I or immediate hypersensitivity (see Chapter 14).

Although parasites stimulate various immune defence mechanisms in their host, they present a major medical problem as immune responses are often ineffective.

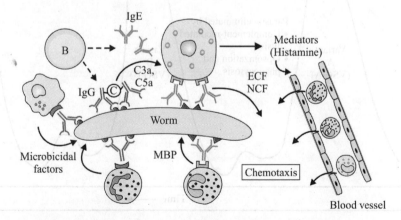

Fig. 12.14   Protective mechanisms against helminths. Immunoglobulin-E, mast cells, and eosinophils have a major role to play NCF, neutrophil chemotactic factor.

Evasion of Immune Responses by Parasites

Some major ways by which parasites escape detection by the host immune system are summarized in the text that follows.

Antigen Masking

Schistosoma mansoni covers its surface with various host proteins such as human leukocyte antigen (HLA) proteins and also ABO blood group substances. Thus, it appears as self and is not recognized as foreign.

Antigenic Variation

Trypanosoma brucei, which causes African sleeping sickness, is able to change its *variant surface glycoprotein* (*VSG*) throughout life. New variants that arise are unaffected by antibodies to previous variants. Thus by producing escape variants, trypanosomes cause chronic infection (Fig. 12.15).

Shedding of Surface Antigens

Plasmodium falciparum, *S. mansoni*, and *Leishmania* spp. shed their surface antigens abundantly. Shed antigens bind to antibodies and block their interaction with the parasite. In other words, immune complexes act as blocking factors.

Inactivation of Complement

Leishmania is able to escape complement-mediated lysis by a unique mechanism. It is able to detach C5b-9 complexes from its surface before MAC disrupts membrane integrity by creating pores in its membrane. *Trypanosoma cruzi* produces proteins that functionally mimic decay accelerating factor (DAF), a regulatory protein that functions to inhibit the complement cascade.

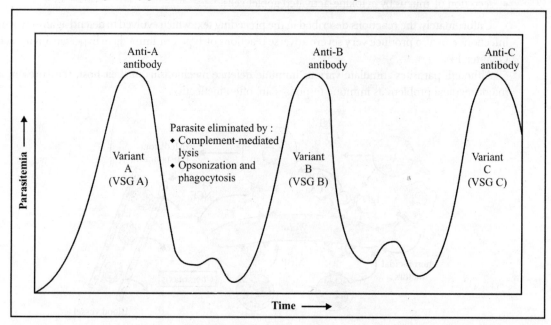

Fig. 12.15 Antigenic variation during chronic trypanosome infection. Antibodies induced by variant A fail to protect against variant B which switches to a new VSG. Hence, it escapes the previous antibody response. As this is a continued process, the organism is not cleared from the blood.

Cleavage of Immunoglobulin Molecules

Trypanosoma cruzi and also roundworms secrete proteases that degrade antibodies.

Immunosuppression

Parasites may suppress T cell subsets to their advantage. *Wuchereria bancrofti*, the agent that causes filariasis, suppresses the TH2 subset in infected people. Such people are thus, unable to mount a protective IgE and eosinophil-associated immune response.

Table 12.4 summarizes some of the evasive strategies that parasites use to escape immune detection.

Table 12.4   Evasion of immune responses by parasites.

Mechanism of evasion	Examples
Antigen masking	*Schistosoma mansoni*
Antigenic variation	*Trypanosoma brucei*
Shedding of surface antigens	*Plasmodium falciparum* and *Schistosoma mansoni*
Inactivation of complement	*Leishmania* spp. and *Trypanosoma cruzi*
Cleavage of Ig molecules	*Trypanosoma cruzi*
Immunosuppression	*Wuchereria bancrofti*

Malaria is a Major Cause of Mortality Worldwide

Malaria caused by *Plasmodium* spp. and transmitted to humans by female anopheles is the most widespread parasitic disease. There are various species of *Plasmodium* that cause malaria in humans, of which *P. falciparum* is the most deadly.

There are approximately 500 million cases annually with 1–2 million deaths, largely young children, every year. Most of the deaths occur in sub-Saharan Africa, the region worst affected by the disease. It is characterized by headache, fever, sweating, chills, and gastrointestinal symptoms. If untreated, the disease can progress to cerebral malaria, anaemia, severe organ failure, and death.

There are various stages in the life cycle of *Plasmodium*—from sporozoite to merozoite to gametocyte —each with its own specific antigens (Fig. 12.16). Bite of an infected female anopheles mosquito injects sporozoites into the dermis which then travel to the liver after penetrating capillaries. Parasites multiply intracellularly for about a week causing infected hepatocytes to rupture releasing merozoites which invade still more red blood cells (RBCs). Some merozoites develop into male and female gametocytes within red cells (sexual reproductive phase). These are taken up by a mosquito during a blood meal. Fertilization occurs in the mosquito gut, forming a zygote and eventually immature sporozoites which travel to the salivary glands where they mature to continue the life cycle.

The pathology in malaria that leads to conditions such as cerebral malaria and anaemia are linked to the erythrocyte stage (Box 12.2).

Host Immune Response to Plasmodium

Immune response mounted by the host against the parasite is complex and poorly understood. The sporozoite is the stage most accessible to antibodies, but it is brief as it takes the sporozoites only about 30 minutes to reach the liver. Even if an antibody response is activated, it is ineffective as the protozoan sheds off its surface *circumsporozoite (CS) protein*. This protein mediates adhesion of sporozoites to liver

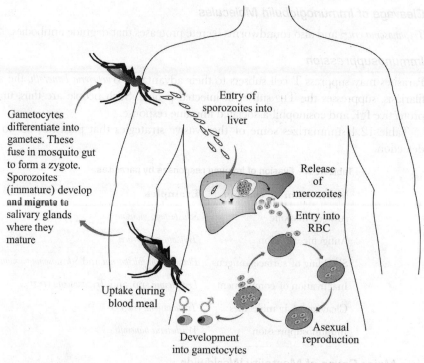

Fig. 12.16 Life cycle of the malarial parasite.

Gametocytes differentiate into gametes. These fuse in mosquito gut to form a zygote. Sporozoites (immature) develop and migrate to salivary glands where they mature

Entry of sporozoites into liver

Release of merozoites

Entry into RBC

Uptake during blood meal

Asexual reproduction

Development into gametocytes

Box 12.2   Pathology in malaria is associated with the erythrocyte stage

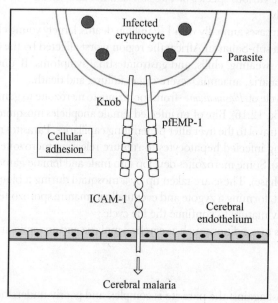

Infected erythrocyte

Parasite

Knob

pfEMP-1

Cellular adhesion

ICAM-1

Cerebral endothelium

Cerebral malaria

Fig. 12.17   *P. falciparum* infected erythrocyte. Infected erythrocytes express the parasite protein pfEMP-1 on their surface. Interaction of this protein with ICAM-1 on cerebral endothelium leads to cerebral malaria.

Plasmodium falciparum erythrocyte membrane protein-1 (*PfEMP-1*), an adhesin, is expressed on the erythrocyte membrane when *P. falciparum* merozoites invade RBCs. It can bind to CR1, a receptor for complement protein C3b, on other infected and uninfected erythrocytes causing red cells to cluster (rosette formation) and agglutinate. It is interesting that the parasite can express many different PfEMP-1 proteins allowing cellular adhesion with various receptors on many different cell types. For instance, binding to receptors on vascular endothelial cells causes sequestration of infected erythrocytes in blood vessels in various tissues leading to obstruction of blood vessels. This can lead to cerebral malaria (Fig. 12.17) in which the patient may lapse into coma, and can also damage many organs leading to organ failure and finally death. Thus, sequestration and agglutination associated with the erythrocyte stage are correlated with much of the pathology seen in malaria. The hepatic phase, however, is short and asymptomatic.

cells. A big obstacle in the design of antimalarial vaccines is that antibodies generated against the sporozoite stage do not react with the erythrocyte stage.

Much of the life cycle of *Plasmodium* is intracellular in RBCs which lack MHC expression, and in liver hepatocytes which express class I MHC molecules. As erythrocytes lack MHC molecules, CTLs do not kill infected erythrocytes but they are protective during the hepatic stage. They recognize malarial sporozoite antigens displayed on the hepatocyte surface associated with class I MHC molecules and kill infected cells by inducing apoptosis (via granzymes and Fas ligand). For optimal protection by CTLs, help from TH cells is essential. There are various factors that regulate CMI but these are not well defined.

Malaria Vaccines

As malaria and also other parasite infections (such as schistosomiasis, leishmaniasis, and sleeping sickness) cause considerable morbidity, and frequent chemotherapy due to continued exposure in those living in endemic areas is not a feasible approach, there is an urgent need to develop prophylactic vaccines. Unfortunately, there are many hurdles in the way of malarial vaccine development which include the following.

1. There are four species of the parasite which are antigenically distinct.
2. The parasite has a complex life cycle involving different stages.
3. The three different forms of the parasite, namely, sporozoites, merozoites, and gametes, are each antigenically distinct from the other; immunization with antigens derived from a particular stage induces immunity only to that stage.
4. Sporozoites and merozoites very rapidly infect liver cells and RBCs, respectively, and are exposed to the immune system for a very brief period.
5. The parasite has evolved various strategies to evade the immune system, for example, by changing its surface antigens.

In view of the above-mentioned obstacles faced by vaccinologists, malaria vaccines have not been easy to develop. However, they continue to be an area of active investigation, especially as strains resistant to drugs, such as chloroquine (and other antimalarials) are emerging. In spite of major challenges, some advances have been made which is encouraging. A combination strategy targeting distinct antigens at different stages of the parasite life cycle is an attractive approach.

As the life cycle of the parasite is complex, there are various targets for vaccination. Invariant antigens of the initial sporozoite stage induce blocking antibodies and are most desirable, as they would prevent infection. Other targets that are well characterized and that are attractive vaccine candidates include *merozoite surface proteins (MSPs)*. Although these proteins exhibit polymorphism, each parasite expresses only one allele. Antibodies to recombinant *MSP-1*, *MSP-2*, and *MSP-3* have been shown to block merozoite invasion of RBCs (blocking antibodies). When children were immunized with this blood stage vaccine, there was a reduction in the parasite load. Parasitized RBCs (pRBCs) express *pfEMP-1* (Fig. 12.17) which has attracted a lot of attention. But 60 variant gene copies occur in each parasite and parasites are able to switch to expression of a different molecule. This extensive antigenic polymorphism is unfortunate and is a big obstacle in the way of designing a vaccine to prevent malaria development. The sexual stage and blocking of transmission are also promising targets for vaccine development.

IMMUNITY TO FUNGI

Protective immune responses to fungi and yeasts, unlike immune responses to bacteria and viruses, are poorly defined. Early innate defences involve neutrophils and macrophages. They phagocytose fungi for intracellular killing and release antimicrobial substances such as reactive oxygen intermediates (ROIs) and lysosomal enzymes. Fungi infecting humans may live extracellularly or in intracellular compartments. Hence, both antibody-mediated and cell-mediated immune responses are induced. Cytokines secreted by TH1 cells activate intracellular killing mechanisms similar to those activated by intracellular bacteria. Protective immunity mediated by TH1 cells and macrophages appears to play a more dominant role than humoral responses. Host tissue injury due to granulomatous inflammation may occur in some intracellular fungal infections, such as by *Histoplasma capsulatum* that resides inside macrophages.

Opportunistic fungal infections such as by *Candida albicans* cause severe disease in immunodeficient individuals. With AIDS-afflicted people alarmingly on the rise, the number of immunocompromised hosts has also risen and opportunistic fungal infections are common. *Candida albicans* infection is also seen to occur frequently in recipients of organ transplants on immunosuppressive therapy and those on corticosteroid or cancer chemotherapy. Administration of antifungals to transplant recipients on cyclosporin can give rise to serious side effects. This is because antifungals are potent inhibitors of hepatic cytochrome P-450 enzymes which metabolize cyclosporin (a drug that is nephrotoxic). Cyclosporin which remains unmetabolized causes severe nephrotoxicity.

SOME DAMAGING CONSEQUENCES OF INFECTION BY PATHOGENS

Sometimes pathogens fail to be eliminated by the host. They persist and enter into an extended chronic phase during which the immune response is continually activated. This can cause considerable damage to host tissues. Various causes for damage are discussed in the following text.

Immune Complexes

As antigens are shed in abundance by persisting pathogens, there is formation of large quantities of immune complexes. Erythrocytes which express complement receptors on their surface have a major role in carrying immune complexes to the liver and spleen where they are phagocytosed by macrophages (Fig. 12.18). But when the scavenging capacity of macrophages is exceeded, or when

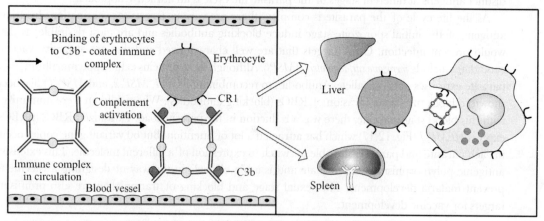

Fig. 12.18 Erythrocytes help in clearance of circulating immune complexes. Erythrocytes carry C3b-coated immune complexes bound to complement receptors on their surface to liver and spleen where these complexes are phagocytosed by macrophages.

immune complexes are too small, they tend to deposit in blood vessels and organs, particularly kidney glomeruli. The inflammatory response that ensues due to increased complement activation by immune complexes causes damage and interferes in the functioning of the organ.

Excessive Cytokines

Cytokines when produced in excess can be highly toxic to the host (see Chapter 7). *Septic shock* is a severe pathologic consequence that occurs in infections by Gram-negative bacteria. Cell wall endotoxins, for example, LPS stimulate macrophages to overproduce IL-1 and TNF-α. Their increased level causes septic shock. Symptoms are severe and include a drop in blood pressure (BP), fever, and widespread blood clotting in various organs. *Superantigens*, such as enterotoxins of staphylococci, stimulate massive T cell proliferation. Activated T cells release abundant cytokines including TNF-β and then die by apoptosis leading to loss of important immune cells. Excess TNF production by T cells also produces symptoms similar to septic shock.

Autoimmune Reactions

Sometimes antibodies induced against a pathogen cross-react with host tissues, particularly when microbial antigens resemble self-antigens (*molecular mimicry*). For example, antibodies to antigens of streptococci (causes throat infections) cross-react with heart valve antigens resulting in the disease rheumatic fever (see Fig. 15.18).

Immunosuppression

Immunosuppression occurs frequently in parasite diseases and leads to increased susceptibility to bacterial and viral infections. There is a strong link between malaria and Burkitt's lymphoma (a lymphoproliferative disorder). This is because the host, infected by the malarial parasite, is unable to mount an effective protective response to EBV. The virus produces a protein vIL-10, a homologue of IL-10 (a macrophage-suppressive cytokine), which is responsible for the immunosuppression.

Granuloma Formation

Some intracellular bacteria, such as *M. tuberculosis*, are resistant to killing mechanisms in phagocytes. Such bacteria persist for long periods causing chronic antigenic stimulation, and T cell and macrophage activation. A *granuloma* is formed around the persisting microbe which serves to localize the microbe and prevent its spread (see Fig. 9.6). There is tissue injury and inflammation due to overactivity of the immune system, referred to as the delayed-type hypersensitivity (DTH) response.

SUMMARY

+ Host defence mechanisms afford protection against various types of infectious agents. The nature of the pathogen is an important determinant of the type of immune response stimulated.
+ Innate antiviral defences include interferons, NK cells, and macrophages, whereas antibodies and CTLs are important components of the specific adaptive immune response.
+ Extracellular bacteria can be eliminated by complement-mediated lysis in presence of or without antibodies, and by phagocytosis. A CMI

response dependent on CD4+ TH1 cells (and also CTLs) is mounted against intracellular bacteria.
+ Parasitic diseases include those caused by single-celled protozoa and multicellular worms. These are a big threat to health, especially in the tropics and the developing world. Many cause chronic infection and have complex life cycles with stage-specific antigens.
+ The type of defence mechanism activated in parasite infections depends on the particular parasite, its location, and developmental stage.

Innate mechanisms are often weak and ineffective. Parasites in the blood stimulate antibody production, whereas those residing in cells activate a cell-mediated immune response.

◆ It is difficult to achieve protection against helminths due to their large size and complexity. Eosinophilia and increased levels of IgE (TH2 responses) are characteristic features of worm infections.

◆ Immune responses to fungal infections are not well understood. Neutrophils and macrophages are the major effectors in early defence. Both cell-mediated and antibody-mediated immune responses occur.

◆ Microbes avoid recognition and destruction by the immune system in various ways. Evasion strategies generally aim at concealment from immune system components or disrupting the immune response.

◆ The immune response itself may be the cause of considerable tissue injury (immunopathology). Chronic persistence of bacterial and parasite antigens leads to granuloma formation, whereas response to some bacterial and viral antigens may trigger autoimmune reactions. Excess formation of immune complexes and overproduction of cytokines also cause damage.

REVIEW QUESTIONS

1. Indicate whether the following statements are true or false. If false, explain why.
   (a) LPS, an exotoxin, is a potent stimulator of macrophages.
   (b) Most of the pathology seen in malaria is linked to the hepatic stage.
   (c) Antigenic shift in influenza virus involves point mutations in the viral genome.
   (d) A TH2 response protects against mycobacterial infections.
   (e) Increased serum IgE levels characterize extracellular bacterial infections.
   (f) Neutralization of a toxin by an antibody is termed attenuation.

2. Self-assessment questions
   (a) Recognition of a protein antigen by B cells does not require MHC. Do you think that a humoral antibody response to the protein antigen injected into mice would be affected by the MHC type? Give reasons to support your answer.
   (b) Can you explain why both CD4$^+$ and CD8$^+$ T cells are needed to protect against *Plasmodium* infection? Are erythrocytes infected by parasites lysed by cytotoxic T cells? Why or why not?
   (c) It was observed experimentally that when mice were treated with specific antibodies to interferons (IFNs), susceptibility to viral infection increased. Explain this observation highlighting the role of interferons.
   (d) What are some of the major obstacles in the way of vaccine development against parasites?

Explain with special emphasis on malarial vaccines.
   (e) How does the host immune system respond to infection by parasitic worms? What strategies do parasites use to avoid being detected by the host?

3. For each question, choose the *best* answer.
   (a) Which of the following is not an evasive strategy used by pathogens to escape the immune system?
   (i) Antigenic variation
   (ii) Molecular mimicry
   (iii) Increasing complement activation
   (iv) Inhibiting phagocytosis
   (b) Viral and bacterial attachment to mucosal surfaces is prevented by
   (i) IgE
   (ii) IgG
   (iii) Defensins
   (iv) Secretory IgA
   (c) Which cytokine pair is particularly important in defence against *M. tuberculosis* infection?
   (i) IL-10 + IL-4
   (ii) IL-4 + IL-6
   (iii) IL-12 + IFN-γ
   (iv) IL-6 + IL-1
   (d) Major basic protein, a product toxic to helminths, is produced by
   (i) Macrophages
   (ii) NK cells
   (iii) Eosinophils
   (iv) Neutrophils

Vaccination and Vaccine Strategies

13

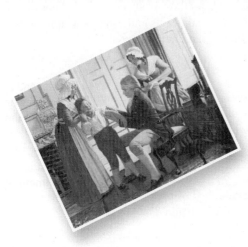

LEARNING OBJECTIVES

Having studied this chapter, you should be able to understand the following:

♦ Use of IVIG and xeno-antisera in passive immunization
♦ The principle behind immunization and how immunological memory protects against re-infection with the same pathogen
♦ Current (whole microorganisms/toxoids/polysaccharides) and developing (anti-idiotype/recombinant vector/DNA/synthetic peptide) approaches to vaccine development
♦ Potential benefits and limitations of various vaccine approaches
♦ That adjuvants administered with vaccines enhance their immunogenicity
♦ The novel approaches being developed for delivery of antigens.
♦ The need for vaccines that stimulate both humoral and cell-mediated immunity

It was the Chinese and the Turks who in the fifteenth century tried to induce immunity to smallpox caused by variola virus. They used a technique called *variolation* in which dried crusts obtained from smallpox pustules were inhaled (see Chapter 1). The credit goes to Edward Jenner for his contribution towards developing an approach for manipulating the immune response by which the patient's own immune system was activated to induce protective immunity. Jenner used cowpox virus (vaccinia) to immunize people against smallpox. Thus, the term *vaccination* was coined (from the Latin word *vacca* meaning 'cow') for the process of inducing acquired immunity. Another big success followed with Pasteur's vaccine against chicken cholera and development of the concepts of *attenuation*. The greatest achievement was when World Health Organization (WHO) announced in 1980 that smallpox had been globally eradicated.

Immunization has now become a very important public health measure. Improvements in sanitation along with vaccination have led to a dramatic reduction in deaths due to infectious diseases. This is seen particularly in those areas of the world where vaccines are available and adequate vaccination programmes are underway. Vaccines for many childhood illnesses are now available, and development of new vaccines continues to be the primary desirable goal in immunology.

Some major problems remain which include the following:

♦ Non-availability of vaccines for some major diseases, such as human immunodeficiency virus (HIV) and malaria; an improved vaccine for tuberculosis is also needed

♦ Failure to eradicate even those diseases for which vaccines are available; it is not an easy task to deliver vaccines to all regions of the world

Unfortunately, millions of children (mostly below 5 years of age) die from infectious diseases each year throughout the world especially in underdeveloped countries. Some infectious diseases which cause significant mortality include whooping cough, diphtheria, measles, and different types of diarrhoea. It is essential that immunization programmes be made more intensive for which tremendous effort is required.

This chapter includes a discussion on passive and active immunization and the principle behind vaccination. The range of vaccines currently being used and those being developed along with their advantages and disadvantages are described. The use of adjuvants and some new approaches for antigen delivery are briefly introduced in the concluding part of the chapter.

TYPES OF IMMUNITY—PASSIVE AND ACTIVE

Broadly, immunity can be of two types: *natural* or *acquired*. Natural or inborn immunity is present even in absence of infection. Phagocytic cells which engulf microbes and help in their elimination form an important part of natural defence mechanisms. There are many more inborn mechanisms which have been introduced in the earlier chapters. Acquired immunity can be *passive* or *active* (Fig. 13.1).

Passive Immunity

Passive immunity in an unprotected individual is established by preformed antibodies which can be acquired *naturally* or *artificially*. Natural passive immunity is acquired by

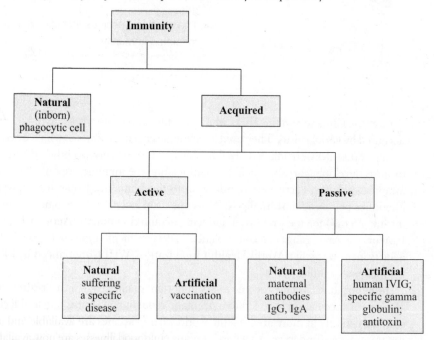

Fig. 13.1   Types of immunity.

- transport of maternal immunoglobulin-G (IgG) antibodies to the foetus via the placenta; and
- transport of IgA antibodies to newborn infants via colostrum and mother's milk; these afford protection against microbes in the gut.

Artificial passive immunity can be acquired in various ways (Table 13.1).

Table 13.1   Passive immunization. The preparations used to acquire passive immunity and the conditions in which they are used are shown.

Preparation	Disease/Condition
Pooled human IVIG	Mumps, measles, and hepatitis A
Specific gamma globulins (hyperimmune sera)	Varicella, hepatitis B, pertussis, rabies, mumps, and tetanus
Horse antitoxin	Snake bites, spider bites, botulism, diphtheria, and tetanus

Pooled Human Intravenous Immune Globulin (IVIG)

This is human IgG prepared from plasma pooled from many healthy blood donors. It contains antibodies to many pathogens that the donors have encountered.

Specific Gamma Globulins (Hyperimmune Sera)

These can be recovered from the sera of patients who are convalescing from a particular disease, such as hepatitis B. Specific antibodies to causative agents of other diseases can be obtained similarly from patients. Sera of vaccinated individuals also, such as those who have received a vaccine for mumps, rabies, or varicella (chickenpox), will contain high titres of antibodies specific for the disease.

Horse Antitoxin

These are antibodies to toxins which cause diseases, such as tetanus, diphtheria, and botulism. They are prepared by immunizing large animals such as horses with the toxin and then recovering the antitoxin antibodies from the serum of the immunized animal.

Passive immunization provides immediate protection to a non-immune individual. However, some serious drawbacks of passive immunization include the following:

1. Horse antitoxins being foreign proteins (*xeno-antisera*) stimulate an immune response which can give rise to complications termed *serum sickness*. Immune complexes increase in the patient's circulation giving rise to a type III hypersensitivity reaction (see Chapter 14). The problem can be avoided by use of antibodies of human origin.
2. As these antibodies are catabolized and gradually removed from the circulation, they are effective for only a short period and need to be administered every 3 weeks or so.
3. Immunity being short lived, it affords no protection on re-exposure to the toxin or microbe, that is, there is no immunological memory.

Passive immunization is used mostly in emergency situations, such as exposure to tetanus toxin or snake venom. Owing to their extreme toxicity, these substances would lead to death of the patient before the immune response is activated. Use of passive immunization provides quick protection. It is also used in pregnancy due to the risk to the foetus of many of the currently used vaccines. Besides the uses described in the preceding text, passive antibody therapy is required for patients suffering from rare congenital defects in antibody synthesis, such as *x-linked agammaglobulinemia* (see Chapter 16).

A major clinical achievement of immunology is the treatment of Rh negative mothers (lacking the Rhesus D antigen on erythrocytes) with IgG anti-RhD antibodies (*Rhogam*) to prevent *haemolytic disease of the newborn (HDN)*. Administration of these antibodies prevents sensitization of the mother's immune system to any foetal Rh positive erythrocytes transferred to the mother's circulation by transplacental haemorrhage. This avoids any adverse effects on subsequent pregnancies. Rhogam is widely used in clinical practice and has resulted in a dramatic reduction in incidence of HDN in the newborn.

Active Immunity

Active immunity is the immunity induced to a foreign antigen in which the person's own immune system actively participates. It is long-lasting, unlike passive immunity. *Natural active immunity* is induced by suffering from a particular disease and surviving it. *Artificial active immunity* is generated by *vaccination* in which a *vaccine* is administered to an individual. A vaccine is a harmless whole organism killed or weakened, or parts of the organism, or even a detoxified toxin. Vaccination is a form of *prophylaxis*, a preventive measure against disease, and its primary goal is to protect against infection.

Principle of Vaccination

The principle on which vaccination is based is illustrated in Fig. 13.2.

Immunization with tetanus toxoid activates a *primary immune response* in which naïve B lymphocytes are activated and memory cells are induced. When the person contacts the wild-type microbe (*Clostridium tetani*), as in a natural infection, a *secondary immune response* is activated which neutralizes the toxin. This response is rapid and more intense than the primary response. It is the activation of long-lived memory B cells which have been earlier generated on exposure to tetanus toxoid that enables the immune system to mount a swifter and more intense immune response when the microbe is encountered a second time. Vaccination with tetanus toxoid does not protect against other diseases. Thus, the two key features in vaccination are *specificity* and *memory*, both of which are elements of *adaptive immunity*. It should be remembered from earlier chapters that the major antibody isotype in the primary response

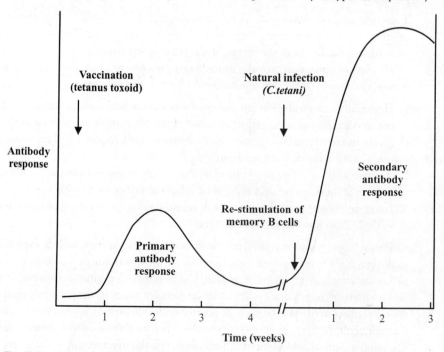

Fig. 13.2   Principle of vaccination.

is IgM, whereas IgG predominates in the secondary response (see Fig. 4.17). Importantly, antibodies produced in the secondary response are of much higher affinity. This is due to an event called *somatic hypermutation* which occurs in germinal centres and generates B cells with high-affinity receptors for antigens (see Chapter 10).

Herd (or Group) Immunity

Herd immunity is the proportion of persons in a community or a population with immunity to a particular infectious disease. If the proportion of immune (vaccinated) persons in a population is large, there is less likelihood of a susceptible individual being exposed to disease, and less chance of transmission of the disease from an infected person to a susceptible member. Thus, high herd immunity due to immunization indirectly protects the population as a whole from disease. Herd immunity applies only to diseases which depend on human transmission.

REQUIREMENTS AND AIMS OF A SUCCESSFUL VACCINE

For a vaccine to be successful, it should be

- safe to administer (should not cause adverse effects, for example, allergic reactions to extraneous components in the vaccine such as egg proteins);
- protective (should generate long-lived memory cells);
- able to induce immunity of the right type (humoral and/or cell-mediated);
- low cost and easily affordable (high cost is a problem especially in under-developed countries);
- stable on storage (live vaccines need to be stored in the cold); and
- immunogenic (acellular vaccines require an adjuvant).

It is relevant to mention here that though a humoral response protects against some infections, a cell-mediated response is advantageous in others. Still other infections are resolved when both arms of the immune system are activated. An ideal vaccine for successful vaccination should, therefore, aim at inducing immunity of the right type: antibody and/or cellular immunity. Antibodies, both induced by immunization and passively administered, protect against extracellular microbes and their products, for example, toxins. Cell-mediated immunity which involves T cells and macrophages is important in preventing intracellular infections—bacterial, viral, and fungal.

The *route of administration* of a vaccine is an important consideration. The usual route for most immunizations is subcutaneous or intramuscular. This provides systemic protection against pathogens once they have gained access into the body. To induce immunity at mucosal surfaces, a vaccine needs to be administered via the oral route. For instance, for inducing immunity to polio virus and *Salmonella typhi*, the vaccine is administered orally which is the route of infection for both. This stimulates secretory IgA (sIgA) which affords protection at mucosal surfaces. Inducing immunity at mucosal surfaces is important as these are the major sites through which many infectious diseases are transmitted. Reference has been made earlier to the enormous area of lymphoid tissue that is found at mucosal sites (see Chapter 3).

Vaccines containing soluble antigens, such as protein antigens, need to be administered along with *adjuvants*, which are described in the concluding section of this chapter.

TYPES OF VACCINES—VACCINES IN CURRENT USE AND IN DEVELOPMENT

Different approaches to vaccination, both current and experimental, are shown in Table 13.2 and are summarized in the following text.

Table 13.2 Vaccine types—current and experimental.

Current	Experimental
Killed (whole organism) vaccines	Anti-idiotype vaccines
Live attenuated (whole organism) vaccines	Recombinant vector vaccines
Subunit vaccines	DNA vaccines
♦ Recombinant proteins	
♦ Capsular polysaccharides	
Conjugate vaccines	Synthetic peptide vaccines
Toxoids	

Vaccines in Current Use

Vaccines currently being used in humans include killed bacteria and viruses, and live attenuated (avirulent) organisms. Purified components prepared by rDNA technology, capsular polysaccharides, and toxoids are also in wide use. The various vaccine types are considered in the following text.

Whole Organism Vaccines

Following are different kinds of whole organism vaccines.

Killed vaccines   These vaccines contain infectious organisms that have been killed by chemicals such as formaldehyde, γ-ray irradiation, or high temperature. The organisms lose their pathogenicity but retain antigenicity. It is important that inactivation be carried out under controlled conditions so that proteins are not denatured and conformational determinants are retained. Some killed bacterial and viral vaccines are shown in Table 13.3.

Table 13.3 Some principal inactivated whole organism vaccines. These vaccines stimulate the humoral branch of the immune system.

Disease	Comments
Bacterial	
Typhoid	Has unpleasant side effects; attenuated and subunit vaccines are now available
Cholera	Killed vibrios may be combined to cholera toxin B subunit
Pertussis	An acellular pertussis vaccine containing purified bacterial proteins, for example, p69 from recombinant sources is less toxic
Viral	
Polio	Salk's inactivated vaccine; recommended for immunocompromised patients
Rabies	Administered with rabies gamma globulin (passive)
Hepatitis A	Attenuated vaccine also available

Live attenuated vaccines   The term *attenuation* refers to weakening of a microorganism's ability to produce disease. It creates an avirulent form of the organism which replicates only poorly in the human host. There are various methods to attenuate virulent organisms such as

♦ by growing them under abnormal culture conditions; polio virus used in Sabin vaccine is attenuated by growing in monkey kidney epithelial cells till it is unable to grow in human cells;

- by modifying growth conditions such as increasing temperature and altering aerobicity; and
- by culturing virulent organisms in unnatural hosts; vaccinia virus used in the vaccine for smallpox was attenuated by passage through calves, sheep, and other animals.

In newer approaches based on rDNA technology, viruses can be attenuated irreversibly by selectively removing genes necessary for virulence. This would eliminate the risk of reversion to virulence that can occur when classical methods of attenuation are used. One strategy for developing an acquired immunodeficiency syndrome (AIDS) vaccine is to use an irreversibly attenuated strain. Live attenuated vaccines, both viral and bacterial, are shown in Table 13.4.

Table 13.4 Live attenuated vaccines. As it is easier to attenuate viruses than bacteria, most attenuated vaccines are viral vaccines. These vaccines are important as they stimulate both humoral and cell-mediated immunity.

Disease	Vaccine/Comments
Viral	
Polio	Oral polio vaccine (OPV); Sabin
Measles ⎫	
Mumps ⎬ MMR	Vaccine simultaneously immunizes against three diseases
Rubella ⎭	
Hepatitis A	Killed vaccine also available
Varicella (chickenpox)	Caused by a human herpes virus
Yellow fever	Vaccines produced from two strains of yellow fever viruses
Bacterial	
Tuberculosis (TB)	BCG (Bacillus Calmette-Guerin)
Typhoid	Ty 21a

Measles is a contagious viral disease caused by rubeola virus which infects through the respiratory tract. It is a potentially fatal disease that causes brain and kidney damage and can lead to blindness. Epidemics affecting a large number of children were common till programmes of immunization were initiated in 1968. Hundreds of children died annually in these epidemics. Immunization against the measles virus has resulted in rapid reduction in number of deaths. The *MMR—measles (rubeola), mumps, rubella (German measles)—vaccine* is a triple vaccine containing live, attenuated viruses. It is now part of the immunization protocol in young children and is administered after 15 months of age, as before that the vaccine is not very effective. German measles is a milder viral disease that also causes skin rash and is highly contagious.

Eradication of polio is an important future goal. There are two types of vaccines—the Salk (killed) and the Sabin (live attenuated) vaccine—in use against polio infection (Box 13.1).

Attenuated viral vaccines are suitable for inducing a cell-mediated immune response which cannot be achieved by a killed viral vaccine. As viruses can replicate within host cells, there is processing of viral proteins and presentation of viral peptides to cytotoxic T cells. A comparison of the major features of killed and attenuated vaccines is given in Table 13.5.

Subunit Vaccines

Some risks associated with whole organism vaccines can be avoided with vaccines that consist of immunogenic molecules derived from pathogens. These are the acellular or subunit vaccines and those in current use include recombinant antigens and capsular polysaccharides.

Box 13.1   Polio vaccines

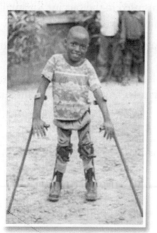

Fig. 13.3   A polio victim.

There are three strains of polio viruses (picornaviruses) that cause poliomyelitis. As the virus exhibits affinity for motor neurons in the spinal cord and the brain, infection, which is rare, spreads to the central nervous system causing paralysis (paralytic poliomyelitis). Jonas Salk was the first to develop a successful inactivated vaccine using a mixture of the three strains of polio virus. He used formalin to inactivate the viral particles. The *injectable polio vaccine* (*IPV*) of Salk became available in 1955. This requires boosters every few years but is safe to administer to immunocompromised people. Sometime later in 1957, Albert Bruce Sabin put in all his efforts to develop a live attenuated vaccine. The *oral polio vaccine* (*OPV*) of Sabin became available for use in 1963. Its administration is easy and costs involved are low. Besides, it induces intestinal immunity (sIgA) and also production of other antibodies. Its limitation is that it may mutate in rare cases to a virulent form and cause disease in vaccinated children or immunocompromised individuals. In 1995, the Center for Disease Control (CDC) recommended use of a combination of inactivated virus and attenuated virus for controlling polio. Although use of the combination vaccine holds promise, the high costs involved would pose a problem especially for developing countries. After smallpox, the first disease to be eradicated by vaccination, it is likely that polio will follow, and will be eradicated in the near future. Figure 13.3 shows a polio victim.

Table 13.5   Killed (inactivated) vaccines versus attenuated vaccines.

Features	Inactivated vaccines	Attenuated vaccines
Reversion to wild type	Cannot revert to virulent type	Virulence may be restored due to further mutation
Requirement for boosters	As the organism cannot replicate, booster injections needed to maintain immunity	A single small dose is sufficient due to capacity for transient growth
Immunity type generated	Mostly humoral immunity	Both humoral and cell-mediated immunity
Stability	Stable during transport and storage	Less stable and require refrigeration
Potential to cause disease	Acceptable for immunocompromised people	Can be administered only to healthy people; not suitable and may cause disease in • T cell immunodeficiency states (AIDS) • immunosuppressed persons
Production	Killed by chemicals, γ-ray irradiation, and high temperature	Attenuated by • growing the pathogen under abnormal culture conditions • growing in unnatural hosts • genetic alteration

Recombinant proteins   Protein antigens can be expressed in unlimited amounts by rDNA technology. The genes that encode for them can be cloned and expressed in many systems. Some examples are given in Table 13.6. The first recombinant subunit vaccine *r hepatitis B surface antigen* (*rHBsAg*), approved for medical use to protect against hepatitis B virus infection, is produced in yeast cells. Processing of donor blood to obtain the protein, as was done earlier, was a costly procedure and out of reach of the public in developing countries. But now by cloning the gene for HBsAg in

Table 13.6   Recombinant protein vaccines.

Organism	Recombinant protein	Expression system
Plasmodium falciparum	Circumsporozoite (CS) protein	*Escherichia coli*
Human immunodeficiency virus (HIV)	Envelope glycoproteins • gp 120 • gp 41 Core antigens • p 24 • p 17	Mammalian and insect cell systems; chinese hamster ovary (CHO), a mammalian cell line
Hepatitis B virus	Hepatitis B surface antigen (HBsAg)	Yeast and mammalian systems
Bordetella pertussis	Surface antigen p69	*Escherichia coli*

yeast supplies have increased and the cost of the vaccine has been brought down. Shanvac B from Shantha Biotech, India, contains rHBsAg.

This approach has several advantages including easy availability, low cost, and safety. Besides, it is useful for generating vaccines for microorganisms that cannot be easily grown in culture (e.g., some hepatitis viruses). A major limitation is that such vaccines induce only humoral immunity.

Capsular polysaccharides   Some bacteria, such as *Haemophilus influenzae*, are resistant to phagocytosis. However, if the capsule is coated with antibodies and/or complement (C3b), macrophages and neutrophils readily phagocytose them (see Fig. 12.9). Capsular polysaccharides are used as vaccines as they promote humoral immunity, the major form of protection against encapsulated bacteria. A vaccine for *Streptococcus pneumoniae* consists of 23 distinct capsular polysaccharides (Table 13.7). The major drawback with this vaccine is that there is no (or poor) formation of memory B cells, whose generation is T_H cell dependent. It is the right time to remind ourselves that polysaccharide antigens are thymus-independent (TI) antigens that function independently of T cells, though T_H cells may augment B cell activation by these antigens. Chapter 10 should be referred for further details on B cell response to TI antigens.

Table 13.7   Capsular polysaccharide vaccines.

Organism	Vaccine type
Streptococcus pneumoniae	23 distinct capsular polysaccharides
Haemophilus influenzae type B	Purified capsular polysaccharides; a more effective conjugate vaccine is now available
Salmonella typhi	Vi capsular polysaccharides; these are without side effects of the killed vaccine

Conjugate Vaccines

Immunogenicity of capsular polysaccharide vaccines can be improved by linking them to a protein carrier to give a conjugate vaccine. A good example is the *H. influenzae* type B (HiB) vaccine in which capsular polysaccharides are linked to tetanus/diphtheria toxoid. This vaccine reduces risk of meningitis in children below 5 years of age. The vaccine activates T_H cells which secrete cytokines resulting in an improved response to the polysaccharide (Fig. 13.4).

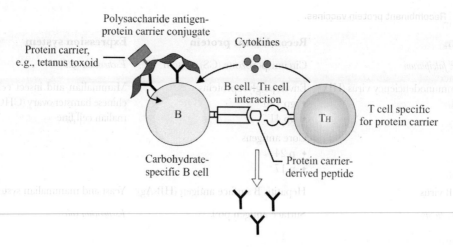

Fig. 13.4 Conjugate vaccines. Immune response to a polysaccharide antigen can be enhanced by conjugating it to a carrier protein. A conjugate vaccine such as the HiB vaccine is, therefore, more effective than a pure carbohydrate vaccine.

Toxoids

The harmful effects of some bacteria are due to the exotoxins they secrete. For instance, the exotoxin of *C. tetani* is a neurotoxin which blocks muscle relaxation causing stiffness of muscles and characteristic muscle spasms. Exotoxins of *Corynebacterium diphtheriae* cause myocardial, nervous, and renal damage. These bacterial products can be modified with chemicals, such as formalin, so that they lose their toxicity but retain their antigenicity. Such a detoxified product is called a *toxoid* (Fig. 13.5). A toxoid stimulates formation of antibodies which neutralize the toxin and facilitate removal by phagocytic cells. The *DTaP* (*diphtheria and tetanus toxoids, and acellular pertussis*) vaccine is a triple-antigen vaccine mandatory in the immunization protocol for children. The earlier vaccine had killed *Bordetella pertussis* which, due to controversies regarding safety, was replaced by its surface antigen *p69*.

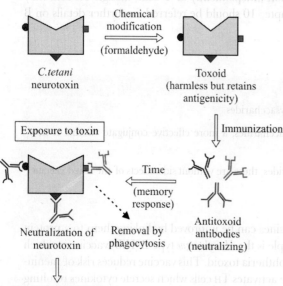

Fig. 13.5 Toxoids as vaccines. *C. tetani* neurotoxin is neutralized by antitoxoid antibodies. The complexes are engulfed by phagocytic cells.

Vaccines in Development

The categories of vaccines at various stages in the development process and which appear promising include anti-idiotype vaccines, recombinant vector vaccines, DNA vaccines, and synthetic peptide vaccines. These are introduced in the following text.

Anti-idiotype Vaccines

Idiotopes are the unique amino acid sequences found in the variable region of an antibody molecule (see Chapter 4). The combined idiotopes found on V_H and V_L regions of an antibody (*Ab-1*) is called *idiotype*. Idiotopes act like antigenic determinants and induce production of *anti-idiotype antibodies* (*Ab-2*). Those generated against the antigen-binding site of Ab-1 mimic the original antigen and may be used as a vaccine in place of it (Fig. 13.6).

Antibodies raised against an immunizing antigen (Antigen X) are selected for high-affinity antibody. This first antibody (Ab-1 or idiotype-1) is protective against the immunizing antigen. Monoclonal antibody technology is then used to make anti-idiotype antibodies against the V region of idiotype-1. Proper screening selects anti-idiotype-1 (Ab-2) which has a three-dimensional shape similar to the epitope on the original immunizing antigen, that is, Antigen X.

Anti-idiotypic antibodies when used as immunogen induce *anti-anti-idiotypes/Ab-3*. These resemble antibodies (Ab-1) induced by a natural infection, and so, can react with antigens and confer protection. Anti-idiotype vaccines have been tested in several animal models and have proved to be effective. Immunization with anti-idiotype antibodies raised against a mouse monoclonal antibody to HBsAg elicit antibodies (Ab-3) which have been shown to protect mice against Hepatitis B virus. Another potential application is in tumour immunotherapy based on administration of anti-idiotypes as surrogate tumour-associated antigens (TAA). The few human trials conducted using anti-idiotype vaccines to stimulate immunity against tumours have shown encouraging results. This approach would be useful for antigens that are not strongly immunogenic, such as polysaccharides or lipids. Also, a protein copy of such antigens (unlike polysaccharides and lipids) would be able to induce a memory response.

Recombinant Vector Vaccines

In this vaccination strategy, the desired gene encoding a major antigen of a virulent pathogen is introduced into an attenuated organism which serves as a vector. Some vectors used include vaccinia

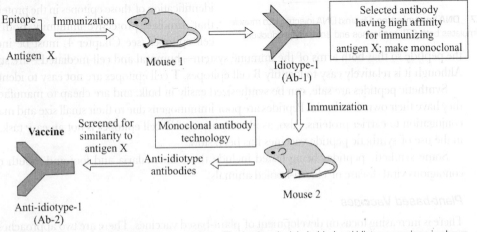

Fig. 13.6 Anti-idiotype antibodies as vaccines. The basic principle behind anti-idiotype vaccines is shown here.

virus and canarypox virus (a large virus related to vaccinia virus). When individuals are vaccinated with genetically engineered vaccinia, it replicates in the immunized host. The gene is expressed and the polypeptide product synthesized serves as the vaccine. This approach to immunization is being experimented on animals for hepatitis B and rabies.

Attenuated *Salmonella typhimurium*, which infects cells of the mucosal lining of the gut, can be engineered with genes from the cholera bacillus. The advantage of this vector is that it induces sIgA, thereby providing effective gut immunity against cholera.

Although recombinant live vaccines are not without limitations, they have an advantage over subunit vaccines in that they induce both a cell-mediated and a humoral antibody response (as do live attenuated vaccines).

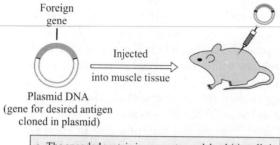

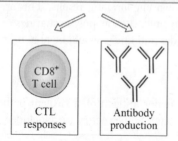

Fig. 13.7   DNA immunization. Plasmid DNA injected into muscle cells stimulates both CTL responses and antibody production.

DNA Vaccines

The gene for a protective antigen is cloned into a plasmid which is injected intramuscularly (Fig. 13.7). Cells in muscle tissue, including myocytes and dendritic cells, take up the plasmid DNA. The protein is expressed in vivo and is processed and presented on the surface in association with major histocompatibility complex (MHC) molecules. Some of the protein produced in muscle cells is secreted and taken up by dendritic cells. The details of the process are under investigation. Both cytotoxic T lymphocyte (CTL) responses and antibody production are stimulated. There are other advantages also. DNA vaccines are cheap and stable, and do not require refrigeration. Some vaccines undergoing clinical trials include those for malaria, AIDS, and tuberculosis.

Synthetic Peptide Vaccines

Synthesizing peptides for use as vaccines requires identification of those epitopes in the protein antigen that stimulate protective immunity. Both B and T cell epitopes (see Chapter 4) must be included in the peptide so that both arms of the immune system—humoral and cell-mediated—are stimulated. Although it is relatively easy to identify B cell epitopes, T cell epitopes are not easy to identify.

Synthetic peptides are safe, can be synthesized easily in bulk, and are cheap to manufacture. But they have their own drawbacks. Peptides are poor immunogens due to their small size and may require conjugation to carrier proteins. Also, as identification of T cell epitopes is not an easy task, progress in the use of synthetic peptide vaccines has been slow.

Some synthetic peptides being tested include those for malaria and foot-and-mouth disease (a contagious viral disease of cloven-hoofed animals).

Plant-based Vaccines

There is increasing focus on development of plant-based vaccines. There are two approaches towards this goal:

- ◆ *Development of edible vaccines*—The gene encoding the protein of interest is expressed in the edible part of the plant. Transgenic tomatoes and bananas are being developed for this purpose.
- ◆ *Production of recombinant antigenic proteins in plants*—The antigenic protein is expressed in the transgenic plant. It is then purified and used as a vaccine.

ADJUVANTS AND NEW APPROACHES TO ANTIGEN DELIVERY

Particulate antigens such as red blood cells (RBCs) and bacteria are generally good immunogens. They can be injected alone into an animal as they induce a potent immune response. But, for soluble material, for example, a protein, a much more improved T and/or B cell-mediated response can be obtained by injecting the immunogen mixed with an *adjuvant* (from the Latin word *adjuvare*, meaning 'to help'). Thus, adjuvants are important as they enhance immunogenicity of vaccines when administered along with them, particularly if the vaccine contains soluble material such as protein. Most acellular vaccines require adjuvants.

The precise manner in which adjuvants enhance immune responses is not clear, but they appear to act in one or more of the following ways:

1. They induce a local inflammatory reaction at the site of injection which stimulates macrophage influx.
2. They form a local depot of antigen in which the antigen is retained in small granulomas from where it is gradually released to the immune system; this mimics a prolonged series of injections and increases time of exposure of the immune system to the antigen.
3. They activate antigen-presenting cells (APCs), particularly dendritic cells and macrophages, both of which are important for initiation of an immune response.

Killed bacteria and microbial components make good adjuvants. By stimulating production of cytokines, they enhance inflammatory reactions and stimulation of APCs. The most commonly used adjuvant is *Freund's complete adjuvant (FCA)*. It is a mixture of oil, detergent, and heat-killed mycobacteria. *Freund's incomplete adjuvant (FIA)* is a mixture of oil and detergent alone without killed mycobacteria. *Muramyl dipeptide (MDP)*, a component of *Mycobacterium tuberculosis,* is a major stimulatory component and can be used in different forms. These adjuvants are not suited for human use but are commonly used in vaccines for experimental animals. Several vaccines being used in humans, such as tetanus and diphtheria toxoid vaccines, have been made particulate with *compounds of aluminium* such as *phosphate* or *hydroxide*. Without them, the toxoid is not sufficiently immunogenic. Efforts are being made to produce improved adjuvants for enhancing T cell-mediated responses in humans.

A lot of interest is focused on *liposomes* as delivery vehicles for antigen presentation to the immune system. They are small lipid membrane vesicles prepared by mixing a soluble protein antigen with amphipathic molecules (having both polar and non-polar portions), such as phospholipids, under conditions that promote vesicle formation. Along with antigens, liposomes can be made to incorporate stimulants also. Besides preventing loss of antigens, they can effectively fuse with APCs delivering antigens intracellularly and facilitating presentation to the immune system.

Another recent approach involves use of *immunostimulating complexes (ISCOMs)*. These are small micelle-like structures containing entrapped protein. They are formed from a mixture of lipids, mainly cholesterol and also phosphatidylcholine, and some plant-derived detergents . *Immunostimulating complexes* can fuse with APCs allowing the antigen to enter the cytosol, thereby mimicking viral infection. The peptides derived from cytosolic proteins are loaded onto newly synthesized class I MHC molecules in the endoplasmic reticulum and transported to the cell surface where they are presented to CD8$^+$

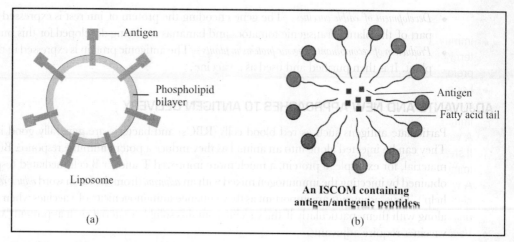

Fig. 13.8 Antigen delivery systems.

CTLs. Immunostimulating complexes are thus able to stimulate a cell-mediated immune response. The two antigen delivery systems described in the preceding text are depicted in Fig. 13.8.

FUTURE GOAL

There are still many diseases for which effective vaccines are not available and are urgently needed (Table 13.8). Developing these vaccines is a major goal in immunology. An effective vaccine must stimulate both arms of the immune system. But most vaccines in current use work by eliciting a humoral immune response alone. Efforts are ongoing to develop vaccines that stimulate cell-mediated immune responses as well. It is hoped that with the many advances in molecular biology and genetic engineering, new and improved vaccines will be made available. An approach that appears promising to vaccinologists is to have a single vaccine that would confer resistance to a wide range of diseases simultaneously. *Vaccines, besides affording protection against various communicable diseases, have the potential to protect against cancer.* Approaches to development of vaccines to fight cancer are reviewed in Chapter 18.

Table 13.8 **Some diseases/pathogens for which effective vaccines are needed.** Vaccines for staphylococcal and streptococcal exotoxins are not available.

Bacteria	Viruses	Fungi	Protozoa	Worms
Leprosy (*Mycobacterium leprae*)	AIDS (HIV)	*Candida* spp.	Malaria (*Plasmodium* spp.)	Schistosomiasis
Syphilis (*Treponema pallidum*)	Hepatitis C	*Pneumocystis* spp.		
Staphylococci	Papilloma virus		Leishmaniasis	
Streptococci (Group A)	Severe acute respiratory syndrome (SARS-corona virus)		Trypanosomiasis	
	Dengue			

SUMMARY

- Immunity is of two types: passive and active. Short-term passive immunization involves administering preformed antibodies and is used in emergencies.
- Long-term active immunization can be achieved by infection or by vaccination. The aim is to induce immunological memory.
- A vaccine should be safe, stable, and of low cost. It should provide long-term humoral and/or cellular immunity.
- A wide range of vaccines currently being used include killed vaccines, live attenuated vaccines, sub-unit vaccines, conjugate vaccines, and toxoids.
- Vaccines in development and which hold promise include anti-idiotype vaccines for polysaccharide and/or lipid antigens, recombinant live vector vaccines, and DNA vaccines. DNA vaccines, like live-attenuated vaccines, stimulate both humoral and cell-mediated immunity.
- Progress in development of synthetic peptide vaccines has been slow.
- Adjuvants are substances that boost the immune response. Soluble protein antigens in a vaccine are mixed with adjuvants and administered.
- Some new approaches to antigen delivery include liposomes and ISCOMs.
- There is urgent need of vaccines for agents that cause AIDS, dengue, SARS, malaria, tuberculosis and for parasitic protozoa and worms besides many others.
- There is increasing focus on development of vaccines to fight cancer.

REVIEW QUESTIONS

1. Indicate whether each of the following statements is true or false. If false, explain why.
   (a) It would be safer to administer an attenuated vaccine rather than a purified subunit vaccine to an immunosuppressed patient.
   (b) BCG is used to protect against Hepatitis B virus infection.
   (c) DNA vaccines are poor inducers of cytotoxic T lymphocyte responses.
   (d) Tetanus toxoid is generally administered to humans with Freund's complete adjuvant (FCA).
   (e) Immunity induced to smallpox virus using cowpox virus is an example of antigenic cross-reactivity.
   (f) Naturally acquired active immunity confers long-lasting immunity to an infectious microbe.

2. Self-assessment questions
   (a) Can you explain why use of human immuno-globulin is preferred to xeno-antisera as a source of antibodies? In what conditions are the two useful?
   (b) What form of vaccine is used for diphtheria immunization? Unlike the influenza vaccine, the vaccine against diphtheria is generally always effective. Can you explain why this is so?
   (c) What requirements should a vaccine fulfil for a vaccination programme to be successful? What are the types of vaccines currently being used in humans and what are their merits and demerits?
   (d) What are the limitations of polysaccharide vaccines? How can their effectiveness be enhanced? Illustrate with an example.
   (e) Explain passive and active immunization and the ways by which the two are achieved. Which vaccines in development would be able to stimulate both arms of the immune system?

3. For each question, choose the *best* answer.
   (a) Vaccines against intracellular microbes should aim at stimulating
      (i) macrophage and/or CTL responses
      (ii) secretory IgA at mucosal surfaces
      (iii) humoral immunity
      (iv) NK cells
   (b) Which of the following vaccines would stimulate both humoral and cell-mediated immunity?
      (i) Killed
      (ii) Live attenuated
      (iii) Synthetic peptides
      (iv) Polysaccharides

(c) A toxoid
  (i) is a harmless toxin
  (ii) is more immunogenic than the toxin
  (iii) exhibits enhanced binding to antitoxin
  (iv) stimulates both branches of the immune system

(d) The vaccine type used for Hepatitis B is
  (i) toxoid
  (ii) attenuated
  (iii) inactivated
  (iv) purified macromolecule

Hypersensitivity Reactions

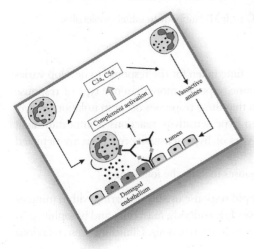

LEARNING OBJECTIVES

Having studied this chapter, you should be able to understand the following:

♦ That exaggerated and inappropriate immune responses lead to hypersensitivity reactions which are of four types

♦ The mechanism of tissue injury varies in different types and is due to antibodies (IgE or IgG/IgM)/immune complexes/inflammatory TH1 cells

♦ Immunological mechanisms that underlie type I allergic responses and that these reactions can be so severe as to be fatal

♦ Approaches to treatment/relief of allergy and their basis

♦ That antibodies either in the free form (type II) or as immune complexes (type III) can cause injury in different ways

♦ How activation of effector mechanisms of type IV or delayed-type hypersensitivity (DTH) by T lymphocytes causes damage

♦ That DTH reactions which take more time than the other types manifest in different ways

The main focus of earlier chapters has been on the protective role of the immune system in defence against harmful agents. But the same responses that are beneficial to the host and contribute to survival may, occasionally, react in ways that are damaging and sometimes even life-threatening. The term *hypersensitivity* is used when immune responses to foreign, often inert and ordinarily harmless substances, mediated by antibodies and/or immune cells, are exaggerated or inappropriate, and cause injury to the host. Autoimmune diseases also represent a form of hypersensitivity in which the immune system of the host sees self-components as foreign and mounts a response against them. Such autoimmune reactions have the potential to cause considerable damage and are discussed in Chapter 15.

This chapter discusses the immunological mechanisms which are involved in different types of hypersensitivity responses. The major features and symptoms associated with some clinical hypersensitivity diseases and their pathogenesis are elaborated. The chapter also briefly summarizes the various approaches that contribute to prevention or relief of type I hypersensitivity reactions and the principles that underlie treatment.

TYPES OF HYPERSENSITIVITY REACTIONS

Coombs and Gell categorized hypersensitivity reactions into four types on the basis of immune components (cells and molecules) involved (Table 14.1).

Table 14.1   Types of hypersensitivity reactions.

Hypersensitivity type	Feature
Type I, Allergy	Antibody-mediated (IgE)
Type II, Cytotoxic	Antibody-mediated (IgG or IgM) (antibody to cell-surface antigens)
Type III, Immune complex	Antibody-mediated (IgG or IgM) (antibody to soluble molecules)
Type IV, Delayed	T cell (TH1)-mediated

The mechanisms leading to pathology and also the time taken for the response to develop varies in the four types. Owing to the complexity of the immune response, more than one type of response may be evoked to a particular antigen, and it is seldom that these responses occur in isolation in vivo. Understanding mechanisms that lead to pathology in hypersensitivity reactions is important as it would help to devise strategies for therapy. The four types of hypersensitivity reactions are depicted in Fig. 14.1.

In brief, the different types of hypersensitivity responses include the following:

IgE-mediated immediate (type I) hypersensitivity   This is a rapid response usually occurring within minutes following re-exposure to the antigen (allergen). It involves IgE antibody, mast cells, and basophils, and is due to release of various mediators that trigger inflammatory reactions. Clinically, these reactions are commonly referred to as *allergy* or *atopy*.

Cytotoxic (type II) hypersensitivity   This is triggered when antibody (IgG or IgM) binds to antigens on the surface of cells. There is activation of complement leading to cell lysis, or phagocytosis by neutrophils and macrophages. In addition, neutrophils or other killer cells attach to antibody- coated targets through their Fc receptors and mediate antibody-dependent cell-mediated cytotoxicity (ADCC). Red blood cells can also be targets. A mismatched blood transfusion is a good example of a type II reaction. The time taken for a type II response to develop is variable and it takes usually hours.

Immune complex-mediated (type III) hypersensitivity   This develops when antigen–antibody (IgG primarily, or IgM) complexes are formed in the circulation (or in tissues) in excess. These immune complexes deposit at various sites and activate complement. Generally, the damage mediated by granulocytes occurs within 6–24 hours. Type III reactions may also be localized.

Cell-mediated (type IV) or delayed-type hypersensitivity   This is a delayed reaction, typically takes 24–72 hours but may take more, and is mediated by T cells (CD4$^+$ TH1 cells) and not antibodies. Cytokines released by T cells recruit mononuclear phagocytes to affected sites. Some triggers that evoke these reactions include allografts (foreign cells/tissues), intracellular pathogens, soluble proteins, and chemicals.

The different types of hypersensitivity responses are described in the following sections.

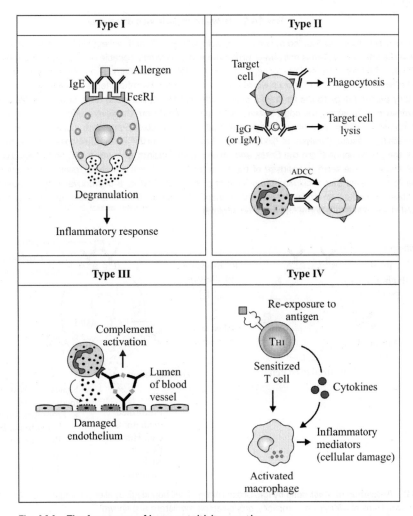

Fig. 14.1   The four types of hypersensitivity reactions.

IGE-MEDIATED IMMEDIATE (TYPE I) HYPERSENSITIVITY

Type I hypersensitivity reactions caused by IgE are major pathological reactions and are commonly known as *allergy* or *atopy*. Atopy refers to the inherent ability of some individuals to produce large amounts of IgE in response to certain environmental antigens and to develop type I immediate hypersensitivity reactions. Such individuals are said to be *atopic*. Type I reactions may be mild or severe (anaphylaxis) and, sometimes, even life threatening (fatal anaphylaxis). Early studies by Portier and Richet (1902) provided the first indication that the immune system can have detrimental effects on the host (Box 14.1).

Type I responses are rapid and exaggerated responses that occur in individuals on exposure to certain antigens called *allergens* to which they have previously been exposed. The response involves production of IgE antibodies (but not other isotypes) on exposure to allergen, followed by binding of IgE to receptors on mast cells. Re-exposure to allergen at a later time cross-links cell-bound IgE and triggers degranulation of mast cells with release of various mediators that cause the symptoms of allergy (Fig. 14.2).

Box 14.1   How anaphylaxis was discovered

Early investigations conducted by two French biologists, Portier and Richet (1902), revealed for the first time that the immune system is not always protective and is, at times, capable of causing harm. They studied the effects of a toxin from sea anemone, a marine invertebrate, on mammalian physiology. Curious to find out whether prior exposure to a toxin would protect against the harmful effects of the toxin at some later time , they exposed dogs to the toxin (in a dose insufficient to kill) a second time, several weeks after an initial exposure. Surprisingly, the dogs, instead of being protected from the severe effects of the toxin by antitoxin antibodies, reacted to it very strongly and died within minutes. Symptoms included excessive salivation, breathing difficulty, paralysis of hind limbs, and diarrhoea. Portier and Richet coined the term *anaphylaxis* for the phenomenon (from the Greek *ana* which means 'against' or 'away from', and *phylaxis* which means 'protection'). The term is opposite of the term 'prophylaxis' which means 'towards protection'. It should be remembered that vaccination is a form of prophylaxis, that is, a preventive measure against disease. Subsequently, further studies revealed that anaphylaxis is the result of a hypersensitivity reaction. Penicillin and insect stings are some causes of anaphylaxis.

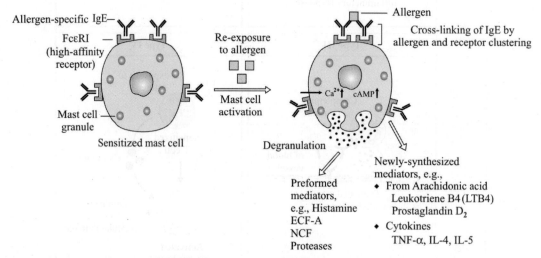

Fig. 14.2   Activation of mast cells by IgE. Cross-linking of cell-bound IgE by allergen triggers degranulation of mast cells causing symptoms of allergy. For simplicity, only selected mediators are shown.
ECF-A, eosinophil chemotactic factor-A; NCF, neutrophil chemotactic factor

Allergens

An allergen is a substance, protein or non-protein, that is normally harmless but evokes a heightened immune response (type I hypersensitivity) in some individuals who are prone to allergy. Instead of ignoring these substances, the immune system in such individuals reacts to them with serious consequences. Following are some common allergens:

♦ Fungal spores
♦ Pollen (e.g., ragweed)
♦ Insect (e.g., wasps and bees) venom
♦ House mites
♦ Household dust
♦ Animal dander
♦ Peanuts
♦ Sea-foods (e.g., shellfish)
♦ Medicines

Phases in Development of Allergy

With the background provided in the preceding text, the chapter proceeds to a discussion of the broad phases in the development of allergic reactions.

Sensitization Phase

This is the initial encounter with allergen which may enter the body via different routes. It may be inhaled, ingested, or it may penetrate through the skin as by an insect bite. The allergen activates B cells which differentiate into plasma cells that secrete allergen-specific IgE into the circulation. Immunoglobulin-E production by B cells requires help from TH2 cell cytokines, such as interleukin-4 (IL-4). Immunoglobulin-E antibodies, through their Fc tails, bind to high-affinity FcεRI on mast cells in tissues, such as in respiratory and gastrointestinal tracts, and on basophils in blood. Once IgE binds to its specific receptors, it stays fixed permanently. These cells with surface-bound IgE are said to be *sensitized*, as shown in Fig. 14.3(a).

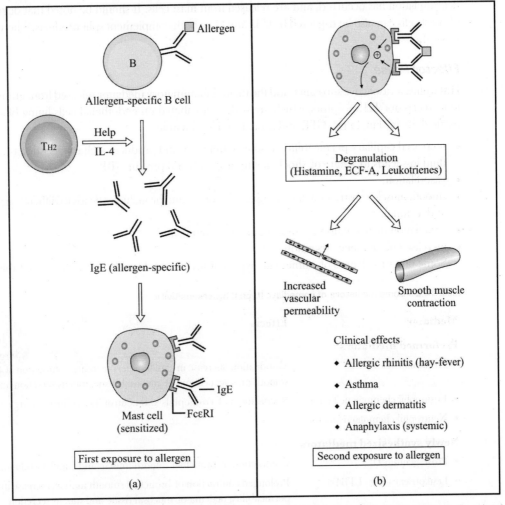

Fig. 14.3 Type I hypersensitivity. On first exposure to allergen, IgE binds to FcεRI on tissue mast cells. On second exposure to the same allergen, adjacent IgE molecules bound to mast cells are cross-linked. Activating signals are delivered leading to mast cell degranulation. The released mediators cause symptoms of type I hypersensitivity.

Levels of IgE are very low in normal individuals ($\sim$0.05 µg ml^{-1} compared to $\sim$13.5 mg ml^{-1} for IgG1-IgG4), but are elevated in an individual who is prone to allergy (and also in parasite infections).

Activation Phase

Binding occurs to cell-bound IgE on second or subsequent encounter with the same allergen as in Fig. 14.3(b). There is cross-linking of adjacent IgE molecules causing FcεRs on the cell surface to cluster. Clustering of receptors delivers signals that cause a change in membrane fluidity allowing Ca^{2+} ion influx with a transient increase in cAMP levels. This promotes entry of water and Ca^{2+} ions into granules stimulating fusion of granules with plasma membrane and exocytosis of granule contents. The release of preformed mediators from granules is called *degranulation. A subsequent fall in cAMP levels is essential for degranulation to continue.* By increasing cAMP levels, certain drugs interfere in degranulation and are useful in the treatment of allergic disorders (described in the following text). Some inflammatory products such as prostaglandins and leukotrienes are synthesized de novo after degranulation has occurred, and are released from mast cells. It should be noted that degranulation of mast cells can also be triggered by C3a and C5a, both complement split products. There are other ways also.

Effector Phase

Histamine, a vasoactive substance and the major inflammatory mediator released from granules, binds to its receptors (H1 receptors) which are widely distributed on endothelial cells lining blood vessels, particularly in skin, lungs, GIT, and nose. Its effects include

- increased capillary permeability (results in fluid loss and produces a characteristic rash; excessive fluid loss leads to a state of shock due to drop in blood pressure (BP)),
- vasodilation,
- smooth muscle constriction, for example, of bronchi and bronchioles (leads to difficulty in breathing and asthma),
- stimulation of nerve fibres (causes pain and itching), and
- increased nasal mucus secretion.
  Some other mediators of immediate hypersensitivity and their effects are listed in Table 14.2.

Table 14.2 Some mediators of immediate (type I) hypersensitivity.

Mediator	Effects
Preformed mediators	
• Histamine	Vasodilation, increase in capillary permeability, contraction of bronchial smooth muscle, oedema of mucosal tissue, mucus secretion and itching
• Eosinophil chemotactic factor	Recruitment of eosinophils and neutrophils to site of allergic response
• Neutrophil chemotactic factor	
Newly synthesized mediators	
• Prostaglandin D$_2$	Contraction of bronchial smooth muscle and capillary dilation
• Leukotrienes (e.g., LTB4)	Prolonged contraction of bronchial smooth muscle, increase in capillary permeability, oedema of mucosal tissue and mucus secretion

Allergic Reactions can Manifest in Various Ways

The dose and route of exposure to allergen, extent of mediator release from mast cells/basophils, and genetic background of the individual are some important considerations which determine the type of reaction that manifests. Clinically, allergic reactions can be localized or life-threatening systemic reactions (anaphylaxis).

Localized Allergic Reactions

The diverse clinical symptoms/pathology seen depends on the characteristics of the target organ (Table 14.3).

Table 14.3   Some common allergic disorders (localized) caused by activation of mast cells at mucosal surfaces.

Allergic disorder	Allergen	Symptoms/Pathology
Hay fever (nose)	Ragweed pollen	Watery eyes Running nose Inflammation of upper airways
Asthma (lung)	Household dust Pollen	Difficulty in breathing Inflammation and tissue damage (late-phase reaction)
Food allergy (gut)	Eggs Shellfish	Urticaria Increased peristalsis (smooth muscle contraction)

Hay fever or *allergic rhinitis* is a common form of localized allergic reaction. It is seasonal and is due to exposure to air-borne pollen such as ragweed pollen and grass pollen. Symptoms include watery eyes, sneezing, nasal congestion, and shortness of breath. There is increased mucus secretion, an effect caused by histamine released from mast cells in the nasal mucosa.

Asthma, also a local reaction, is due to certain allergens which, when inhaled, stimulate mast cell degranulation in bronchi. Leukotrienes are released which cause prolonged contraction of bronchial smooth muscle, oedema, and mucus secretion. Shortness of breath results due to airway obstruction. Other symptoms include coughing and wheezing. Accumulation of a large number of eosinophils in the bronchial mucosa is a feature of chronic asthma and is a *late-phase response* that is discussed in the following text.

Certain foods when ingested cause allergy (*food allergy*). Such food allergens cause inflammation of the mucous membranes of the digestive tract resulting in abdominal pain and diarrhoea. A swelling or redness due to leakage of fluid and protein (urticaria) caused by degranulating mucosal mast cells may also be seen in some cases. Shellfish, wheat, eggs, and peanuts are some common food allergens.

Atopic dermatitis is an inflammatory disease of the skin involving TH2 cells, unlike TH1 cells in contact dermatitis (described in a later section), and eosinophils. Mediators released by degranulating mast cells recruit inflammatory cells, particularly eosinophils, to the site of allergen contact. If bacterial infections occur, eruptions which appear on the skin are filled with pus.

Systemic Anaphylaxis

This is the severest form of hypersensitivity which occurs after a sensitized individual is re-exposed to systemically absorbed allergen. Being a systemic reaction, there is extensive mast cell degranulation at multiple sites. The response is characterized by oedema in various tissues including laryngeal oedema. The widespread oedema causes a fall in BP leading to a state of shock called *anaphylactic shock* which can lead to death. Airways are severely constricted and filled with mucus. Due to airway obstruction, the patient may die of suffocation. It is reminded here that complement-derived peptides C3a and C5a, called *anaphylatoxins*, also elicit mast cell degranulation with similar effects. Besides exposure to insect (wasps and bees) venom, a second contact with horse antitoxin can also lead to systemic anaphylaxis in a sensitized individual. Anaphylactic shock requires immediate treatment and epinephrine is the quickest to act. It restores BP to normal and reduces swelling in the airways.

Late-phase Response

This occurs some hours after the immediate reaction and is associated with influx of T cells, monocytes, eosinophils, and neutrophils. The inflammatory response is intensified causing tissue damage (Fig. 14.4).

Chemotactic factors released by mast cells draw eosinophils and neutrophils to the site. Interaction between adhesion molecules expressed on endothelial cells and immune cells is essential for exit of immune cells from the circulation. On activation by the binding of antibody-coated allergen to their Fc receptors, these cells release biologically active substances that cause tissue damage. For instance, neutrophils release powerful lysosomal enzymes which have potential to cause considerable injury to tissues. Eosinophils release major basic protein (MBP) which damages the epithelium of the respiratory tract in chronic asthma. Lymphocytes also enter the area and promote further sensitization of the host. Besides, by releasing cytokines, they permit activation of eosinophils and other cells that have been drawn to the site. It is unfortunate that the events described in the preceding text, which protect against foreign invaders, also cause unwanted damage in some individuals on activation by ordinarily harmless substances.

Wheal and Flare Reaction

Atopic reactions occur at the site of allergen entry into the body. When an allergen is introduced intradermally, as also happens during a mosquito bite, histamine is released from mast cells in skin. This dilates blood vessels increasing blood flow to the area causing a *flare* or *redness*. Capillary permeability

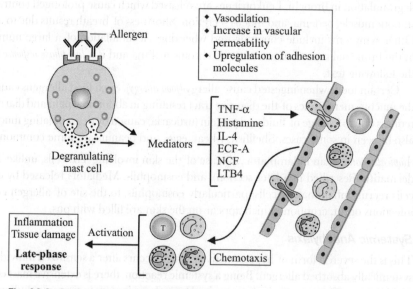

Fig. 14.4 **Late-phase localized inflammatory reactions.** The reactions shown cause damage in chronic asthma.

also increases causing fluid to leak from vessels resulting in a *wheal* or *swelling*. The flare is seen rapidly within seconds or minutes followed by the wheal. It should be noted that if the antigen is introduced systemically, there is widespread degranulation with release of histamine, consequences of which would be very severe as has been discussed in the preceding text. The *wheal* and *flare reaction* forms the basis of the classical diagnostic skin test for allergy (Fig. 14.5). A positive response to an allergen injected into the skin shows oedema, redness, and itching. The reaction disappears in about an hour but due to the late-phase reaction a lump can be seen to form 4–6 hours later.

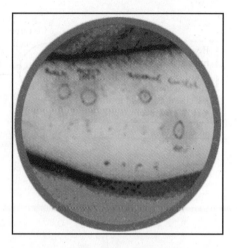

Fig. 14.5 Skin test for allergy. An allergen introduced intradermally causes redness and swelling. This is called *wheal* and *flare reaction*. A range of antigens can be tested to find out to which substance an individual is allergic (atopic) to.

Treatment

There are different approaches to treatment of allergy (type I hypersensitivity reactions). These include inhibiting mast cell degranulation, blocking effects of mast cell mediators, preventing inflammation, allergen avoidance, and desensitization (Fig. 14.6).

Epinephrine is an effective treatment for anaphylactic shock. By increasing levels of cAMP, it decreases mast cell degranulation and relaxes bronchial smooth muscles. *Theophylline*, by inhibiting an enzyme phosphodiesterase (which converts cAMP to 5′-AMP), helps to maintain increased cAMP levels. It is commonly administered to asthmatics (orally or through inhalers). *Sodium cromoglycate* inhibits Ca^{2+} influx into mast cells and, hence, their degranulation. *Cortisone*, an anti-

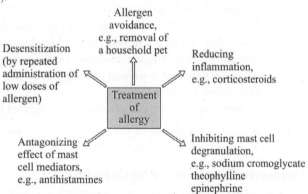

Fig. 14.6 Treatment of type I hypersensitivity.

inflammatory agent, is used in treatment of chronic asthma. *Antihistamines* block H1 receptors on target cells and prevent histamine from binding. This reduces vasodilation and permeability induced by histamine. An immunological approach called *desensitization* is based on repeated administration of low doses of allergen. Although the mechanism is not clear, this form of treatment has shown benefit in some patients.

CYTOTOXIC (TYPE II) HYPERSENSITIVITY

Type II or cytotoxic hypersensitivity reactions are triggered when antibodies (IgG or IgM) see antigens that are part of the cell membrane, such as on the membrane of RBCs, as foreign and bind to them. This triggers activation of complement via the classical pathway. The product C3b opsonizes the target cell and enhances phagocytosis. Complement can also mediate direct lysis of the target cell through the membrane attack complex (Fig. 14.7).

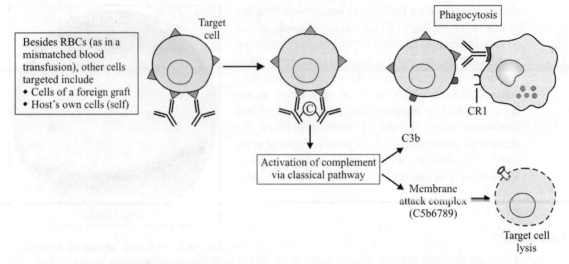

Besides RBCs (as in a mismatched blood transfusion), other cells targeted include
 • Cells of a foreign graft
 • Host's own cells (self)

Target cell

Phagocytosis

CR1

C3b

Activation of complement via classical pathway

Membrane attack complex (C5b6789)

Target cell lysis

Fig. 14.7 Type II hypersensitivity reaction. Target cell is phagocytosed after opsonization with antibody and/or C3b. It can also be directly lysed by membrane attack complex (MAC).

By binding to antibody-coated targets through their Fc receptors, cytotoxic cells, for example, neutrophils, eosinophils, or other killer cells, may cause damage by a process called ADCC. A type II response when mounted against an invading pathogen is beneficial, but not when the response is directed against red blood cells in a blood transfusion reaction/transplanted foreign cells/surface receptors on self-cells (autoimmune). Sometimes by binding to cell surface receptors, autoantibodies affect cell functioning without causing cell damage or inflammation as is seen in autoimmune thyroid disease (see Chapter 15).

Some typical type II reactions are exemplified by

 • haemolytic disease of the newborn (HDN) and
 • mismatched blood transfusion.

Haemolytic Disease of the Newborn (HDN)

An Rh negative mother (lacking the Rhesus or the D antigen on the RBC membrane) may carry an Rh positive foetus if the father is Rh positive. Some of these Rh positive foetal cells may leak into the maternal circulation at the time of delivery and sensitize the mother's immune system which sees the RhD antigen as foreign. Complications do not occur in the first pregnancy. However, in a second pregnancy, a small number of positive foetal red cells may enter the maternal circulation. These stimulate a memory response leading to production of anti-RhD antibodies (IgG). These cross the placenta and bind to foetal erythrocytes (opsonization). A type II reaction develops resulting in their destruction (Fig. 14.8). This is the cause of *haemolytic disease of the newborn*. Due to anaemia (haemolytic anaemia) and accumulation of toxic compounds (bilirubin) released from destruction of RBCs, the child in severe cases may even be stillborn. Haemolytic disease of the newborn can be avoided by giving an injection of *Rhogam* (anti-RhD antibodies) to Rh negative mothers just after delivery of an Rh positive child. These react with any RhD positive foetal erythrocytes that may have entered the circulation and destroy them. This prevents sensitization of the mother's immune system, that is, prevents memory cell formation.

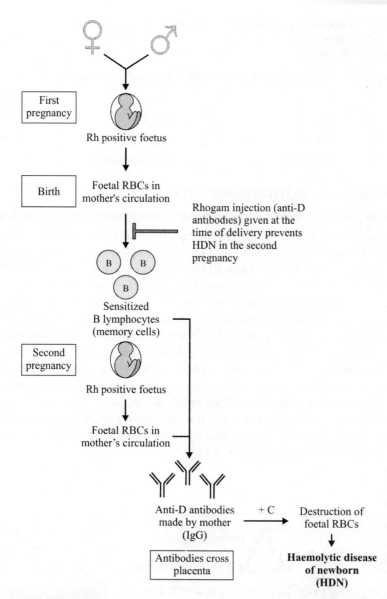

Fig. 14.8 **Haemolytic disease of the newborn (type II hypersensitivity).** Rhogam along with mother's complement destroys any foetal RBCs that escape into the maternal circulation at the time of delivery. This prevents sensitization of the mother's immune system and prevents HDN.

Transfusion Reactions

Natural antibodies (IgM) are present in our circulation against the major blood group antigens A and/or B expressed on the surface of RBCs (Table 14.4).

A blood group A individual will have antibodies to the B antigen and not to the A antigen. Their presence would cause clumping of red cells in blood. Hence, it is necessary to match blood (blood-typing) before transfusion, a procedure that is commonly performed when an individual has suffered severe blood loss. An incompatible or mismatched blood transfusion, in which RBCs carry a different blood group antigen, can be life threatening for a recipient. Complications arise due to pre-existing antibodies when the same blood is transfused a second time. There is clumping of foreign cells followed by phagocytosis, and massive haemolysis inside the blood vessels (type II reaction). Symptoms include fever, vomiting, drop in BP, and back and chest pains.

Table 14.4 The ABO blood group system. There are four blood types which include A, B, AB, and O. These are determined by presence or absence of antigens A and B on the red blood cell surface.

Blood group	Antigens on red blood cells	Antibodies in serum
A	A	anti-B
B	B	anti-A
AB	A and B	Neither
O	Neither	anti-A and anti-B

IMMUNE COMPLEX-MEDIATED (TYPE III) HYPERSENSITIVITY

A type III reaction is triggered by presence of immune complexes (antigen–antibody complexes) in the circulation or in tissues. Normally, these immune complexes do not cause damage as they are engulfed and destroyed by phagocytic cells. But, when immune complexes are formed continuously and in large amounts, they persist and initiate a type III hypersensitivity response. Microbial antigens, self-antigens, and foreign components in serum can stimulate a type III response. The damage caused by immune complexes may be localized within a tissue, as in the *Arthus reaction* or may be systemic.

The classic *Arthus reaction* is due to local deposition of immune complexes within and near walls of small blood vessels. It develops when an antigen is injected subcutaneously or intradermally into a previously sensitized individual. Preformed antibodies react with antigens and form local immune complexes in high concentration. These activate complement, generating products which recruit neutrophils to the site where immune complexes have deposited. Activation of complement is very essential for the Arthus reaction to take place. When unable to completely phagocytose immune complexes, neutrophils release lysosomal enzymes and reactive oxygen intermediates extracellularly. This triggers an inflammatory response 6–24 hours after injection causing localized tissue and vascular damage with consequent functional impairment (Fig. 14.9).

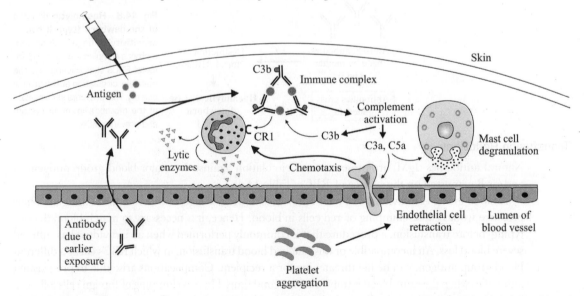

Fig. 14.9 The Arthus reaction. This is induced by intradermal injection of antigen into a sensitized individual. Local deposition of immune complexes triggers inflammatory reactions which cause damage.

The local pulmonary damage due to inhaled antigens is mediated by an Arthus-type reaction. This is exemplified by *Farmer's lung* which is caused by inhaled bacterial spores found in hay.

A systemic reaction develops during passive antibody therapy using horse antiserum to protect against tetanus/diphtheria toxin. Administration of antitoxins affords protection against the microbial toxins, but as they are foreign proteins, the initial contact with horse antitoxin sensitizes the person. On second exposure to horse antitoxin, the sensitized individual forms antibodies against horse proteins forming immune complexes which deposit at various sites and cause injury. *Serum sickness*, the term used for this condition, develops about 10 days after initial exposure to the antigen. Use of passive antibody therapy has declined because of these complications and is used only in certain conditions, such as in pregnancy and in individuals in whom the immune system is suppressed, besides a few others.

The deposited complexes attract neutrophils which, due to failure to phagocytose immune complexes adhering to the basement membrane, release lysosomal enzymes and reactive oxygen intermediates causing tissue damage as seen in Fig. 14.10(a).

Deposition of immune complexes occurs in renal vessels leading to *glomerulonephritis* in which filtration by glomeruli is impaired. This causes proteins and blood cells to be excreted in the urine. Besides kidney, immune complexes also deposit in blood vessels and in joints causing *vasculitis* (inflammation of walls of blood vessels) and *arthritis* (inflammation of joints), respectively (Fig. 14.10b).

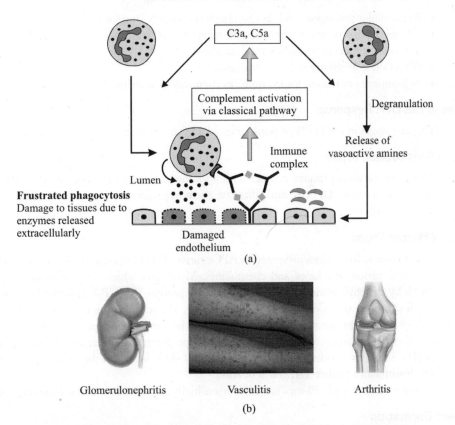

Fig. 14.10   Inflammation in type III hypersensitivity. (a) Immune complexes in the circulation can cause widespread damage (systemic reaction). (b) Complications due to immune complex deposition. Note that small complexes are not readily cleared and so persist.

There are other causes also for systemic disease, including streptococcal infection (streptococcal nephritis), and immune complexes formed in autoimmune disorders, such as rheumatoid arthritis and systemic lupus erythematosus. Immune complexes play a major role in pathology in these diseases (see Chapter 15). The pathology associated with complement deficiencies is due to decreased removal of immune complexes. Lack of opsonization of immune complexes by C3b fails to eliminate them through C3b receptors on phagocytic cells.

CELL-MEDIATED (TYPE IV) OR DELAYED-TYPE HYPERSENSITIVITY

Type IV cell-mediated hypersensitivity is a localized inflammatory reaction, also referred to as *delayed-type hypersensitivity*. It is called so as the response typically takes hours (generally 24–72 hours) to develop—a much longer time compared to other hypersensitivity reactions. T cells, specifically TH1 cells, also called T cells of delayed-type hypersensitivity (DTH) or TDTH play a pivotal role in the response. Other key cells are macrophages and dendritic cells. It is to be noted that in a type III response, described in the preceding text, it is neutrophils, and not macrophages, that are recruited. Although there is no involvement of antibodies, cytokines released by TH1 cells and other immune cells play an important role.

Some stimuli for DTH reactions include the following:

♦ Intracellular pathogens such as mycobacteria, viruses, and fungi
♦ Chemicals that penetrate the skin and conjugate to tissue proteins, for example, nickel, chromium, and other agents in cosmetics and hair dyes
♦ Allografts (foreign organ/tissue transplant)
♦ Self-antigens in tissues, for example, in rheumatoid arthritis

Stages in the DTH Response

The two stages in the DTH response (Fig. 14.11), introduced in Chapter 9, are described here.

Sensitization Phase

This is initiated on primary contact with an antigen. Antigen-presenting cells (APCs) process and present antigens to TH cells, and stimulate them to proliferate and differentiate into TH1 cells and secrete cytokines.

Effector Phase

Re-exposure to the antigen presented by APCs elicits a DTH response. Sensitized TH1 cells are activated to release various cytokines and chemokines. Monocytes which are drawn to the site from blood vessels by the chemokine monocyte chemotactic protein-1 (MCP-1) differentiate into macrophages which are the major effector cells in the response. Macrophages on activation by interferon-gamma (IFN-γ) and tumour necrosis factor-beta (TNF-β) show increased capacity to phagocytose and destroy microbes. Additionally, activated macrophages upregulate class II major histocompatibility complex (MHC) molecules under the influence of IFN-γ. This increases their antigen-presenting function which stimulates further TH1 cell activation.

Some examples of cell-mediated hypersensitivity are described in the following text.

Contact Dermatitis

This is initiated by various small molecules called haptens which, because of their small size, are able to penetrate the skin. Agents which give rise to contact hypersensitivity include certain metals (e.g., nickel or chromium present in metal fasteners in watch straps), oil from poison ivy, dyes, soaps, cosmetics,

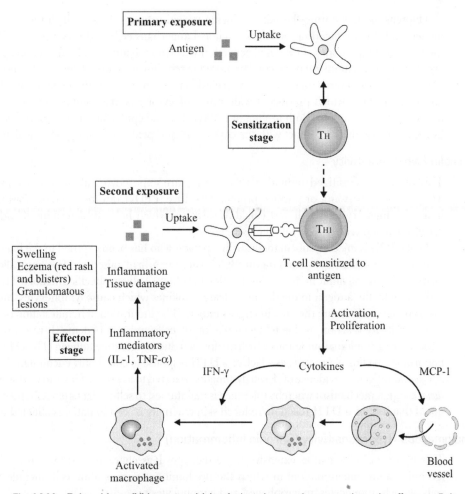

Fig. 14.11 Delayed (type IV) hypersensitivity. Activated macrophages are the major effector cells in the DTH response. B cells do not have any role unlike other hypersensitivity types.
MCP-1, monocyte chemotactic protein-1

and rubber products. Uroshiol, the oil from poison ivy, is a major cause of contact dermatitis in the United States (Fig. 14.12).

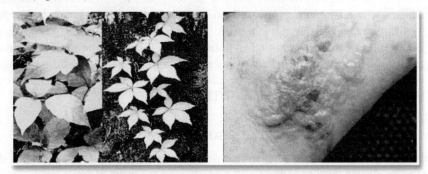

Fig. 14.12 Contact hypersensitivity. Poison ivy is a major cause of contact dermatitis in which blisters form in the skin.

Haptens on penetrating the skin conjugate to skin proteins due to which their immunogenicity increases. They are taken up by APCs, such as Langerhans cells and presented to CD4$^+$ T cells in the regional lymph nodes. This initial activation sensitizes the individual. On second contact with the agent, a rapid and more intense secondary immune response is mounted due to activation of sensitized TH1 cells. Further events that occur have been described in the preceding text. Langerhans cells and also keratinocytes, which produce a wide range of cytokines, have important roles in the contact hypersensitivity response. Both are major cell types in the epidermis. The response is characterized by localized eczema on contact with the compound and peaks at 72 hours after which it subsides.

Tuberculin Hypersensitivity

This occurs in sensitized individuals when they are exposed to tuberculin, a lipoprotein from *Mycobacterium tuberculosis*, or purified protein derivative (PPD) from the same organism. It forms the basis of a memory or 'recall' test called *Mantoux test* which helps to determine if individuals have T cell-mediated reactivity to tuberculosis.

When PPD is injected subcutaneously in a person who has been exposed to the bacterium, or has received the Bacillus Calmette-Guérin (BCG) vaccine, a firm raised red swelling called induration forms which is maximal in 48–72 hours after injection. Antigen-specific memory TH1 cells, on re-acti-vation by the antigen in the dermis, release cytokines which cause lymphocytes, monocytes, and macrophages to infiltrate the area in large numbers. The induration, a manifestation of delayed-type hypersensitivity reaction, is due to accumulation of cells and also oedema. It resolves in about 5–7 days, unlike granulomatous lesions which are formed due to persisting antigen. The DTH reaction has importance in clinical practice, as a lack of a DTH response to commonly encountered antigens, such as *Candida* antigens is evidence of T cell dysfunction referred to as *anergy*. This is to be distinguished from *clonal anergy*, a mechanism whereby tolerance is maintained to self-antigens (see Chapter 15). It is to be noted that lack of a DTH reaction/reduced skin reactivity is seen in patients afflicted with AIDS.

Granulomatous Hypersensitivity (Chronic Inflammation)

This hypersensitivity causes extensive tissue damage. It is characterized by chronic inflammation (granulomatous inflammation) in which the predominant participating cells include mononuclear cells, namely, monocytes, macrophages, and lymphocytes.

Some pathogens/antigens engulfed by macrophages are not easily degraded. For instance, intracellular microbes such as mycobacteria have devised escape mechanisms due to which they stay protected inside macrophages and even multiply. As they persist, they continually stimulate CD4$^+$ TH1 cells to produce cytokines (chronic stimulation). This results in the formation of a *granuloma* which serves to isolate the foreign agent from the rest of the body (see Fig. 9.6). A chronic inflammatory state arises which is seen in both tuberculosis and tuberculoid leprosy, and also in infection by *Schistosoma mansoni*.

Granulomas show extensive necrosis. They may even rupture due to re-activation of dormant bacilli and spread infection to other tissues. It should be borne in mind that although CD4$^+$ TH1-mediated cell-mediated immunity is critical for defence against intracellular pathogens, an overactive cell-mediated immune response, as has also been discussed earlier in Chapter 9, can result in injury to tissues and functional impairment (DTH response).

SUMMARY

• Hypersensitivity responses are exaggerated and inappropriate immune responses that cause considerable tissue injury and even disease. They are classified into four main types depending on the mechanism of tissue injury.

• Type I hypersensitivity or immediate hypersensitivity,

commonly known as allergy, involves production of IgE against environmental antigens or drugs (allergens). It also involves mast cells/basophils and the mediators released by them, such as histamine.

- Initial contact with allergen results in mast cell sensitization in which IgE binds to FcεRI on the mast cell surface. Symptoms appear only on subsequent exposure to allergen and include massive tissue oedema and smooth muscle contraction.
- Anaphylactic shock is a very rapid and severe type I response which can sometimes be fatal.
- The inflammatory response in the late phase reaction, seen in chronic asthma, causes tissue damage.
- Although IgE-mediated type I reactions can produce severe damaging effects, the protective role of IgE in defence against parasite infections is of immense benefit to the host.
- Treatment of allergies aim at inhibiting production of mediators or antagonizing their effects.
- Type II or cytotoxic hypersensitivity is mediated by antibodies (IgG or IgM) that bind to cell and tissue antigens to cause injury and disease. Antibodies mediate damage by activating the complement cascade. Cytotoxic cells bearing Fcγ receptors cause damage by ADCC.
- Cell destruction by type II reactions occurs in a mismatched blood transfusion, and also in a transplanted organ/tissue. These reactions also underlie the harm due to rhesus incompatibility.
- Type III hypersensitivity involves binding of antibodies (IgG or IgM) to antigen, to form immune complexes which are normally phagocytosed.
- An Arthus reaction is initiated when immune complexes deposit at the site of antigen entry. There is localized tissue damage due to neutrophils and complement.
- Immune complexes when formed in excess in circulation deposit at various sites, such as glomerular basement membrane of kidney, in blood vessels, and synovial membrane and cartilage of joints. These activate complement and induce the acute inflammatory response. Lytic enzymes released by neutrophils while ingesting immune complexes cause damage which is widespread.
- Type IV hypersensitivity is a delayed T cell-mediated response. It involves activation of antigen-specific inflammatory TH1 cells in a sensitized individual. TH1 cells release cytokines which cause macrophages to accumulate at the site. Macrophages are activated by antigen-specific TH1 cells to release lytic enzymes that cause injury to tissues.
- Delayed-type hypersensitivity responses are of different types. Inability of macrophages to eliminate pathogens results in formation of granulomas (granulomatous hypersensitivity). This is the most severe form of type IV hypersensitivity and causes significant pathology in tuberculosis and leprosy.

REVIEW QUESTIONS

1. Indicate whether the following statements are true or false. If false, explain why.
   (a) IgE binds to mast cells through its Fab region.
   (b) The injury in systemic lupus erythematosus (SLE) is due to a type III hypersensitivity reaction.
   (c) Tuberculosis is characterized by granulomatous inflammation.
   (d) Haemolytic disease of the newborn is due to transplacental passage of IgM anti-RhD antibodies.
   (e) Leukotriene B4 (LTB4) is a preformed mast cell mediator.
   (f) A positive tuberculin test is an example of a type I hypersensitivity reaction.

2. Self-assessment questions
   (a) What is Rhogam? Can you give reasons why it is administered to an Rh negative woman just after delivery of an Rh positive baby and not earlier?
   (b) What is the sequence of events in type I hypersensitivity reactions? Explain why epinephrine treatment is an effective treatment for anaphylactic shock.
   (c) Give two different mechanisms of antibody-mediated injury in type II hypersensitivity. Illustrate with a clinically important example of a cytotoxic reaction.
   (d) An antigen is injected into the skin of an animal presensitized to it. Which type of hypersensitivity

reaction develops and what type of cells/molecules are involved? Explain the reasons for decline in use of passive antibody therapy.

(e) What is granulomatous hypersensitivity? Give examples of diseases involving such reactions.

3. For each question, choose the *best* answer.

(a) Which one of the following stimulates IgE production by B cells?
   (i) IFN-γ
   (ii) Epinephrine
   (iii) IL-4
   (iv) IFN-γ + IL-4

(b) Which cell type shows intense infiltration in an Arthus reaction?
   (i) Basophils
   (ii) Polymorphonuclear neutrophils (PMNs)
   (iii) Dendritic cells
   (iv) T cells

(c) An intradermally injected antigen showed a positive skin test for delayed-type hypersensitivity. It indicates that
   (i) antibodies to the antigen are present
   (ii) B cells are functionally active
   (iii) mast cells have been activated by IgE
   (iv) a cell-mediated immune response has occurred

(d) Antihistamines act by
   (i) complexing with histamine
   (ii) blocking IgE binding to basophils and mast cells
   (iii) binding to H1 receptors
   (iv) regulating activity of prostaglandins

Immunologic Tolerance and Autoimmunity

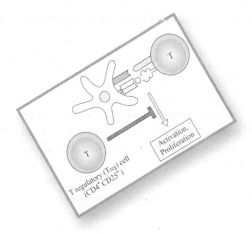

T regulatory (Treg) cell (CD4$^+$ CD25$^+$)

Activation, Proliferation

The immune system is remarkable in that it protects us from attack by an enormous variety of foreign organisms and avoids mounting immune responses to our own antigens (referred to as *autoantigens* or *self-antigens*). This is because of the ability of the immune system to distinguish between self and non-self antigens, a cardinal feature which is acquired during developmental processes in the central lymphoid organs. *Immunological tolerance* is a state of unresponsiveness of lymphocytes to an antigen which can be induced by prior exposure to that antigen. Other factors, such as a high dose of antigen can also lead to a state of tolerance. When unresponsiveness or tolerance of the immune system is to self-antigens, the term *self-tolerance* is used.

It is inevitable that lymphocytes with receptors capable of recognizing self-molecules (autoreactive lymphocytes) will be generated during the random process of receptor gene-rearrangements that occurs during lymphocyte maturation. It is important that mechanisms exist to prevent these autoreactive cells from reacting against self-components. A failure in these mechanisms to control undesirable autoreactive clones will result in an immune attack on the host's own cells/tissues leading to *autoimmunity*.

This chapter focuses on the phenomenon of self-tolerance and starts with a discussion of the various mechanisms involved in maintenance of tolerance to self-antigens, both in central lymphoid organs and in the periphery. The importance of these mechanisms in prevention of autoimmunity is emphasized. The categories of autoimmune disease and the criteria used to define a disease as autoimmune are discussed in the second half of the chapter. Effector mechanisms responsible for tissue damage in autoimmune disease and factors implicated in disease development are described. Some common autoimmune diseases and likely mechanisms that could lead to loss of self-tolerance are briefly reviewed. The concluding part of the chapter focuses on various therapeutic strategies and their basis.

SELF-TOLERANCE INDUCTION IN T AND B LYMPHOCYTES

Mechanisms for tolerance induction exist in both central lymphoid organs, namely thymus and bone marrow (*central tolerance*), and the periphery (*peripheral tolerance*). The various mechanisms involved in establishing tolerance to self-antigens in T and B lymphocytes are considered in the following text.

Central T Lymphocyte Tolerance

Immature T lymphocytes (thymocytes) undergo tolerance induction in the thymus wherein self-reactive clones undergo *deletion* (clonal deletion) by apoptosis. Achieving central tolerance in T lymphocytes is a two-stage education process in which thymic stromal cells and also epithelial cells, macrophages, and dendritic cells play a major role. This is represented diagrammatically in Fig. 15.1. The random nature of rearrangements of T cell receptor gene segments generates receptors that recognize not only various foreign antigens but also self-antigens. In *stage I*, thymocytes with receptors that bind to class I and class II major histocompatibility complex (MHC) molecules survive (*positive selection*), whereas those that do not bind die by apoptosis. In *stage II*, those thymocytes that bind with high affinity to self-peptide–MHC complexes undergo death by apoptosis (*negative selection*). Thus, selection processes allow survival of only those T cells bearing receptors that recognize antigenic peptides derived from foreign antigens, and which are displayed by self-MHC molecules. These mature into $CD4^+$ or $CD8^+$ T cells which are released from the thymus into the circulation.

Peripheral T Lymphocyte Tolerance

As all self-antigens are not expressed in the thymus, self-reactive T cells with receptors for these antigens would fail to be eliminated allowing them to escape into the periphery. These mature cells have the potential to evoke an autoimmune response. Hence, peripheral tolerance mechanisms are needed to prevent these autoreactive T cells (that have escaped central tolerance) from responding to self-antigens. Mechanisms which help to keep autoreactive T cells under control, in the periphery, are discussed in the following text.

Anergy

The reader by now must be well aware of the concept that T cells receiving only signal 1 (through T cell receptor, TCR, interaction with a specific peptide–MHC complex on antigen-presenting cells, APCs) without the costimulatory second signal fail to respond to antigen, that is, they are functionally inactivated (see Fig. 8.7). Normally, in absence of infection, APCs display mostly self-antigens and lack costimulatory B7 molecules. Self-reactive T cells which survive negative selection and escape into the periphery are rendered anergic on receiving only signal 1 from APCs. This functional inactivation of autoreactive T cell clones or non-responsiveness on contact with a self-antigen is called *clonal anergy*.

Cytotoxic T lymphocyte antigen-4 (CTLA-4), the inhibitory ligand on activated T cells for B7 molecules, which was introduced in Chapter 8, has an important role in tolerance induction. It functions to maintain T cell anergy to self-antigens, thereby helping to keep autoreactive T cells under control

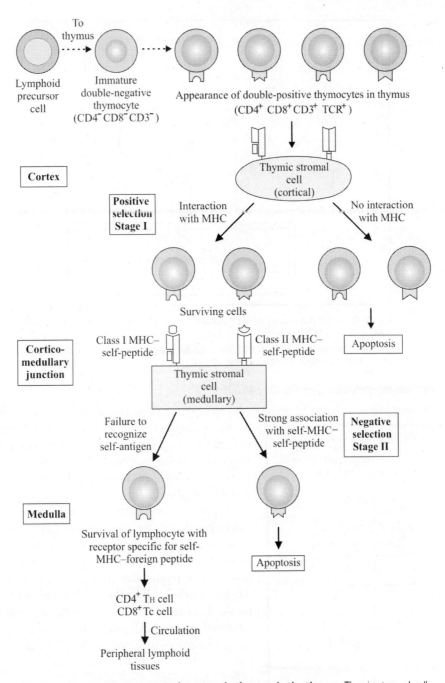

Fig. 15.1 The two-stage process for central tolerance in the thymus. Thymic stromal cells have an important role in the selection process. Principles similar to those depicted in Fig. 8.5 are represented here.

(Fig. 15.2). Knockout mice lacking CTLA-4 show uncontrolled activation of lymphocytes which infiltrate into various organs as in systemic autoimmunity.

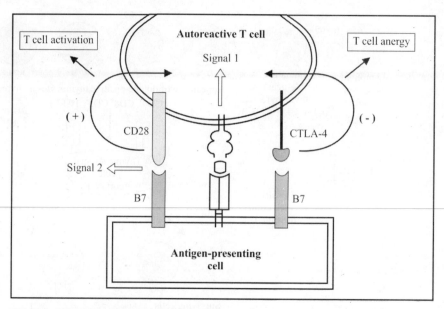

Fig. 15.2 CTLA-4 downregulates T cell activation. Mutation in the gene encoding CTLA-4 could increase susceptibility to autoimmune disease.
Source: Simmonds, M.J. and S.C.L. Gough (2005), 'Genetic insights into disease mechanisms of autoimmunity', *British Medical Bulletin*, 71, 93–113.

Activation-induced Cell Death (AICD)

On repeated stimulation by antigen (due to presence of persisting antigen such as self-antigen, and

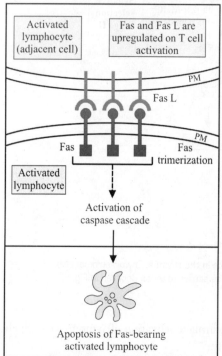

foreign antigen in chronic infection), T cells are activated but do not continue to proliferate. Rather, the pathway of cell death is triggered resulting in apoptosis of the activated T cell. Binding of *Fas*, a monomer expressed on activated T cells, to the trimeric membrane protein *Fas L* causes Fas to trimerize (Fig. 15.3). Fas L is co-expressed with Fas mainly on activated T cells and can engage Fas on the same or even a different cell. Activation of a series of events which finally lead to activation of *caspases* results in T cell apoptosis. Caspases are cytoplasmic cysteine proteases—enzymes that contain cysteine in their active site. Their name derives from the fact that they cleave their substrates on the *C*-terminal side of an aspartic acid residue. Fas–Fas L mediated apoptotic cell death eliminates autoreactive T cells in the periphery, thereby limiting autoimmune reactions. As this mechanism of cell death is a consequence of activation, it is called *activation-induced cell death*.

Fig. 15.3 Peripheral T lymphocyte tolerance by AICD. Binding of Fas receptor to Fas L results in trimerization of Fas. Death signals are transduced inside activating the caspase cascade and leading to apoptosis of the activated Fas-bearing T cell. Fas L-Fas binding can also occur on the same T cell. *Note:* This mechanism is employed by Tc cells to kill their targets.

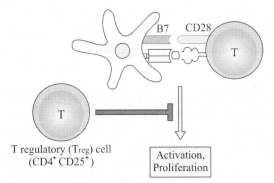

T regulatory (Treg) cell
(CD4$^+$ CD25$^+$)

Activation,
Proliferation

Fig. 15.4   T regulatory (Treg**) cells.** T**reg** cells downregulate
T cell (both CD4$^+$ and CD8$^+$) function, including self-reactive
T cells. They play a key role in prevention of autoimmunity.

T Regulatory (Treg) Cells and Peripheral Tolerance

T regulatory (Treg) cells represent approximately 5–10 per cent of all peripheral T cells. As they develop in the thymus in absence of antigen exposure, they are called *natural Treg cells*. These thymus-derived CD4$^+$ CD25$^+$ T cells populate peripheral lymphoid organs where they suppress activation and function of T cells, including self-reactive T cells such as those specific for self-antigens not expressed in the thymus (Fig. 15.4). As currently, there is a lot of attention focused on Treg cells, there is more to this population of T cells in Box 15.1. Regulatory T cell populations, other than natural Treg cells, may also be extra-thymically generated, that is, in the periphery.

Box 15.1   T Regulatory (CD4$^+$ CD25$^+$ Treg**) Cells**

T regulatory (T**reg**) cells like other T cells express TCR and CD4. They constitutively express high levels of CD25, the interleukin-2 (IL-2) receptor α chain which is also expressed on activated and effector T cells, and CTLA-4. These cells have some interesting characteristics. They do not proliferate in response to ligation of TCR and CD28. Nor do they secrete IL-2, but they do require IL-2 for their maintenance. T**reg** cells exert their suppressor function by direct cell-to-cell contact with APCs or with responding T cells and their action may not involve cytokines. For instance, they do not depend on IL-10 for biological activity. Interleukin-10, as mentioned in the following text, is a requirement for activity of other types of regulatory T cells. T**reg** cells are involved in

* downregulating both CD4$^+$ and CD8$^+$ T cell function (including self-reactive T cells that escape negative selection in the thymus);
* regulation of peripheral tolerance; and
* protection from autoimmune disease.

Although regulation of immune responses by T**reg** cells is essential, it is not always advantageous to the host. As we shall see in Chapter 18, T**reg** cells downregulate host anti-tumour immunity, thereby creating a favourable environment for growth of tumours. In view of their crucial role, T**reg** cells may be manipulated for clinical use (Fig. 15.5).

Besides natural T**reg** cells which are generated in the thymus, there are other categories of regulatory T lymphocytes that differ in origin and effector function. These include *T*R1 cells which develop in the periphery and secrete the immunosuppressive cytokine IL-10. Unlike natural T**reg** cells, these cells express CD25 only after receiving activating signals. Like natural T**reg** cells, they regulate adaptive immune responses. *T*H3 cells represent another category. These are gut-derived and were initially identified in studies on *oral tolerance* which is discussed in a section that follows. They secrete transforming growth factor-beta (TGF-β) and mediate antigen-specific IgA production. Both categories, namely TR1 and TH3 cells, are inducible and are generated after naïve T cells encounter antigens presented on dendritic cells (DCs) in the periphery. The different types of regulatory T cells and their possible relationship to each other are currently under investigation.

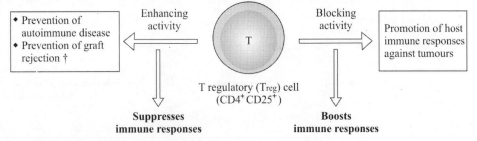

Fig. 15.5   Manipulation of Treg** cells for clinical use.**
† this is done by establishing donor-specific transplantation tolerance

Central B Lymphocyte Tolerance

The mechanisms important for induction of tolerance to self-antigens in B lymphocytes and which occur in the bone marrow (central tolerance) are briefly summarized in the following text.

Clonal Deletion

Immature B lymphocytes undergo negative selection in the bone marrow when their receptors interact strongly with self-antigens (see Chapter 6). The principle of B cell deletion by apoptosis is similar to that seen in T cell tolerance and results in elimination of the autoreactive B cell. B cells undergo positive selection, too, though it is not as well understood as in T lymphocytes.

Receptor Editing

Sometimes, initially generated B lymphocyte antigen receptors are self-reactive and can recognize self-antigens in the bone marrow. These receptors can be changed in a process referred to as *receptor editing*. In this process, B cells undergo a second rearrangement using unrearranged *V* and *J* gene segments to express a new immunoglobulin (Ig) light chain. This creates a different receptor that may be more desirable (not autoreactive), and involves re-activation of recombination activating genes RAG-1 and RAG-2. Due to receptor editing, immune responses to self are avoided.

Peripheral B Lymphocyte Tolerance

Peripheral mechanisms that help to maintain tolerance to self-antigens in mature B lymphocytes are explained in the following text.

Anergy

B cells require two signals to be activated by T-dependent (TD) antigens. Signal 1 is delivered by antigen binding to mIgM and the second signal when CD40 L on the T cell surface interacts with CD40 expressed on the B cell. In absence of this second costimulatory signal, self-reactive B cells exposed to self-antigens are rendered anergic (Fig. 15.6). Failure of self-reactive B cells to receive full signals may occur if tolerance has been induced in self-reactive T lymphocytes, or because they may have been deleted. Lack of the necessary T cell help renders B cells anergic. They are unable to re-enter follicles where further activation events occur. There is no autoantibody (antibody directed at self-antigen) production as a result of B cell anergy and they may undergo death by apoptosis due to lack of survival stimuli.

Many autoimmune diseases due to autoantibodies may be because of a failure in mechanisms leading to B cell tolerance. Due to dependence of B cells on T cells for activation signals, failure in maintenance of T cell tolerance also may lead to generation of autoantibodies.

Thus, several different mechanisms contribute to the maintenance of self-tolerance in lymphocytes. These mechanisms are essential for keeping potentially harmful self-reactive lymphocytes in check.

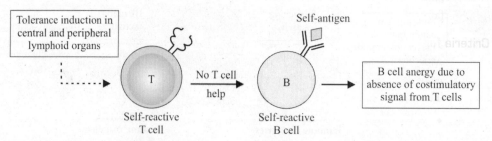

Fig. 15.6 Peripheral B lymphocyte tolerance.

Box 15.2   Artificial tolerance induction in vivo

Tolerance induction can be artificially induced in vivo in different ways that can be clinically important. For instance, it may be used to prevent rejection of transplanted organs/tissues and also to manipulate autoimmune disease. Tolerance induction is important in context of transplantation as immunosuppressive protocols in current use are not specific and induce generalized immunosuppression of the immune system. Hence, there is increasing focus on inducing donor-specific transplantation tolerance (see Chapter 17).

Artificial tolerance induction to prevent autoimmune disease involves feeding self-antigens that are the targets of autoimmune attack. Exposure to protein antigens by oral feeding can lead to immunological tolerance known as *oral tolerance*. Importantly, the dose of antigen is a critical factor in tolerance induction. Oral tolerance implies that if one feeds an antigenic protein and then subsequently injects the protein, immune responses (both humoral and cell-mediated) to the protein antigen are suppressed. To cite an example, when mice are fed *myelin basic protein (MBP)*, the target autoantigen in multiple sclerosis , there is suppression of immune responses and mice do not develop *experimental autoimmune encephalomyelitis (EAE)* when they are later injected with MBP. EAE, as we will see later, is a disease very much like multiple sclerosis, an autoimmune desease in humans. Antigens that are administered orally encounter gut-associated lymphoid tissue (GALT) which has certain unique properties that favour tolerance induction. Mechanisms involved include

- anergy in antigen-specific T cells and
- release of immunosuppressive cytokines such as TGF-β by regulatory T cells (T$_{H3}$).

Encouraging results of oral tolerance have been obtained in mice, but human clinical trials are still in early stages. It is due to oral tolerance that immune responses to food antigens and to commensals (bacteria that normally reside in the intestinal lumen) are avoided.

A better understanding of these mechanisms and the way they fail will help to understand aetiology of human autoimmune diseases, the cause of many of which is still unknown. In this context, it is relevant to mention here that tolerance can also be induced artificially in vivo in various ways that can be exploited for clinical use (Box 15.2).

The chapter now proceeds to a description of the nature of autoimmunity and autoimmune disease, including mechanisms that are likely to be involved.

AUTOIMMUNITY AND AUTOIMMUNE DISEASE

The term *autoimmunity* refers to immune responses mounted against antigens of the host itself. Although many autoimmune responses do not cause tissue injury, sometimes the response is harmful with pathological consequences. In such cases, the response results in *autoimmune disease*. The self-antigens that the immune system responds to are called *autoantigens*. Although normally the immune system does not target self-components, the potential to react with self does exist. But these potentially autoreactive lymphocytes, as has been explained earlier, may be prevented from responding to host components due to self-tolerance mechanisms established in the thymus and the bone marrow (central tolerance), and in the periphery (peripheral tolerance). When these self-tolerance mechanisms break down or fail, autoimmunity results.

Criteria for Autoimmune Disease

Although autoantibodies and autoreactive T cell clones can be detected in patients with various evidence of disease, there are some criteria that have been set for establishing a disease as autoimmune. These include

- *ability to reproduce the disease by transferring autoantibodies or self-reactive lymphocytes to a human host (direct evidence)*. This provides definite proof, but due to ethical reasons, it is difficult to obtain. However, direct evidence is available in a few cases called *experiments of nature*. Placental transfer of autoantibodies to the foetus from mothers suffering from Graves' disease, or from myasthenia gravis, results in a transient form of the disease in newborn infants. As maternal IgG is catabolized, symptoms disappear;

♦ *reproducing the disease in experimental animals (indirect evidence).* This is by transfer of autoantibodies or autoreactive T cell clones and looking for disease development in animals;

♦ *beneficial effect of immunosuppressive therapy; and*

♦ *infiltration of lymphocytes in the affected tissue as revealed by biopsy.*

Categories of Autoimmune Disease

The categories of autoimmune disease need to be defined before the chapter proceeds to a description of the mechanisms underlying pathology of autoimmune diseases, factors which are involved in their development, and some of the better understood specific autoimmune diseases.

Organ-specific

When autoantibodies or T cells respond to self-antigens localized in a particular organ or tissue, it leads to organ-specific disease. Tissue damage is largely limited to that particular organ, for example, Hashimoto's thyroiditis (HT), myasthenia gravis, and others.

Non-organ-specific or Systemic Disease

Here, the immune response is directed against a broad range of target antigens that are distributed systemically (throughout the body). Tissue damage is widespread, as in rheumatoid arthritis (RA) and systemic lupus erythematosus (SLE).

The spectrum of autoimmune disease is shown in Fig. 15.7. The two diseases HT and SLE represent the two extremes of the autoimmune spectrum.

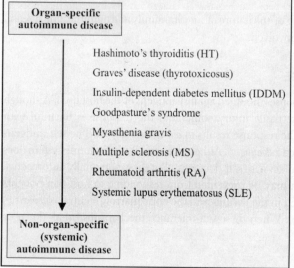

Fig. 15.7 Spectrum of autoimmune disease. The spectrum ranges from organ-specific disease to non-organ-specific disease. Distinct effector mechanisms underlie diseases at the extreme ends of the spectrum.
Note: The spectrum does not represent the complete spectrum and many autoimmune diseases have not been included.

Mechanisms of Autoimmune Pathology

Tissue damage in a majority of autoimmune diseases is mediated by autoantibodies, whereas in some diseases, T cells (T$_H$1) of delayed-type hypersensitivity (T$_{DTH}$) and cytotoxic T lymphocyte (CTL) responses elicit damage. Deposition of immune complexes also can cause considerable injury. The different mechanisms of pathology in autoimmune disease are shown in Fig. 15.8. When immune complexes are produced in excessive amounts and clearance is inefficient, they tend to deposit in tissues, particularly in renal glomeruli, synovia of joints, and also in arteries. This results in *glomerulonephritis, arthritis,* and *vasculitis,* respectively. Immune complex-mediated disease tends to be systemic with little or no specificity for a particular organ or tissue.

Target autoantigens and effector mechanisms that cause pathology in some selected autoimmune diseases are shown in Table 15.1.

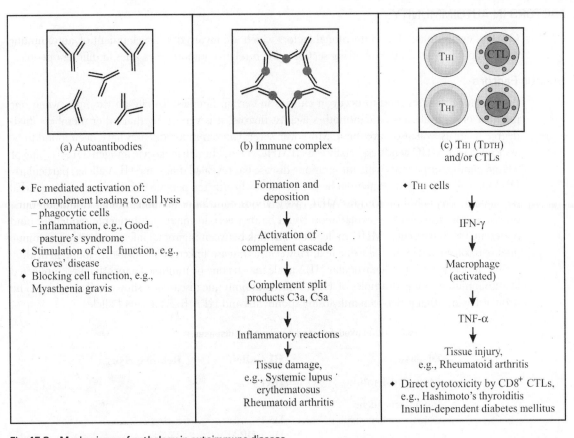

(a) Autoantibodies

(b) Immune complex

(c) TH1 (TDTH) and/or CTLs

- Fc mediated activation of:
  – complement leading to cell lysis
  – phagocytic cells
  – inflammation, e.g., Good-pasture's syndrome
- Stimulation of cell function, e.g., Graves' disease
- Blocking cell function, e.g., Myasthenia gravis

Formation and deposition

↓

Activation of complement cascade

↓

Complement split products C3a, C5a

↓

Inflammatory reactions

↓

Tissue damage, e.g., Systemic lupus erythematosus Rheumatoid arthritis

- TH1 cells

↓

IFN-γ

↓

Macrophage (activated)

↓

TNF-α

↓

Tissue injury, e.g., Rheumatoid arthritis

- Direct cytotoxicity by CD8+ CTLs, e.g., Hashimoto's thyroiditis Insulin-dependent diabetes mellitus

Fig. 15.8 Mechanisms of pathology in autoimmune disease.

Table 15.1 Target autoantigens and effector mechanisms in selected autoimmune diseases.

Disease	Target autoantigen	Effector mechanism
Graves' disease	TSH receptor	Stimulating autoantibodies
Insulin-dependent diabetes mellitus (type I)	Insulin, glutamic acid decarboxylase, and others	TH1 cells (TDTH); CTLs; autoantibodies
Goodpasture's syndrome	Non-collagen protein in lung and renal basement membrane	Autoantibodies
Myasthenia gravis	Acetylcholine receptor	Blocking autoantibodies
Multiple sclerosis	Myelin basic protein (MBP)	TH1 (TDTH); CTLs; autoantibodies
Autoimmune haemolytic anemia	Red blood cell surface antigens	Autoantibodies
Rheumatoid arthritis	Unknown cartilage antigen; IgG	Immune complexes; autoantibodies; TH1 (TDTH)
Systemic lupus erythematosus	dsDNA, histones, and others; RBC and platelet membrane antigens	Immune complexes; autoantibodies

FACTORS IN AUTOIMMUNITY

Genetic, environmental, and hormonal factors which are involved in development of autoimmune disease are discussed in the following sections. Their relative importance varies in different people.

Genetic Factors

Autoimmune diseases tend to occur in clusters in certain families. To cite an example, when one member of a family has autoantibodies against thyroid, it is very likely that other members (first-degree relatives) will also have them. Moreover, several autoimmune diseases have been found to be associated with MHC genes, especially class II MHC genes. Human leukocyte antigen (HLA) typing of a large number of patients with autoimmune disease has revealed that some HLA alleles, particularly HLA class II alleles, are prevalent in higher frequency in afflicted persons as compared to the general population. Precisely how certain MHC associations contribute to susceptibility to autoimmune disease is not clear. A likely explanation could be that certain microbial antigenic sequences bind preferentially to particular MHC molecules. The link between microbial infection and autoimmune disease is considered in the following text. However, as disease-linked HLA alleles are found in healthy people also, expression of a particular HLA allele may be one of multiple factors that are implicated in autoimmunity. Some examples of HLA-linked autoimmune disease are shown in Table 15.2. The strongest association is between ankylosing spondylitis and HLA B-27, a class I allele.

Table 15.2 HLA-linked selected autoimmune diseases.

Disease	HLA allele	Relative risk‡
Rheumatoid arthritis	DR4	4
Insulin-dependent diabetes mellitus (type I)	DR3	5
	DR4	5–6
	DR3/DR4 (heterozygotes)	25
Multiple sclerosis	DR2	4
Systemic lupus erythematosus	DR2 DR3	5
Ankylosing spondylitis†	B27 (class I allele)	90–100

‡, this is quantified by typing the HLA alleles in individuals with disease and in healthy people and dividing the frequency of the alleles in the two sets

†, an inflammatory disease of the vertebral joints which affects mostly males

It is relevant to mention here that although the major contribution in many autoimmune diseases is from MHC genes, other genes also, some of which influence self-tolerance, contribute to development. The importance of CTLA-4 in inducing anergy in self-reactive cells has been explained in a preceding section. A mutation in the gene encoding this molecule tilts the balance towards autoimmunity (Fig. 15.2).

Environmental Triggers

Infectious organisms are considered the major environmental factors which, together with genetic susceptibility, may be important for initiating autoimmune disease. Microbes may contribute to disease development by stimulating increase in expression of B7 costimulators on APCs. This will enable

APCs, which normally in the resting state are presenting self-antigens in absence of B7 costimulators, to stimulate self-reactive T cells. In other words, infection leads to breakdown in T cell tolerance to self-antigens (see Fig. 5.11). Cross-reactivity between microbial antigens and self-antigens is also a contributory factor. Rheumatic fever following streptococcal infection provides a direct link between a specific infection and autoimmune disease (described in the following text).

Sex-based Differences in Autoimmune Disease—Hormonal Factors

The development of autoimmunity shows a gender bias, women being more susceptible to disease than men. Systemic lupus erythematosus is 10 times more common in females than in males. Although the causes are not fully understood, it is believed that sex steroids, mainly estrogens, progesterone, and testosterone, influence function and development of various lymphocyte populations. The tendency of females to mount stronger proinflammatory T_{H1} responses may be a reason why females are more prone than men to develop autoimmune disease.

Most autoimmune diseases occur in adults and are more common in the third and fourth decade of life. It is to be noted that presence of autoantibodies does not always result in disease. A significant finding is that autoantibodies such as *anti-nuclear autoantibodies (ANAs)* and *rheumatoid factors (RFs)* are prevalent in older people over the age of 80, but they show no signs of disease.

SOME COMMON AUTOIMMUNE DISEASES

Some selected examples of organ- and non-organ-specific autoimmune diseases are described in the following sections. It is emphasized here that there are other ways, too, of classifying autoimmune diseases, such as on the basis of effector mechanism involved. However, whatever the basis of classification, the distinctions are far from perfect.

Organ-specific Autoimmune Disease

Some common examples of organ-specific autoimmune disease and their significant features are highlighted in the following text.

Graves' Disease

In this disease, autoantibodies to the thyroid-stimulating hormone (TSH) receptor chronically stimulate the thyroid, leading to oversecretion of thyroid hormones (T3 and T4). The normal negative feedback control does not operate (Fig. 15.9).

These autoantibodies have a stimulatory effect and do not cause organ damage. *Graves' thyrotoxicosus* is a form of hyperthyroidism associated with inflammation and protrusion of the eyes (Fig. 15.10). The disease was named after R. Graves, an Irish physician, who was the first to describe it.

Myasthenia Gravis

Autoantibodies to the acetylcholine receptor block the binding of the neurotransmitter acetylcholine to its receptor. Transmission of nerve impulses across the neuromuscular junction is blocked resulting in muscle weakness. It is to be noted that here, unlike Graves' disease, autoantibodies block functioning of the receptor (Fig. 15.11). There is no associated tissue damage.

Autoimmune Haemolytic Anaemia

In autoimmune haemolytic anaemia (AIHA), IgG autoantibodies bind to antigens on the red blood cell (RBC) surface and activate complement. As RBCs are very vulnerable to complement-mediated lysis, there is premature destruction of erythrocytes. Opsonization of RBCs by antibodies or C3b

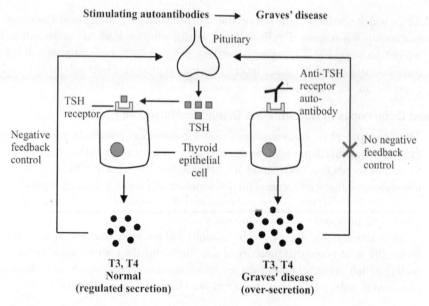

Fig. 15.9 Graves' disease. Chronic stimulation of the thyroid by anti-TSH receptor autoantibodies leads to over-secretion of thyroid hormones (T3 and T4).

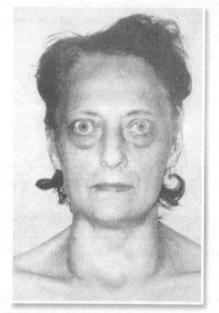

Fig. 15.10 Graves' thyrotoxicosus. In this disease, hyperthyroidism is associated with inflammation and protrusion of the eyes.

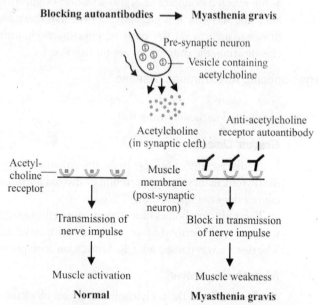

Fig. 15.11 Myasthenia gravis. Blocking of acetylcholine receptor by anti-acetylcholine receptor autoantibodies prevents transmission of nerve impulses across the neuromuscular junction.

with subsequent phagocytosis can also occur. Some drugs, for example, penicillin, can induce AIHA. Penicillin, like haptens, binds to proteins on the RBC surface and elicits production of autoantibodies which cause lysis. The anti-hypertensive drug α-methyl dopa acts similarly. *Drug-induced AIHA* is reversible and symptoms generally disappear when the drug is withdrawn.

Goodpasture's Syndrome

This disorder is caused by autoantibodies to kidney and lung basement membrane protein. Autoantibodies deposit in renal glomeruli and alveoli of lungs, and activate complement (type III hypersensitivity reaction). The complement split products that are generated trigger inflammatory reactions in the kidney and the lungs, causing damage to glomerular and alveolar basement membranes, respectively. There is progressive kidney damage (glomerulonephritis) and pulmonary haemorrhage, outcome of which can be fatal. Common epitopes on epithelial cells in kidney and lung basement membrane may explain why both sites are the targets of autoimmune attack.

Insulin-dependent Diabetes Mellitus (Type I)

Insulin-dependent diabetes mellitus (IDDM; type I) is due to an autoimmune attack on the pancreas which specifically destroys the β-islet cells. T cells, both $CD4^+$ and $CD8^+$ cells, and also macrophages, infiltrate into the pancreas. A delayed-type hypersensitivity (DTH) response is activated resulting in inflammatory destruction of the islet cells. This, and also direct cytolysis by CTLs, results in decreased insulin secretion causing blood glucose to rise. An environmental agent, probably measles or a mumps virus, appears to trigger the disease. The increased production of local interferon-gamma (IFN-γ) upregulates class II MHC expression on β cells allowing recognition by TH cells. Autoantibody responses, though not common, occur against self-antigens such as insulin, and the enzyme glutamic acid decarboxylase which is located on the β islet cell membrane.

Systemic Autoimmune Disease

Systemic (non-organ-specific) autoimmune diseases are characterized by widespread lesions as the autoimmune response targets a broad range of autoantigens which are distributed in many organs/tissues. The major examples are discussed here.

Rheumatoid Arthritis

Rheumatoid arthritis is a well-known autoimmune disorder characterized by a chronic inflammatory reaction in the joint synovium which eventually leads to damage of synovial joints (Fig. 15.12).

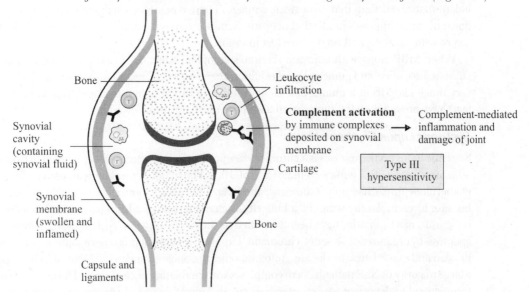

Fig. 15.12 A synovial joint in rheumatoid arthritis. Deposition of immune complexes in the joint synovium and leukocyte infiltration cause joint inflammation.

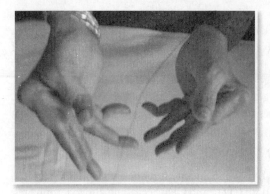

Fig. 15.13   Rheumatoid arthritis. Deformities in the small joints of the hands of a rheumatoid arthritis patient (*Source:* Photograph kindly provided by S. Singh and Prof. D.N. Rao, Department of Biochemistry, AIIMS, New Delhi).

The disease involves the small joints of the extremities (Fig. 15.13), and also larger joints including knees, shoulders, and elbows. Symptoms include morning stiffness, fatigue, pain, and weight loss.

Approximately 75 per cent of adults with chronic disease produce IgM autoantibodies called *rheumatoid factors* (*RFs*), which react with antigenic determinants in the Fc region of self-IgG. Large amounts of immune complexes (RF-IgG complexes) can be detected in the joint fluid. These trigger inflammatory reactions (type III hypersensitivity) by activating the classical pathway of complement. Circulating immune complexes may lead to systemic vasculitis.

Both cell-mediated and humoral mechanisms contribute to disease pathology. CD4$^+$ TH1 cells (TDTH), dendritic cells, macrophages, and neutrophils infiltrate into the joint synovium. Macrophages, which are stimulated by cytokines from activated T cells, mediate erosion of cartilage and bone. Cytokines detected in synovial fluid include interleukin-1 (IL-1), IL-8, tumour necrosis factor-alpha (TNF-α), and IFN-γ. An imbalance in the cytokine network, and neutrophils, contributes to the disease in a major way.

Multiple Sclerosis

Multiple sclerosis (MS) is a common inflammatory disease in young adults which affects the central nervous system (CNS). It is characterized by demyelination and chronic neurological disability (Fig. 15.14). Immune system components, for example, autoreactive T cells, macrophages, and to a lesser extent, B cells gain access from blood into CNS by crossing the blood–brain barrier (BBB). Autoreactive T lymphocytes attack specific proteins in CNS myelin such as *myelin basic protein* (*MBP*). Activated macrophages secrete numerous cytokines, for example, IL-1 and TNF-α which trigger non-specific inflammatory reactions that cause tissue damage. There is neurological dysfunction leading to slowing down of nerve impulses in affected neurons. Symptoms may be mild with numbness in the limbs or severe with paralysis and progressive loss in vision.

When MBP along with adjuvant (Freund's complete adjuvant, FCA) is injected into laboratory animals (rats, mice, and guinea pigs), it results in *experimental autoimmune encephalomyelitis* (*EAE*), a disease very much like MS in humans (Box 15.2). Studies on this animal model (described in the following text) have provided useful information about the mechanisms involved in the disease process.

Systemic Lupus Erythematosus

Systemic lupus erythematosus is a chronic systemic disease that affects mostly women between 20 and 40 years of age, with a female-to-male ratio of 10:1. The major clinical signs are skin rashes, arthritis, glomerulonephritis, haemolytic anaemia, and fever. The reddish 'butterfly rash' on the cheeks, so called because it resembles the wings of a butterfly, is characteristic of SLE (Fig. 15.15). Nucleosomes, the basic units of chromatin, have been identified as the major target in SLE. These are formed during apoptosis by organized cleavage of chromatin. Exposure to sunlight promotes apoptosis of neutrophils in the skin and exacerbates the disease. Autoantibodies to double-stranded (ds) DNA, which are present in a large majority of SLE patients, form complexes with circulating nucleosomes. The immune complexes formed tend to deposit at various sites, particularly kidney, due to which many patients develop renal complications. Other sites of deposition include joints, skin, arteries, and lungs.

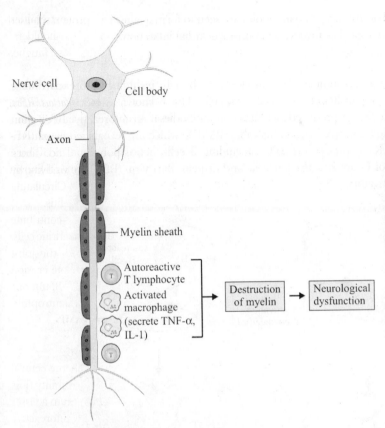

Nerve cell

Cell body

Axon

Myelin sheath

Autoreactive
T lymphocyte

Activated
macrophage
(secrete TNF-α,
IL-1)

Destruction
of myelin → Neurological
dysfunction

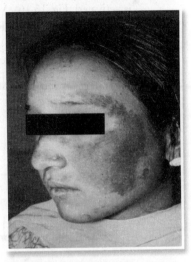

Fig. 15.15 An SLE patient with the characteristic butterfly rash over the cheeks.
(*Source:* Photograph kindly provided by S. Singh and Prof. D.N. Rao, Department of Biochemistry, AIIMS, New Delhi).

Fig. 15.14 Multiple sclerosis affects the CNS. Autoreactive T cells along with activated macrophages attack specific proteins in nerve cell myelin, such as myelin basic protein (MBP) resulting in myelin destruction.

Also commonly found in SLE are autoantibodies to RBCs and platelets. These cause complement-mediated lysis resulting in anaemia and thrombocytopenia. *Autoantibodies in serum are helpful in diagnosis of some autoimmune disorders. Detection of anti-nuclear antibodies against ds DNA helps in diagnosis of SLE, whereas presence of RFs assists in diagnosis of RA. Common laboratory tests for autoantibodies include screening of serum by immunofluorescence microscopy, agglutination tests (for RFs), and ELISA* (see Appendix 1).

MECHANISMS LEADING TO AUTOIMMUNITY

Some likely mechanisms that could lead to loss of self-tolerance and which may contribute to the development of autoimmunity are considered in the following sections.

Exposure of Hidden or Sequestered Antigens

Developing T cells in the thymus become self-tolerant to only those antigens to which they are exposed. They may not be exposed to some antigens such as late-developing antigens or those that are sequestered in organs such as eyes, brain, and testes. But sometimes these hidden tissue antigens are exposed, structurally altered or released due to damage to tissues (for instance, by an infectious agent, ischemic injury, radiation or chemicals). They would then be the target of an autoreactive T cell response/autoantibodies. For instance, autoantibodies are seen to form against lens protein released after eye damage, and against cardiac myocytes in post-myocardial infarction.

Polyclonal B Cell Activation

Certain viruses and bacteria can stimulate several clones of B cells, including autoreactive ones, in a non-specific manner without help from specific TH cells. This is known as *polyclonal activation*. Antibodies of many specificities are produced including autoantibodies if an autoreactive B cell clone is activated (Fig. 15.16). Molecular patterns on microbes (PAMPs) which are recognized by pattern-recognition receptors (PRRs) expressed on APCs, including B cells, act as polyclonal activators. Lipopolysaccharide (LPS) of Gram-negative bacteria, and Epstein–Barr virus (EBV) are well-known examples of polyclonal activators.

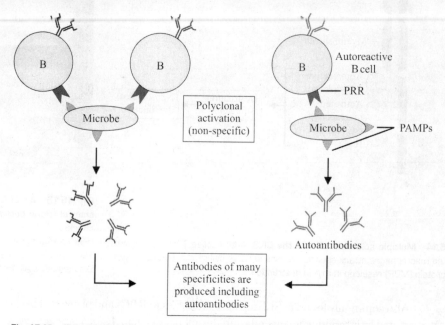

Fig. 15.16   Polyclonal activation of B cells by microbial PAMPs.

Carrier Effect

Sometimes microbial proteins or drugs may interact with self-antigens. A self-reactive B cell endocytoses the complex and presents microbial peptides to a microbe-specific T cell. The specific TH cell then provides help to the self-reactive B cell, and causes it to proliferate and produce autoantibodies (Fig. 15.17). This effect is called the *carrier effect*. It is also referred to as the *T cell bypass mechanism* as autoreactive T cells have been tolerized and are unable to collaborate with self-reactive B cells to generate autoantibodies.

Molecular Mimicry

Many epitopes in microbial antigens are identical or similar to epitopes in self-molecules. This cross-reactivity between microbial and self-molecules is referred to as *molecular mimicry*. Rheumatic fever, which follows streptococcal infections of the throat, is due to anti-streptococcal antibodies that cross-react with myocardial proteins (Fig. 15.18). Short similar sequences have been identified in myocardial proteins and streptococcal protein. At some later time, there is cardiac inflammation (myocarditis)

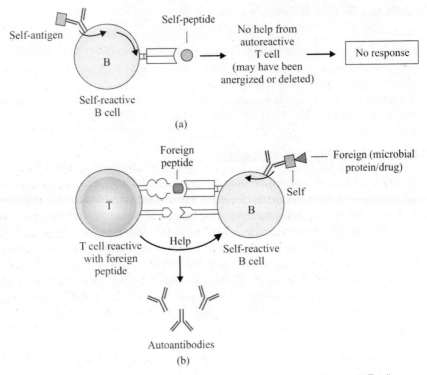

Fig. 15.17 **The carrier effect.** The mechanism bypasses help from self-reactive T cells.

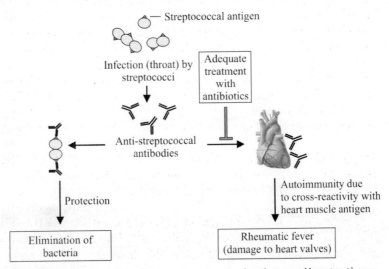

Fig. 15.18 **Cross-reactivity between streptococcal antigens and heart antigens causes rheumatic fever.**

which weakens heart muscle, causing breathlessness and fatigue in patients. Rapid treatment of the infection at the start with antibiotics helps to clear the infection before the immune response is activated to produce autoantibodies. However, as autoimmune disorders have a long asymptomatic period, evidence for the role of microbes as initiating agents is not easy to find. Hence, the role of molecular mimicry in autoimmunity is, as yet, unclear.

CD4⁺ Tн Cells and Tн1/Tн2 Balance in Autoimmunity

Studies conducted on animal models of autoimmune disease (described in the following text) have provided a wealth of information. Such studies have shown that CD4⁺ Tн cells have a major role to play in disease development and progression. For instance, transfer of autoreactive T cell clones from diseased animals to normal animals has been shown to induce disease. The Tн1/Tн2 balance is a critical factor in determining whether autoimmunity develops or not. While Tн1 cells favour development of autoimmune disease, the Tн2 subset is protective and blocks disease development.

TREATMENT OF AUTOIMMUNE DISEASE

Strategies for treatment of autoimmune disease are similar to approaches used to prevent graft rejection. These are summarized in Fig. 15.19 and are briefly considered in the following text.

Symptoms in many organ-specific autoimmune disorders can often be corrected by *metabolic control*, such as by use of anti-thyroid drugs in Graves' disease. *Replacement therapy* using insulin helps to correct the defect in type I IDDM. In a technique called *plasmapheresis*, plasma is removed from the patient's blood by continuous-flow centrifugation. The RBCs are resuspended in a suitable medium and returned to the patient. Removal of circulating immune complexes and antibodies with plasma results in short-term reduction of symptoms in diseases such as SLE, RA, myasthenia gravis, and others.

Corticosteroids, for example, *prednisone* are potent anti-inflammatory agents and have shown benefit in RA, SLE, and immune complex nephritis. A compromise dose is used that reduces tissue injury without disturbing protective immunity. *Cyclosporin*, an immunosuppressive drug, blocks T cell activation by inhibiting IL-2 synthesis by T cells. Only antigen-activated T cells are inhibited, whereas non-activated T cells are spared. The drug has shown benefit in early IDDM and SLE.

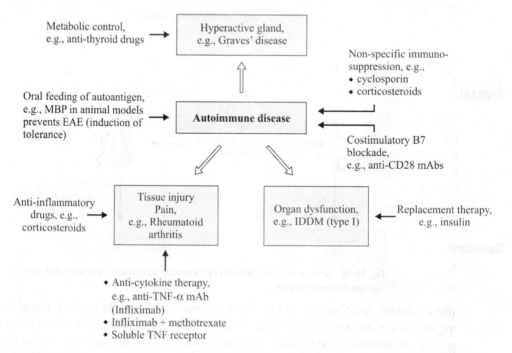

Fig. 15.19 Various strategies for treatment of autoimmune disease. Some additional approaches which are in the experimental stage are included in the main text and have not been shown.

The *cytokine IFN-β* has antiviral effects and has been approved for the treatment of multiple sclerosis. The possible role of virus in triggering MS may explain why IFN-β has a beneficial role. It reduces myelin destruction slowing the progression of physical disability. Severity and duration of attacks are also reduced.

Anti-cytokine therapy has also shown benefit in patients. *Infliximab*, a chimeric anti-TNF-α monoclonal antibody, neutralizes TNF-α, a pro-inflammatory cytokine and has been approved for treatment of RA in the United States and Europe. It has been observed in clinical settings that within a day of infliximab therapy, IL-6 levels, which are elevated in RA patients, return to normal. Symptoms such as morning stiffness, pain, and tiredness disappeared within hours of infusion. A major disadvantage is the need for repeated injections and high cost. Synergistic treatment with infliximab and methotrexate, an antifolate drug, shows significant improvement in symptoms and a more lasting benefit. *Soluble TNF receptors* which bind with high affinity to TNF-α and neutralize its pro-inflammatory activity have been approved for treatment of RA (see Fig. 7.14).

Experimental Approaches

Treatment with *anti-CD4 monoclonal antibodies* reverses multiple sclerosis and arthritis in animal models. The approach, however, suffers from the drawback that it depletes all CD4$^+$ T cells which, in turn, affects immune responsiveness of the recipient. Another experimental approach aims at *B cell depletion* considering that autoantibodies have a major role in autoimmune diseases such as RA and SLE. This can be achieved by targeting the B cell transmembrane protein CD20 with monoclonal antibodies. Encouraging results have been obtained.

Preventing interaction of B7 molecules with CD28 by *blocking the B7 costimulatory signal* interferes in activation of T cells and has shown benefit in RA. *Blocking the CD40–CD40 L interaction* by using antibodies to CD40 L also holds promise. Feeding autoantigen with the aim of inducing *oral tolerance*, introduced earlier, is also being explored.

Further studies are needed to establish the efficacy of these newer approaches. It is important that the strategy being investigated should not interfere with protective immunity of the patient.

ANIMAL MODELS OF AUTOIMMUNE DISEASE

There are certain inbred strains of mice which are genetically programmed to develop some auto-immune diseases spontaneously. These diseases can also be induced experimentally by injecting appropriate animals with the inducing antigen in FCA. The inducing antigen used corresponds to self-antigens associated with the human disease. The autoimmune diseases that develop in these animal models show close resemblance to their human counterparts. It is through these animal models that tremendous valuable information has been obtained about mechanisms that are likely to lead to autoimmunity. They also allow evaluation of potential therapies (Table 15.3).

Spontaneous Animal Models

Some spontaneous animal models which have proved helpful in understanding the nature of human autoimmune disease are briefly introduced here.

(NZB x NZW) F₁ Mouse

This is a valuable model for studying the pathogenesis of SLE. The incidence of the disease in these hybrids is greater in females as for human SLE. These mice develop autoantibodies directed against nuclear components, erythrocytes, platelets, and immune complex glomerulonephritis as in humans.

Table 15.3 Some selected animal models of autoimmune disease.

Animal model	Equivalent human disease	Method of induction
(NZB x NZW) F$_1$ mouse	Systemic lupus erythematosus	Spontaneous
Non-obese diabetic (NOD) mouse	Insulin-dependent diabetes mellitus	Spontaneous
Experimental autoimmune encephalomyelitis (EAE) [rats, mice, and guinea pigs]	Multiple sclerosis	Immunization with MBP in FCA†
Experimental autoimmune myasthenia gravis(EAMG) [rats and guinea pigs]	Myasthenia gravis	Immunization with acetylcholine receptor in FCA†

† FCA, Freund's complete adjuvant

Non-obese Diabetic (NOD) Mouse

The non-obese diabetic (NOD) mouse is a useful animal model that spontaneously develops autoimmune diabetes resembling human IDDM. Valuable information has been obtained through these mice regarding various non-MHC genes that contribute to disease development.

Animal Models of Induced Autoimmune Disease

In addition to the spontaneous animal models introduced in the preceding text, two animal models in which autoimmunity is induced experimentally are also listed here.

Experimental Autoimmune Encephalomyelitis Model

Experimental autoimmune encephalomyelitis, a demyelinating disease of the CNS, can be induced in rats about 1–2 weeks after immunization with MBP in FCA. Exposing immature T cells to MBP injected directly into the thymus (where normally this self-antigen is not present) during the neonatal period leads to tolerance to MBP, and EAE can be prevented. The EAE model is valuable for testing therapeutic strategies in MS. Studies have shown that MBP administered orally to mice makes MBP-specific T cell clones in the periphery (which might have escaped negative selection in the thymus) self-tolerant. This significant observation has led to initiation of clinical trials in humans.

Experimental Autoimmune Myasthenia Gravis Model

It was through studies on this animal model (rats/guinea pigs) that it was revealed that autoantibodies to the acetylcholine receptor are the cause of myasthenia gravis in humans.

SUMMARY

- Immunological tolerance is a state of unresponsiveness of lymphocytes to an antigen. Tolerance to self-antigens (self-tolerance) prevents damaging reactions to body's own cells and tissues.
- Tolerance is induced in both immature (central tolerance) and mature (peripheral tolerance) lymphocytes. Several mechanisms contribute to tolerance to self-antigens in T and B lymphocytes.

- Central tolerance relies on selection processes and results from deletion of self-reactive lymphocytes. Peripheral tolerance results from functional inactivation of autoreactive clones (clonal anergy) that have survived the negative selection process.
- Activation-induced cell death and also CD4$^+$ CD25$^+$ T regulatory (T$_{reg}$) cells play a crucial role in maintaining peripheral T cell tolerance.

- Tolerance can be artificially induced in vivo to prevent rejection of foreign grafts and to manipulate autoimmune disease.
- When mechanisms that ensure self-tolerance break down, the immune system attacks host components. This is referred to as autoimmunity. An autoimmune response to self-antigens that causes tissue damage results in autoimmune disease.
- Besides the presence of autoantibodies and autoreactive T cell clones in patients, certain criteria which establish a disease as autoimmune include transmissibility to humans and animals, infiltration of T and/or B lymphocytes in affected tissues, and clinical improvement with immunosuppressive drugs.
- Autoimmune diseases can be organ-specific or non-organ-specific (systemic).
- Pathology in autoimmune disease is mediated by autoantibodies, Tcells (TDTH), CTLs and immune complexes. More than one effector mechanism may contribute to damage in a particular autoimmune disease.
- There is a strong genetic association between specific autoimmune diseases and certain MHC alleles. Environmental factors such as microbes also play an important role.
- Incidence of disease is higher in females than in males; sex hormones, too, are contributory factors.
- Tests based on autoantibodies (e.g., ANAs in SLE) are helpful in diagnosis.
- Some mechanisms proposed for induction of autoimmune disease include exposure of hidden antigens, polyclonal B cell activation, carrier effect, and molecular mimicry.
- CD4$^+$ TH cells are key players in development of autoimmunity. TH1 subset of T cells favours development, whereas the TH2 subset has a protective role.
- Metabolic control is generally the usual mode of therapy of organ-specific diseases. Systemic diseases involve use of immunosuppressive and anti-inflammatory drugs.
- Use of cytokines, and anti-cytokine therapy that neutralizes TNF-α, has shown beneficial results.
- Newer experimental immune-based approaches are under investigation.

REVIEW QUESTIONS

1. Indicate whether the following statements are true or false. If false, explain why.
   (a) Graves' disease is a systemic autoimmune disease.
   (b) There is strong association between ankylosing spondylitis and HLA B-8.
   (c) Myasthenia gravis in neonates is due to transplacental passage of maternal autoantibodies (IgG) against the TSH receptor
   (d) Self-proteins do not undergo processing/presentation as do foreign proteins.
   (e) TH1 cells promote development of autoimmunity.
   (f) A defective Fas gene prevents a cell from undergoing apoptosis.

2. Self-assessment questions
   (a) How are self-reactive lymphocytes that have survived central tolerance mechanisms in thymus and bone marrow prevented from causing harm to the host?
   (b) What are some possible ways by which a viral infection contributes to the development of organ-specific autoimmune disease?
   (c) Experimental autoimmune encephalomyelitis (EAE) animal model is a very useful model of an autoimmune disorder. Explain how it has proved useful?
   (d) What is the cause of the vasculitis seen in SLE patients? Which laboratory test is helpful in diagnosis of SLE and what does it detect?
   (e) Briefly explain a strategy being explored for inducing tolerance artificially in vivo. How can this be exploited for clinical use?

3. For each question, choose the *best* answer
   (a) Which of the following autoimmune diseases is non-organ specific?
      (i) Hashimoto's thyroiditis
      (ii) Systemic lupus erythematosus (SLE)
      (iii) Graves' disease
      (iv) Insulin-dependent diabetes mellitus

(b) Autoantibodies that help in diagnosis of rheumatoid arthritis are
   (i) antinuclear
   (ii) anti-acetylcholine receptor
   (iii) anti-TSH receptor
   (iv) anti-IgG Fc

(c) Which of the following is an animal model for insulin-dependent diabetes mellitus (IDDM) type I?
   (i) SCID mouse
   (ii) EAE mouse
   (iii) NOD mouse
   (iv) (NZB x NZW) F_1

(d) Goodpasture's syndrome is characterized by autoantibodies to
   (i) IgG
   (ii) basement membrane protein
   (iii) RBC antigens
   (iv) acetylcholine receptor

Immunodeficiency Diseases

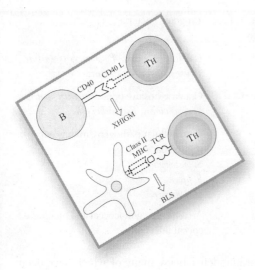

LEARNING OBJECTIVES

Having studied this chapter, you should be able to understand the following:

♦ Genetic defects in immune system components that lead to primary immunodeficiency
♦ Various causes that later in life lead to secondary immuno-deficiency disorders
♦ That increased susceptibility to infections is a sign of a faulty immune system
♦ Various options available to treat immunodeficiency and that gene therapy is in its experimental stage
♦ Some tests available for evaluation of immunodeficiency and which help in diagnosis
♦ Structure of HIV and its replication cycle
♦ Clinical progression of AIDS
♦ How HIV causes immunosuppression
♦ Therapeutic management of AIDS patients
♦ Vaccine development against HIV and the difficulties faced

The immune system is complex and has evolved to provide defence against a wide range of infectious organisms and their toxic products. Sometimes there are defects in function of immune system components. This can result in serious and often fatal immunodeficiency diseases which can be classified into two types: *primary* and *secondary*. *Primary immunodeficiency diseases* are due to genetic defects in components of the immune system and are, generally, congenital (inborn) and rare. Some of these diseases are caused by defects in genes on the X chromosome and, hence, are seen mostly in males. Sometimes, primary deficiency may be due to a developmental abnormality in immune system maturation as is seen in DiGeorge syndrome (DGS). For reasons that are not very clear, patients with primary deficiencies show a tendency to develop autoimmune disease.

Primary immunodeficiency diseases are very instructive and have helped in understanding the functional importance of the deficient component(s). We first learned about B and T cells and their respective roles in humoral and cell-mediated immunity from inherited deficiency disorders. Now, many immunodeficiency states have been created in mice with the use of targeted gene knockout techniques. These are adding considerably to our knowledge.

Secondary immunodeficiencies are not due to genetic defects but are acquired during life. They may be a consequence of infection, other diseases, or the treatments that are given.

The main consequences of a faulty immune system are increased susceptibility to infections and also increase in incidence of certain cancers. The type of infections occurring in patients is a useful clue to the type of immunodeficiency disorder and helps in diagnosis (Table 16.1).

Table 16.1 Nature of infection(s) in patients with selected congenital diseases in various arms of the immune system.

Defective component	Disease	Nature of infection
B and T cells	Severe combined immunodeficiency (SCID)	Bacteria, viruses, fungi, and protozoa
B cell	X-linked agammaglobulinemia (X-LA); other hypogammaglobulinemias	Pyogenic bacteria
T cell	DiGeorge syndrome	*Candida albicans, Pneumocystis carinii,* viruses, and mycobacteria
Phagocyte	Chronic granulomatous disease (CGD)	Catalase-positive organisms, e.g., *Staphylococcus aureus, Escherichia coli*
Complement proteins	C1, C4, C2, and C3	Extracellular pathogens, mainly encapsulated bacteria: *S. pneumoniae* *S. pyogenes* *H. influenzae*
	C5, C6, C7, C8, and C9	*Neisseria* spp. (gonococcal and meningococcal infections)

The chapter describes some selected congenital immunodeficiencies, many of which have been referred to in earlier chapters Various approaches to treatment of primary immunodeficiency disorders are considered and some experimental animal models are described. Among the acquired immunodeficiencies, the main focus is on acquired immunodeficiency syndrome (AIDS), a global concern.

PRIMARY IMMUNODEFICIENCY DISEASES

The overall cellular development of the immune system showing the sites of involvement of selected primary immunodeficiencies is depicted in Fig. 16.1.

The functional defects of some B and T cell deficiency states are summarized in Table 16.2 and are discussed in the following text.

B Cell Immunodeficiency

Patients with B cell disorders show increased susceptibility to pyogenic bacterial infections (Table 16.1), but immunity to viral and fungal infections is generally unaffected (as these are dealt with by CMI).

X-linked Agammaglobulinemia

This was first described in 1952 by a physician O. C. Bruton during investigations conducted on a young boy who suffered frequent and severe bacterial infections. X-linked agammaglobulinemia is

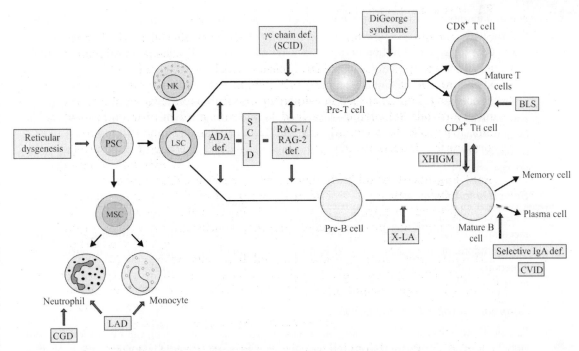

Fig. 16.1   Location of defects that give rise to primary immunodeficiency disorders. Some selected congenital diseases are indicated here in boxes. Reticular dysgenesis is due to a stem cell defect; affected infants die early as a result of frequent and very severe infections. BLS, due to lack of class II MHC expression on DCs, affects T cell activation. The pro-T and pro-B cell stage is not shown.
PSC, pluripotent stem cell; LSC, lymphoid stem cell; MSC, myeloid stem cell

Table 16.2   Some selected primary immunodeficiency diseases affecting B and T cells.

Immune component affected	Disease	Functional defect
B cell	X-linked agammaglobulinemia (X-LA)	Mutation in B cell-specific tyrosine kinase (Btk); mature B cells lacking; serum Ig isotypes low or absent
	Selective IgA deficiency	IgA decreased or absent; B cell numbers normal
	Common variable immunodeficiency (CVID)	Failure of B cells to mature to plasma cells; most Ig isotypes reduced in serum; precise defect unknown
T cell	DiGeorge syndrome (DGS)	Defect in embryogenesis; thymic hypoplasia; decreased mature T cells but B cells normal; serum Ig level reduced or normal
	X-linked hyper immunoglobulin M syndrome (XHIGM)	Mutation in CD40 L; TH cell-dependent B cell and macrophage activation blocked; IgM increased; other isotypes lacking
	Bare lymphocyte syndrome (BLS)	Lack of class II MHC expression due to mutation in genes encoding transcription factors; T cell activation signals lacking; both cellular and humoral immunity impaired

due to a mutation in the gene which encodes *B cell-specific tyrosine kinase (Btk)*. This is associated with the pre-BCR and delivers downstream activating signals for B cell maturation. Due to mutation in the gene for Btk, maturation of B cells is arrested at the pre-B cell stage, due to which number of mature B cells is reduced. Consequently, Immunoglobulin-G (IgG) levels are lowered in serum, whereas other isotypes are usually absent. Due to lack of opsonization and phagocytosis, the child suffers from recurrent bacterial infections, such as by *Staphylococcus aureus* and *Streptococcus pneumoniae*, and patients generally die young. Reduction in the number of B cells in patients can be revealed by flow cytometric analysis (see Appendix 1). As seen in Chapter 10, Btk is also involved in BCR-mediated signalling in mature B cells.Its phosphorylation activates a series of signalling events which are essential for B cell activation.

Selective IgA Deficiency

This is a common defect in which patients have low or no serum IgA due to a fault in the switch mechanism to IgA-producing plasma cells. Patients show variable clinical symptoms, though many are asymptomatic and entirely normal. Some patients suffer from respiratory and genitourinary tract infections and diarrhoea owing to lack of secretory IgA on mucosal surfaces. As levels of isotypes other than IgA are normal or increased, the disorder is referred to as *selective IgA deficiency*.

Common Variable Immunodeficiency

Patients show lack of antibody-producing B cells (plasma cells). There are low levels of most immuno-globulin isotypes in the circulation, and patients suffer frequent bacterial infections notably of upper and lower respiratory tract (as is seen in males with X-LA). Infections by *S. aureus*, *Haemophilus influenzae*, and *S. pneumoniae* are common, and occur in early childhood and even in late life. Some patients present with T cell dysfunction. Hence, this disorder manifests variably.

T Cell Immunodeficiency

T cells play a key role in adaptive immune responses to many pathogens by providing help to B cells to make antibodies and enhancing killing ability of macrophages. This is the reason why patients with defects in T cell development or function are very vulnerable to different types of infectious agents (Table 16.1).

DiGeorge Syndrome

DiGeorge patients show defects in embryogenesis due to which there is incomplete development of the thymus (thymic hypoplasia) and the parathyroid glands. There is T cell deficiency and hypocalcaemia, whereas B cell numbers are normal. Cell-mediated immunity to viruses and fungi is especially compromised in this condition and newborns suffer from heart problems. Patients show characteristic facial features such as unusually small jaws, prominent low-set ears, and increase in distance between the eyes.

The use of live attenuated vaccines such as measles or Bacillus Calmette-Guérin (BCG) is contraindicated in such infants as they lack T cells and fail to generate normal immune responses. The nude mouse described in the later part of the chapter is a valuable animal model of DGS.

X-linked Hyper IgM Syndrome

X-linked hyper IgM (XHIGM) syndrome is caused by a mutation in the activated TH cell surface molecule CD40 ligand (CD40 L) whose gene is located on the X chromosome. This, as was learned in Chapter 10, normally interacts with CD40 on the B cell and provides a costimulatory signal for

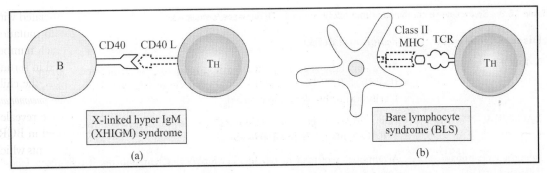

Fig. 16.2   Defects in CD40 L and class II MHC molecule expression (primary immunodeficiency). (a) Defective CD40 L on activated T helper cells results in XHIGM. (b) Lack of expression of class II MHC molecules on APCs results in BLS.

B cell activation, and induces isotype switching. In CD40 L deficiency, CD40 on B cells is not engaged, though B cells themselves are normal as in Fig.16.2(a).

Although response of B cells to T cell-dependent antigens is blocked, response to T-independent antigens is unaffected. Hence, there is increased IgM but other isotypes—IgG, IgA, and IgE—are deficient or very low. Additionally, TH cells are unable to deliver activating signals to infected macrophages (which also express CD40). This helps to explain why cell-mediated immunity is defective in these patients.

Bare Lymphocyte Syndrome

It is a rare form of inherited deficiency due to absence of class II MHC expression on dendritic cells (Fig. 16.2b) and also on B cells and macrophages, and is the result of mutations in genes whose products regulate transcription of class II MHC molecules. Cellular, as well as humoral immunity to foreign antigens is severely impaired. In absence of class II MHC molecules, protein antigens cannot be presented to CD4$^+$ T cells. Failure of TH cell activation results in reduced B cell and DTH responses, and inability to generate cytotoxic T cells. This is not surprising considering the central role of class II MHC molecules in the development and activation of CD4$^+$ T cells. Infections are common in the first year of life leading to early death.

Severe Combined Immunodeficiency

This is a very severe form of primary immunodeficiency as there is almost complete failure in T cell development. Due to extreme reduction in number of T cells (*lymphopenia*) in the circulation, which may extend to B cells and also NK cells, both cellular and humoral immunity is compromised in infants. They are susceptible to almost every type of infection—bacterial, viral, protozoal, and fungal—which can have a fatal outcome in the very first year of life. Early diagnosis and haematopoietic stem cell (HSC) transplantation is needed for all patients with severe combined immunodeficiency (SCID). For this, a suitable donor needs to be identified after proper human leukocyte antigen (HLA) matching of donor and recipient. Vaccinating infants with live attenuated organisms (such as Sabin polio vaccine) can lead to death due to progressive infection.

Mutations in at least nine different genes can give rise to various types of SCID, some of which are summarized in Table 16.3.

X-L SCID

Mutation in the interleukin-2 (IL-2) Rγ chain gene located on the X chromosome leads to a defect in the γ chain of the IL-2 receptor. The γ chain is a signal transducing protein and is a component

Table 16.3 Some severe combined immunodeficiency (SCID) diseases/deficiencies.

Disease/Deficiency	Functional defect
X-L SCID	Mutation in the gene for γc chain of IL-2 receptor (also a component of receptors for IL-4, IL-7, IL-9, IL-15, and IL-21); T cells decreased due to lack of maturation signals; B cells normal but serum Ig reduced
RAG-1/RAG-2 deficiency	Failure to rearrange antigen receptor (TCR and BCR) genes due to mutation in RAG-1/RAG-2; mature B and T cells absent
Adenosine deaminase (ADA) deficiency	Accumulation of toxic metabolites in lymphocytes; lymphopenia (T cells affected most); serum Ig levels low
Reticular dysgenesis	Stem cell deficiency; maturation of all leukocytes affected; fatal soon after birth

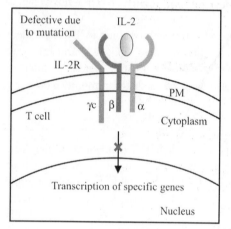

Fig. 16.3 X-L SCID. A defect in the γc chain of the IL-2 receptor (IL-2R) leads to X-L SCID.

of receptors for numerous other cytokines including IL-4, IL-7, IL-9, IL-15, and IL-21, the reason why it is called common γ (γc) chain. While receptors for IL-2 and IL-15 are comprised of three chains, receptors for IL-4, IL-7, and IL-9 are dimeric. Binding of IL-2 to the receptor fails to transduce signals and activate transcription of specific genes in T cells. Responses to all other cytokines which have the γc chain as a part of their receptors are also affected. The immunodeficiency is due to a severe reduction in the number of mature T cells and faulty signalling by several cytokine receptors (Fig. 16.3).

RAG-1/RAG-2 Deficiency

In one form of SCID, there is a specific defect due to mutation in the genes RAG-1/RAG-2. As was discussed in Chapter 6, the products of these two genes are necessary for rearrangement of antigen receptor genes in B cells and also T cells, and without which there is early arrest of B and T lymphocyte development. Lymphocytes fail to mature in patients who, as a consequence, are severely immunodeficient.

Adenosine Deaminase Deficiency

Deficiency of adenosine deaminase (ADA), an enzyme involved in breakdown of purines, results in accumulation of deoxy ATP. This is a toxic purine metabolite which inhibits DNA synthesis and cell proliferation (Fig. 16.4). Early lymphoid progenitor cells which proliferate actively during maturation are the most affected cells. T cell maturation particularly is blocked and most patients show severe lymphopenia. Deficiency of ADA can be diagnosed prenatally by amniocentesis. Clinical trials are on for gene therapy, though bone marrow/HSC transplantation, till now, is the best option.

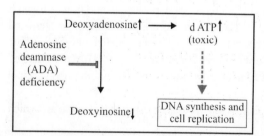

Fig. 16.4 SCID due to ADA deficiency. In ADA deficiency, deoxy ATP (dATP), a toxic product, accumulates due to which development of lymphoid stem cells is blocked at an early stage and there is lymphopenia.

The abnormalities discussed in the preceding text affect adaptive immunity. Some disorders of innate immunity are described in the section that follows.

Immunodeficiencies of Innate Immunity

Sometimes defects in components of the innate immune system, such as in phagocytes and complement proteins can cause severe immunodeficiency (Table 16.4).

Table 16.4   Some immunodeficiencies of innate immunity.

Immune component affected	Disease	Functional defect
Phagocyte	Chronic granulomatous disease (CGD)	Mutation in the gene encoding gp91 phox (subunit of NADPH oxidase) due to which there is lack of reactive oxygen intermediates (ROIs) and defective intracellular killing of microbes
	Leukocyte adhesion deficiency (LAD)-type1	Mutation in genes encoding integrins on leukocytes due to which neutrophils fail to extravasate to infected sites
Complement proteins	C1,C4, C2, and C3	Mutation in genes leads to defects in complement activation; defective opsonization of pyogenic bacteria
	C5, C6, C7, C8, and C9 (terminal components)	MAC formation affected; increase in infection by *Neisseria* spp.

Phagocyte Defects

Phagocytes are important components that participate in both innate and adaptive immunity. Patients with defects in phagocyte function suffer from recurrent bacterial infections of varying severity. While certain patients show defects in killing mechanisms, there are some with defects in other phagocyte processes, such as in adhesion of neutrophils to vascular endothelium and subsequent migration to infected sites in tissues. Two immunodeficiencies due to defects in phagocyte function are described here.

Chronic granulomatous disease   Due to a mutation, chronic granulomatous disease (CGD) patients have a *non-functional NADPH oxidase*, as a result of which there is defective intracellular killing of microorganisms. Phagocytosis of microbes is the major stimulus for activation of NADPH oxidase. Activation involves assembly of cytosolic and membrane components to form a multisubunit enzyme complex. The active enzyme catalyzes univalent reduction of O_2 to $\cdot O_2^-$. Various microbicidal agents are then generated. The most common form of CGD which occurs in approximately 70 per cent of patients is X-linked and is due to a defect in the subunit gp91 phox (*ph*agocyte *ox*idase). Such patients are unable to form microbicidal reactive oxygen intermediates following phagocytosis of microbes (Fig. 16.5). Chronic granulomatous disease is characterized by abscesses and recurrent bacterial infections mainly by catalase-positive organisms such as *S. aureus* (catalase destroys the small amounts of H_2O_2 generated). Due to persistence of bacteria and bacterial products in phagocytes, cell-mediated responses are activated and granulomas form in skin, lungs, and lymph nodes (see Chapter 9). Chronic granulomatous inflammation is a feature of CGD. Standard treatments include antibiotic treatment and surgical drainage of abscesses. Now, commonly used is interferon-gamma (IFN-γ) therapy which stimulates production of $\cdot O_2^-$, reducing both frequency and severity of infections. There are some more forms of CGD, in which components other than gp91 phox are defective, which are autosomal recessive.

Leukocyte adhesion deficiency   Migration of leukocytes from blood vessels to sites of infection (extravasation) involves adhesion of leukocytes to endothelial cells. This occurs through binding of

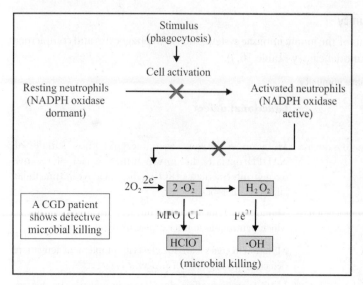

Stimulus
(phagocytosis)

Cell activation

Resting neutrophils
(NADPH oxidase
dormant)

Activated neutrophils
(NADPH oxidase
active)

$2O_2 \xrightarrow{2e^-}$ | $2 \cdot O_2^-$ | → | H_2O_2

A CGD patient
shows defective
microbial killing

MPO | Cl^- Fe^{2+}

$HClO^-$ $\cdot OH$

(microbial killing)

Fig. 16.5 CGD patients show defects in NADPH oxidase. Due to non-functional NADPH oxidase, there is failure to generate microbicidal substances. This results in defective microbial killing. Various microbicidal agents are shown in blue boxes.
MPO, myeloperoxidase

leukocyte integrins (see Chapter 2) to receptors (ICAM-1) on endothelial cells. Defects in integrins interfere in binding of leukocytes to the endothelium and results in *LAD-type 1*. Patients show impaired neutrophil chemotaxis to sites of infection and inflammation.

Complement Proteins

The role of complement in opsonization of bacteria which is dependent on generation of C3b has been described in Chapter 11. This is the reason why deficiency of early components of the classical pathway (C1, C4, and C2) or C3 deficiency leads to increased susceptibility to infections by encapsulated organisms which are phagocytosis-resistant (Table 16.1). Deficiency of C3 which is present in the highest concentration leads to very severe consequences.

Deficiencies of late complement components, C5–C9, fail to generate the completed *membrane attack complex* (MAC). This undermines defence against Gram-negative bacteria, particularly *Neisseria* species.

Some tests routinely performed to evaluate immunodeficiency diseases are briefly summarized in Box 16.1.

TREATMENT OF PRIMARY IMMUNODEFICIENCY DISEASES

Patients need to be totally isolated to avoid exposure to microbial agents, but practically, this is a difficult and extreme option. Other options include

Antibiotic Treatment

This is the standard treatment for infections.

Intravenous Immune Globulin

This is prepared from human plasma collected from a large pool of healthy donors and contains antibodies (IgG) to most pathogens. It partially protects against infections when antibody production is affected. Administration of IVIG to X-LA patients helps to keep bacterial infections in check.

Cytokine Administration

Many cytokine genes have been cloned and expressed, and recombinant products are available. Administration of rIFN-γ is used to restore normal phagocyte function in CGD.

Haematopoietic Stem Cell Transplantation

Haematopoietic stem cell transplantation (HSCT) is now an important form of therapy for inherited (and also acquired) diseases of the haematopoietic system. For instance, immune function in all forms of SCID can be restored by HSCT if done in the first few years of life. Due to absence of T cell function in SCID infants, they cannot reject allografts. The success of HSCT depends on the availability of an HLA-matched allogeneic donor. Use of T cell-depleted and affinity-purified allogeneic stem cells is the preferred treatment for all SCID patients as it helps to avoid graft-versus-host disease (GVHD). Haematopoietic stem cell transplantation and its salient features are revisited in greater detail in Chapter 17.

Gene Therapy

This can be a treatment option when a single gene defect has been identified as in different molecular forms of SCID. Some characteristics of stem cells, such as capacity for self-renewal and maintaining specific functions over the life time of an individual, make them well suited for gene therapy purposes. The early gene therapy trials were initiated for ADA-SCID. The normal ADA gene is inserted into a retroviral vector which is used to transfect the patient's own stem cells (autologous stem cells) that are ADA deficient. These transfected cells are then returned to the patient. Due to many adverse effects, improvements need to be devised and worked on.

ANIMAL MODELS OF IMMUNODEFICIENCY

Two well-studied animal models include the *SCID mouse* and the *athymic* or *nude mouse* (Fig. 16.6). These have been used by immunologists for various experimental purposes.

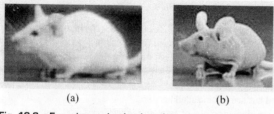

(a)   (b)

Fig. 16.6   Experimental animal models of immunodeficiency.
(a) SCID mouse and (b) athymic or nude mouse.

SCID Mice

Severe combined immunodeficiency mice possess an autosomal recessive mutation designated *scid* and are homozygous for the *scid* gene (*scid/scid*). These animals have to be housed in a germ-free environment or they die early in life. They show T and B cell lymphopenia and so cannot mount T cell or antibody responses. Being immunodeficient, they are unable to reject transplanted foreign tissue and show tolerance to tumours. Various cancer immunotherapies can also be analyzed using SCID mice. Hence, these animals are valuable research models. Adult SCID mice can be manipulated by transplanting human foetal thymus and lymph nodes into them. These *SCID-hu (human) mice* serve as an important in vivo model of the human immune system. In an important application, these chimeric SCID-hu mice can be infected with human immunodeficiency virus-1 (HIV-1; unlike normal mice which are resistant to infection) and candidate vaccines can be tested.

Athymic or Nude Mice

Some mice have a genetic trait designated *nu*. Mice homozygous for this recessive mutation (*nu/nu*) have a vestigial thymus (thymic hypoplasia) and lack fur (hairlessness). They serve as a valuable animal model of T cell immunodeficiency (e.g., DGS). Cell-mediated immunity (CMI) responses cannot occur in these mice and they are unable to make antibodies to most antigens. They are useful experimentally, especially to cancer researchers.

Knockout Mice

Genetically altered mice in which a gene has been knocked out are also being used to gain information about the role of specific genes. For instance, RAG knockout mice have been developed by deleting RAG-1 and RAG-2 genes. Such mice have provided a wealth of information.

SECONDARY IMMUNODEFICIENCY—HIV AND AIDS

Secondary immunodeficiency diseases are due to defects that are acquired during life. They are relatively more common, unlike the primary immunodeficiency diseases which are rare. The various causes that contribute to secondary immunodeficiency are listed in Table 16.5. The entire focus of this section is on the immunology of human immunodeficiency virus (HIV) infection and AIDS. This is both essential and important as AIDS is a world-wide problem and a cause of growing concern. Its study is also highly significant as it brings to light some important immunological principles.

An Introduction to HIV and AIDS

The initial cases of AIDS, first described in 1981, were homosexual men and intravenous drug addicts. When these first cases were described, the cause was not known. The causative agent HIV, a retrovirus, was identified and described in 1984 by Francoise Barre-Sinoussi and Luc Montagnier for which they were awarded the Nobel Prize for Physiology or Medicine in 2008. A retrovirus is an RNA virus which with the help of the enzyme *reverse transcriptase (RT)* converts its RNA genome into DNA. Of the two types described, HIV-1 is the most common cause of AIDS. It has a limited host range; only chimpanzees support infection but infected chimpanzees rarely develop AIDS. Human immunodeficiency virus-2 which is endemic in West Africa is less pathogenic than HIV-1 in

Table 16.5 Some causes of secondary immunodeficiency and associated defect(s).

Cause	Defects
Viral infections, e.g., human immunodeficiency virus (HIV)	Infects $CD4^+$ T_H lymphocytes; T cell depletion (lymphopenia)
Protein-calorie malnutrition	Blocks lymphocyte maturation and function; a major cause of immunodeficiency in under-developed countries
Irradiation, cancer chemotherapy (cytotoxic drugs)	Decrease bone marrow precursors for lymphocytes and neutrophils; increased risk of infections
Chronic infections (e.g., malaria, leprosy, and tuberculosis)	Immunosuppression (e.g., malarial parasite suppresses T cell function)
Malignancy (e.g., lymphoma and leukaemia)	Interferes in development of lymphocytes and other immune cells
Removal of spleen	Affects phagocytosis of microbes
Immunosuppressive drugs (e.g., corticosteroids)	Suppression of T cell responses as in transplant recipients; increased risk of infections

humans and infects certain non-human primates not infected by HIV-1. It is more closely related to simian immunodeficiency virus (SIV) from sootey mangabeys (SIVsm) rather than to HIV-1. Simian immunodeficiency virus causes no disease in its normal host but produces immunodeficiency similar to AIDS when it infects other species such as macaques. Although HIV-1 differs in genomic structure and antigenicity from HIV-2, life cycle of the two is similar.

Some characteristic features of HIV include the following:

♦ A long latent period
♦ Tropism for haematopoietic and the nervous system
♦ Severe immunodeficiency
♦ High mutation rate

Human immunodeficiency virus enters the victim's body through infected blood and body fluids containing free virus or cells harbouring the virus. Some major ways of transmission include the following:

♦ Through sexual contact
♦ Sharing of intravenous drug needles, as in heroin addicts
♦ Transfusion of infected blood or blood products, for example, Factor VIII needed by patients with haemophilia (transmission through this route can be avoided through testing of collected blood)
♦ Transmission from infected mothers to unborn babies through placental transfer or to newborn babies through breast milk

The following discussion is centered on HIV-1, the major cause of AIDS.

HIV—STRUCTURE, GENETIC ORGANIZATION, AND LIFE CYCLE

The structure of HIV-1, the genes which make up the viral genome (both typical retroviral genes and genes unique to HIV) and their functions, and the various steps in the life cycle of the AIDS virus are described here.

Structure

Human immunodeficiency virus is an enveloped human retrovirus that infects cells of the immune system, mainly CD4⁺ TH lymphocytes. The major structural features of HIV-1 are illustrated in Fig. 16.7. The viral particle consists of a phospholipid bilayer or viral envelope which is derived from the host cell membrane. This displays two viral glycoproteins which form knob-like projections and include *gp120* (extracellular) and *gp41* (transmembrane). The two proteins, which are bound non-covalently, enable HIV to enter CD4⁺ TH cells using CD4, a cell surface molecule on TH cells, as virus receptor. The viral core (nucleocapsid) is composed of *p24* capsid protein. It is surrounded by *p17* matrix protein. Two identical RNA strands (the HIV genome) and associated enzymes—reverse transcriptase, integrase, and protease—are packaged inside the viral core. In the process of budding from the host cell, the virus carries with it part of the host cell membrane and proteins (e.g., MHC proteins).

Antibody responses to capsid, matrix, and envelope proteins are determined in sera of patients and are important diagnostically.

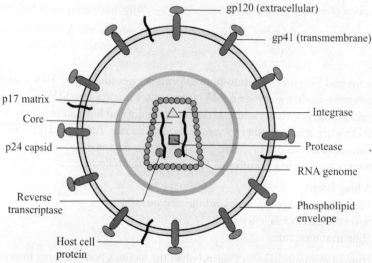

Fig. 16.7 HIV structure.
gp120, glycoprotein 120 kilodalton (kDa)

Genetic Organization

The HIV genome contains nine genes as is shown in Table 16.6. The three standard retroviral genes found in all retroviruses include *env*, *gag*, and *pol*. Besides, there are six regulatory genes unique to HIV which control viral reproduction and infectivity in various ways. Of these, *vpu* enhances budding and release of virus from host cells and downregulates CD4 expression. Knowing the important role that CD4 plays in T cell responses, it should be clear that downregulation would lead to a block in signal transduction and decline in T cell function. In HIV-2 and SIV genomes, vpu is replaced by *vpx*. Proviral DNA transcription is enhanced by *tat* and to some extent by *vpr*, whereas *vif* promotes infectivity of the virus, and *rev* facilitates transport of RNA into the cytoplasm. The product of the *nef* gene downregulates class I MHC molecules on infected cells. This effect of nef is in favour of the virus as viral peptides fail to be displayed to cytotoxic T cells – a very clever strategy deployed by the virus to evade host immune responses. The high genetic variability of HIV which resides mainly in the env gene also favours virus survival.

Table 16.6   HIV genes and their products. Human immunodeficiency virus RNA encodes structural proteins, various enzymes, and other critical proteins that regulate transcription of viral genes and HIV life cycle (see accompanying text).

Genes	Products	
Structural		
env	Envelope glycoproteins	
	gp120	
	gp41	
gag	Matrix and core proteins	
	p17	
	p24	
	p9	
	p7	
Enzymes		
pol	p10 (protease)	
	p32 (integrase)	
	p64 (reverse transcriptase and ribonuclease activity)	
	p51 (reverse transcriptase)	
Regulatory proteins		
tat	p14	Involved in activation and regu-
rev	p19	lation of viral reproduction and
nef	p27	infectivity in various ways
vpr	p15	
vpu	p16	
vif	p23	

Note: env, gag, and *pol* encode polyprotein precursors that are cleaved to smaller protein products indicated here

Life Cycle

The life cycle of HIV is depicted stepwise in Fig. 16.8.

Human immunodeficiency virus infection begins when gp 120 binds with high affinity to CD4 molecule on TH lymphocytes (*step 1*). Macrophages and dendritic cells which express low levels of CD4 (which acts as receptor for the virus) are also infected by HIV. Binding to chemokine receptors is also essential before HIV gains entry. Some chemokine receptors identified that act as co-receptors for HIV include *CXCR4* (on TH cells) and *CCR5* (on macrophages). Different cell populations may be infected by slightly different strains of the virus due to expression of different chemokine receptors.

♦ Conformational changes occur on binding to receptors and co-receptors enabling gp41 to mediate fusion of HIV with host cell membranes. This allows viral RNA to enter the cell's cytoplasm (*step 2*). Inside the host cell, a complimentary DNA (cDNA) copy of viral RNA is synthesized by the viral enzyme reverse transcriptase (*step 3*). The cDNA enters the nucleus where it integrates with host cell DNA as a provirus with the help of viral integrase establishing life-long infection (*step 4*). Within the cell, the provirus stays hidden from the immune system in a latent form till the T cell is activated. *It is due to integration with host cell DNA that the currently employed antiviral therapies fail to eliminate the provirus from infected cells, a big hurdle to a complete cure for HIV.* There may

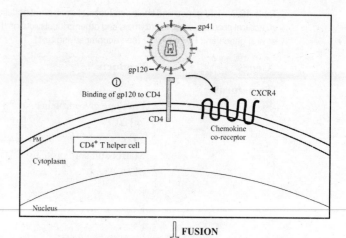

FUSION

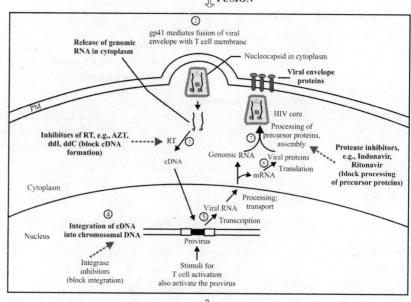

BUDDING

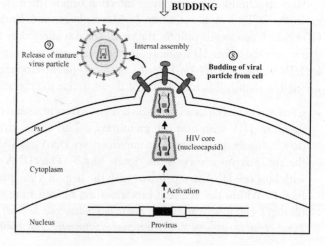

Fig. 16.8   Life cycle of HIV. The details of the steps (numbered 1–9) from initial infection of a CD4⁺ Tн cell to release of a mature virus particle are given in the accompanying text. Three sites targeted by therapeutic drugs are indicated by dashed arrows (red), though there are other susceptible points also in the HIV life cycle.

be latency for months or years or active viral replication depending on the state of activation of the infected cell. The long asymptomatic phase of HIV infection corresponds to this period of latency inside the T lymphocyte (Fig. 16.9). Although stimuli for re-activation of the provirus are not precisely known, infectious microbes/microbial products and cytokines such as IL-1 which activate host T cells, may also re-activate the provirus. On T cell activation, many of its genes are transcribed. Proviral DNA is also transcribed leading to the production of viral RNA (*step 5*) and synthesis of proteins (*step 6*). The viral protease processes precursor proteins before they assemble into new virus particles (*step 7*) which bud from the cell surface (*step 8*). The cell thus serves as an HIV factory releasing viral particles which can start a new round of infection (*step 9*).

The drugs used to manage AIDS patients target various points in the life cycle of HIV, namely, reverse transcriptase, integrase, and protease. These targeted sites are indicated in the figure and are discussed again in a later section.

CLINICAL COURSE OF HIV DISEASE

This can be divided into three phases which are represented in Fig. 16.9. The major features of each phase are summarized in the following text.

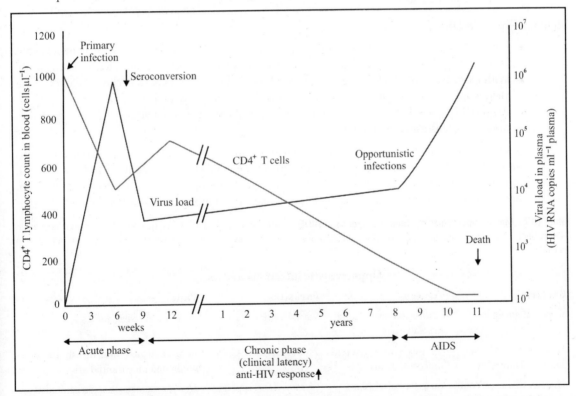

Fig. 16.9 Course of HIV-1 infection. HIV infection progresses through three stages—an acute phase, a long chronic phase, and the terminal phase AIDS. Anti-HIV antibodies in blood peak between 9 and 12 weeks after infection. These can be detected by ELISA and western blotting.
Source: Pantaleo, G., C. Graziosi, and A.S. Fauci (1993), 'The immunopathogenesis of human immunodeficiency virus infection', *New England Journal of Medicine*, 328, pp. 327–335.

Early or Acute Phase

♦ Flu-like illness generally occurring 2–4 weeks after first exposure to HIV
♦ Viraemia (high HIV titre in peripheral blood)
♦ Activation of the adaptive response with generation of virus-specific cytotoxic T lymphocytes (CTLs), and antibodies (*seroconversion*)
♦ Initial viraemia followed by a decrease in viral load
♦ Dissemination of virus to the lymphoid tissue by infected macrophages and dendritic cells

Asymptomatic Phase (Clinical Latency)

♦ Dendritic cells infect naïve T cells by cell-to-cell contact in lymphoid tissues.
♦ Not a truly silent period as viral replication persists.
♦ Slow decline in T cell count in the circulation due to gradual T cell destruction in the lymph nodes.
♦ Immune system competent to handle infections; virus-specific antibodies and CTLs remain at high levels (clinical latency).
♦ Viral load in plasma low for many years.
♦ Infections by various *opportunistic pathogens* (described in the following text) start setting in when the CD4$^+$ T cell count (normal count is ~1,200 cells μl^{-1}) falls to below 500 cells μl^{-1}.
♦ Period typically lasts between 2 and 15 years.

Terminal Phase (AIDS)

♦ Opportunistic infections become more frequent with further decline in CD4$^+$ T cell count to below 200 cells μl^{-1} resulting in profound immunodeficiency which is an indicator of full-blown AIDS.
♦ With lowering of the CD4$^+$ T cell count, levels of antibodies and CTLs decline while infectious virus (viral load) in the circulation increases (can be measured by PCR-based assays).
♦ Acquired immunodeficiency syndrome patients usually survive no longer than 2 years even with the most sophisticated treatment.

Opportunistic pathogens present in the environment cause no disease in normal healthy hosts but in an immunodeficient AIDS patient, due to decline in CD4$^+$ T cell numbers and loss of CMI, opportunistic infections are frequent (Table 16.7). The term 'opportunistic' relates to the fact that these pathogens take opportunity of the host's weakened immunity and cause disease.

Table 16.7 Major opportunistic infectious agents in AIDS. Due to decline in CD4$^+$ T cell numbers to a critical level in an AIDS patient, CMI is defective and opportunistic infections are common. Sites of infection of various pathogens are indicated in brackets.

Opportunistic infectious agents			
Bacteria	**Viruses**	**Parasites**	**Fungi**
Salmonella spp. (gut)	Cytomegalovirus (lungs, gut, and eyes)	*Giardia lamblia* (gut)	*Pneumocystis carinii*‡ (lungs)
Mycobacterium tuberculosis (lungs and other sites)	Herpes simplex virus (mucocutaneous)	*Toxoplasma gondii* (CNS)	*Candida albicans* (oral thrush and disseminated mucocandidiasis)
Mycobacterium avium complex† (disseminated)	Varicella-zoster (skin)	*Cryptosporidium* spp. (gut)	*Histoplasma capsulatum* (disseminated)
	Polyoma virus (CNS)	*Isospora belli* (gut)	*Coccidiodes immitis* (disseminated)
			Cryptococcus neoformans (CNS)

‡a major cause of pneumonia in immunocompromised patients
† *M. avium* complex has two species—*M. avium* and *M. interacellulare*

Besides infections by opportunistic pathogens, neoplasms also develop in AIDS patients. *Kaposi's sarcoma*, a unique neoplasm caused by human herpes virus 8—HHV8—develops which is characterized by lesions in skin, mouth, and gastrointestinal and respiratory tracts. These lesions are seen as blotches or nodules which may be red, purple, black, or brown. Epstein–Barr virus (EBV)-induced *B cell lymphomas* are also common. A large number of AIDS patients show symptoms of the CNS. The AIDS-related *dementia* and *encephalopathy* seen is due to the transport of HIV to the CNS by macrophages and subsequent damage to neurons induced by HIV.

The steps leading from primary infection by HIV to AIDS are summarized in Fig. 16.10.

Role of Macrophages, Dendritic Cells, and Follicular Dendritic Cells in HIV Infection

Although monocytes, macrophages, and dendritic cells express CD4 and are targets for HIV infection, these cells unlike CD4$^+$ T cells are not generally killed by HIV. In epithelia, dendritic cells capture the virus and carry it to the lymph nodes where they may pass HIV to naïve CD4$^+$ T cells by direct cell-to-cell contact. These cells, thus, play an important role in dissemination of HIV into the lymphoid tissues.

Follicular dendritic cells (FDCs) trap large amounts of antibody-coated HIV through Fc receptors on their surfaces and are able to infect macrophages and CD4$^+$ T cells in the lymph nodes. It should be recalled that these are special unique cells with extensive dendritic extensions on their surfaces and which unlike other dendritic cells do not bear class II MHC molecules (see Chapter 10). Human immunodeficiency virus can induce death of FDCs, an effect that can disrupt the entire architecture of peripheral lymphoid tissues which, in turn, cripples immune system functioning.

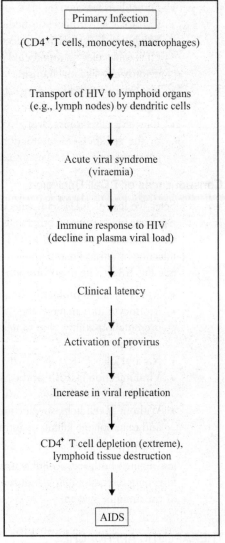

Fig. 16.10 Progression from primary infection by HIV to AIDS.

IMMUNE DYSFUNCTION IN AIDS

Many immune abnormalities attributed to a decline in CD4$^+$ T cell count induced by HIV-1 infection are associated with AIDS. Mechanisms leading to T cell depletion and the consequent immune-system dysfunctioning that arises are now considered.

T Cell Depletion in AIDS

A decline in the CD4$^+$ T cell count is the hallmark of AIDS. Various causes that contribute to T cell depletion and immunodeficiency are summarized here.

- Direct lysis induced by HIV (cytopathic effect).
- Cytotoxic T lymphocyte-mediated killing.
- Soluble gp120, shed from infected CD4$^+$ T cells, complexed to anti-gp120 antibody binds to surface CD4 molecules on uninfected cells. These may be killed by an antibody-dependent cell-mediated cytotoxicity-like mechanism.
- Importantly, binding of gp120 to CD4, besides being a critical step in viral entry, interferes in signal transduction and promotes CD4$^+$ T cell apoptosis.
- Infected cells express viral glycoproteins on their surface which allows binding to uninfected cells by the gp120–CD4 interaction. Lymphocyte fusion leads to formation of multinucleated giant cells and syncytia, and eventually to death of the entire unit.

Consequences of T Cell Depletion

Selective loss of CD4$^+$ TH cells due to HIV infection and absence of cytokines (IL-2 and IFN-γ) dampens functioning of other cells of the immune system. As TH1 cells are more sensitive to apoptotic death induced by HIV, the TH1/TH2 balance is tilted in favour of TH2. This increases susceptibility to infection by intracellular pathogens as TH2 cytokines inhibit cell-mediated immunity by cross-regulation (see Fig. 8.12). The major immune abnormalities are outlined in the following text.

- As CTLs fail to proliferate in absence of IL-2, immune responses to viruses are undermined.
- Monocyte and macrophage function is altered in absence of IFN-γ. There is poor antigen presentation ability (due to decreased expression of MHC class II molecules) and reduced IL-1 secretion.
- Natural killer (NK) cell activity is diminished.
- Viral infection by EBV and CMV (both polyclonal B cell activators) leads to non-specific increase in immunoglobulins (Igs) of various specificities with little functional antibody.
- Without T cell help, specific antibody responses to bacterial infections (extracellular) are lacking and macrophage killing of intracellular microbes is deficient.

Due to multiple effects of loss of CD4$^+$ TH cells caused by HIV infection, the patient is left defence-less against both extracellular and intracellular microbes. Additionally, as has been stated in the foregoing discussion, HIV-induced death of FDCs has very severe consequences on the functioning of the immune system.

THERAPEUTIC APPROACHES

Although there is no effective cure, many agents are used for managing AIDS and its associated symptoms (Fig. 16.8). They include the following.

- Standard antibiotic treatment for infections.
- *3'-azido 3'-deoxythymidine (AZT)* is chemically similar to thymidine and interferes with reverse transcription of viral RNA into cDNA. After incorporation into the growing cDNA chain, it prevents further extension. As cDNA is not formed, replication of the virus is prevented and viral load decreases. However, if treatment is stopped, viral load increases again. Besides, side effects are there on long-term use. 3'-Azido 3'-deoxythymidine is especially toxic to reproducing cells in the bone marrow. White blood cells (WBCs) are reduced, and also red blood cells (RBCs) which results in anaemia. 3'-Azido 3'-deoxythymidine is not a cure as it cannot eliminate the viral nucleic acid integrated into host cell DNA.
- *Dideoxyinosine (ddI)* and *dideoxycytosine (ddC)* are both nucleoside analogs which, like AZT, block

production of proviral DNA. A serious problem is that new variants emerge with a RT resistant to the drugs being used. It is once again reminded here that the enzyme RT converts the viral RNA genome into a cDNA copy (double-stranded) of the viral genome.

Besides blocking reverse transcription, there are other therapeutic approaches also. Inhibition of *viral integrase* prevents integration of HIV genome into that of the host cell, whereas inhibiting *viral protease* interferes with assembly of new virus particles. Inhibiting binding to receptors and co-receptors and fusion of viral and host cell membranes are other strategies being investigated. A peptide *enfuvirtide* that interacts with the extracellular protein gp41 and inhibits fusion has been approved by the Federal Drug Administration (FDA), USA. It is the first therapy to inhibit the entry of HIV-1 into host $CD4^+$ T lymphocytes.

Another treatment makes use of a *triple agent therapy* called *highly active antiretroviral therapy (HAART)*. This includes drugs that block the activity of reverse transcriptase, viral protease, and integrase. It may delay the appearance of mutant strains and also the drug resistance that arises as a consequence. Such a treatment decreases the patient's viral load to very low levels and prevents infection of new cells. However, its potential needs to be evaluated and may take several years.

Some major problems associated with the therapies discussed in the preceding text include high expense, complicated administration schedules, and serious side effects. Unfortunately, none of the above therapies eradicate the reservoirs of latently infected virus.

Vaccine Development

A prophylactic vaccine for HIV-1 is urgently needed. So a highly desired future goal is the development of an effective and safe vaccine against HIV to deal with the AIDS problem. Although this presents many challenges, a lot of active work in this direction is ongoing. Some difficulties that are faced include

- ability of the virus to mutate and vary its surface coat proteins. The high mutation rate of HIV is even more than that of the influenza virus;
- lack of a suitable animal model system in which candidate vaccines, including plasmid DNA and live recombinant vectors can be tested. Although the SIV macaque models are valuable for studies, a better understanding of these models is required. However, with the development of the SCID-hu mouse, referred to earlier in the text, an important animal model has been provided for HIV research;
- the crucial role of cytotoxic T lymphocytes (CTLs) in controlling viral spread; and
- the provirus is able to escape detection by the immune system, by establishing latent infection.

Some approaches to vaccine development include the use of the following.

Live attenuated virus A serious concern is reversion to the virulent form if the virus is not completely attenuated, as can happen when classical methods of attenuation are used. One strategy for developing an AIDS vaccine based on rDNA technology is to use an irreversibly attenuated strain. Selective deletion of one or more parts of the viral genome necessary for virulence, for example, the *nef* gene would eliminate the risk of reversion to virulence.

Recombinant proteins The glycoprotein gp 120 is an important component of the envelope spikes that decorate the HIV-1 surface and is a major target for neutralizing antibodies. But the use of gp120 has not met with much success as the virus envelope evades neutralizing antibodies. Still, a vaccine that can stimulate such antibodies offers hope as studies have shown that neutralizing antibodies offer protection against SIV in macaques.

DNA vaccines These contain one or more HIV genes cloned into a plasmid which is injected into muscle.

Live recombinant viral vectors Use of recombinant poxviruses carrying HIV genes are being explored.

The development of an HIV vaccine remains a big challenge. Although effective and safe protection against HIV infection using traditional vaccine approaches is unlikely, novel strategies including plasmid DNA and live recombinant vectors for eliciting CTL responses are being actively investigated. The encouraging results obtained in non-human primate model systems have led to evaluation of these vaccine strategies in human clinical trials.

DIAGNOSIS

Enzyme-linked immunosorbent assay (ELISA), a highly sensitive immunoassay, can be used to detect HIV antibodies using the core protein p24 or envelope proteins gp41 or gp120 (see Fig. A.7). To confirm HIV infection, the *western blot analysis* (see Appendix 1) is used. Assays for HIV antibody are negative from the time of initial infection till about 6–7 weeks, after which the first antibodies appear when the patient is said to be *seroconverted*. However, infection during this period can be detected by measuring *HIV viral load* (the number of copies of viral genome in the plasma) by sensitive PCR assays. This is also of value in monitoring response to antiviral therapy and is a major way of assessing a patient's status and prognosis.

Quantitation of *CD4$^+$ T$_H$ cells* also holds importance in monitoring AIDS progression and can be achieved through *FACS analysis* (see Appendix 1). Due to selective loss of CD4$^+$ T$_H$ cell subset, a CD4:CD8 ratio of 0.5 is not uncommon in AIDS patients (the normal ratio is close to 2). A falling ratio indicates disease progression.

AIDS can also be monitored by *skin test reactivity* to common recall antigens, for example, tuberculin, tetanus toxoid, or *Candida* antigens (see Chapter 14). Delayed-type hypersensitivity (DTH) responses to such antigens to which an individual normally reacts are lowered as AIDS progresses.

SUMMARY

- Genetic defects in immune system components results in primary immunodeficiency disorders. The defective genes have been identified in several diseases. Some mutations are X-linked affecting only males.
- Primary immunodeficiencies are classified on the basis of defects in B cells, T cells, both B and T cells, phagocytes, and complement proteins. Patients show increased susceptibility to infection with certain classes of pathogens depending on the immune defect. The pattern of infection is often suggestive of the nature of the defect.
- Defects in B cells, phagocytic cells, and complement proteins increase susceptibility to infection by bacteria which need to be opsonized for enhancing phagocytosis.

- T cell-deficient individuals suffer from frequent viral and fungal infections which are eradicated by CMI.
- A drastic block in T cell development leads to severe combined immunodeficiency (SCID), different molecular types of which have been identified.
- Myeloid immunodeficiency results in impaired phagocyte function as in CGD. This can lead to severe bacterial infections.
- Some useful experimental animal models for immunodeficiency include the SCID and the nude mouse. Besides, availability of knockout mice has enabled study of the role of specific genes in immune function.
- Administration of human intravenous immune globulin and antibiotics are common treatments. Haematopoietic stem cell (HSC) transplantation can

help to restore immune function in genetic defects. Gene therapy meanwhile is being explored.

• Infection with opportunistic organisms that usually do not cause disease such as *Candida* and *Pneumocystis* arouse suspicion that immunity is defective. Also, a history of repeated infections suggests a diagnosis of immunodeficiency.

• Human immunodeficiency virus (HIV), a retrovirus, is the causative agent of acquired immunodeficiency syndrome (AIDS). Binding of HIV to CD4 and chemokine co-receptors on T$_H$ cells helps the virus to gain entry and establish life-long infection. HIV gp41 mediates fusion of viral and host cell membranes.

• The provirus integrates into host cell DNA and remains in a latent form for months or years. On cellular activation, the provirus, too, is activated and viral RNA and proteins are produced. This is followed by release of new viral particles from the infected cell.

• There are many possible causes to explain T cell depletion and the consequent severe immuno-deficiency in AIDS: direct lysis, CTL and antibody-mediated mechanisms, apoptosis (other than by CTLs), and lymphocyte fusion due to syncytia formation, besides others.

• Due to severe CD4$^+$ T cell lymphopenia, AIDS patients are prone to various opportunistic infections.

• Although there is no effective cure for AIDS, numerous agents have been developed which block different points in the viral life cycle. An effective vaccine is what is needed and work in this direction is ongoing.

REVIEW QUESTIONS

1. Indicate whether each of the following statements is true or false. If false, explain why.
   (a) Macrophages are resistant to infection by HIV.
   (b) Enumerating CD4$^+$ T cells in blood is helpful in monitoring AIDS progression.
   (c) Primary B cell immunodeficiency increases susceptibility to infection by viruses and molds.
   (d) DiGeorge patients have normal B cells and respond to T-independent antigens.
   (e) HIV-1 is more closely related to SIV than HIV-2.
   (f) Administering intravenous immune globulin (IVIG) is used as therapy in X-LA patients.

2. Self-assessment questions
   (a) Explain causes for primary and acquired immunodeficiencies. Why do T cell deficiencies have greater impact than deficiencies in B cells?
   (b) What is the defect in CGD and how does it impair cell function? What is the overall effect on the host?
   (c) Explain the basis of the immunodeficiency disorder with elevated IgM. Why is there failure to produce other antibody isotypes?
   (d) How does HIV infect T helper lymphocytes? Do you think chemokines could be used to block infection of cells by HIV?
   (e) What are the likely mechanisms that lead to depletion of CD4$^+$ T$_H$ cells in an HIV-infected person? Can you explain how CD4$^+$ T cell lymphopenia affects functioning of cells of the immune system?

3. For each question, choose the *best* answer.
   (a) Mutations in common gamma (γc) chain of receptors for IL-2, IL-4, IL-7, IL-9 and IL-15 causes
      (i) leukocyte adhesion deficiency
      (ii) DiGeorge syndrome
      (iii) hyper IgM syndrome
      (iv) X-L severe combined immunodeficiency (X-L SCID)
   (b) The genetic defect in SCID mice prevents development of
      (i) NK cells
      (ii) haematopoietic stem cells
      (iii) polymorphonuclear neutrophils
      (iv) both B and T cells
   (c) The anti-HIV drug AZT inhibits
      (i) viral protease
      (ii) viral integrase
      (iii) reverse transcription
      (iv) viral entry into host cells
   (d) The polymerase chain reaction can be used in HIV-infected individuals to
      (i) enumerate CD4$^+$ T cells in blood
      (ii) detect antibodies to HIV
      (iii) monitor skin test reactivity
      (iv) detect HIV proviral DNA in latently infected cells

Transplantation and Graft Rejection

17

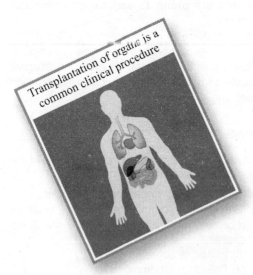

Transplantation of organs is a common clinical procedure

LEARNING OBJECTIVES

Having studied this chapter, you should be able to understand the following:

♦ The types of transplants and nature of transplantation antigens
♦ The direct and indirect pathways of allorecognition
♦ Immune responses that mediate rejection of a foreign graft
♦ How graft rejection reactions can be reduced by use of immunosuppressive drugs
♦ How typing of RBC and MHC antigens helps to avoid graft rejection
♦ The advantage of donor-specific tolerance over general immunosuppressive therapies
♦ Bone marrow transplantation and complications due to GVHD

Transplantation or grafting of organs in an individual is a clinical procedure used for treatment of most end-stage organ failure. It is successful in those rare cases when it is performed between identical twins. But transplantation is usually performed between individuals who differ genetically. In such cases, an adaptive immune response is triggered against the grafted tissue which is seen as foreign leading to its *rejection* (in just the same way the immune system responds to microbes). This is the major barrier to successful transplantation and is due to certain *foreign proteins* (*alloantigens*) present in the graft which, due to genetic differences, differ in individuals within a species. These include the *major histocompatibility complex (MHC) molecules* that were focused on earlier in Chapter 5 and whose prime role is in presentation of antigen to T cells during immune responses to foreign molecules. Their role as alloantigens in transplantation is incidental. Greater the genetic disparity, faster will be the rejection. These molecules were first described through studies on mouse skin graft rejection and have a central role to play in graft rejection responses. Due to the ease of preparation of skin grafts and easy detection of rejection, they have been widely used for understanding mechanisms behind allograft rejection. Other categories of alloantigens are the *minor histocompatibility (MIH) antigens* and the blood group antigens; these can also trigger rejection reactions against the graft.

To reduce rejection responses, immunosuppressive therapies are needed. There have been considerable improvements in this direction. With the release of cyclosporin in 1983, and other immunosuppressive drugs after 1990, rejection episodes have been reduced significantly. Due to these developments and with improved technical skill, transplantation has become a common clinical procedure, and many different organs and tissues are now routinely transplanted (Table 17.1).

Table 17.1   Organs/Tissues/Cells transplanted to treat various conditions. The most commonly transplanted organ is the kidney.

Transplant	Examples of disease
Routinely transplanted	
Kidney	End-stage renal failure
Heart	Cardiac failure
Lung/Heart–lung	Cystic fibrosis, emphysema, and pulmonary hypertension
Cornea	Dystrophy and keratitis
Liver	Cirrhosis and cancer
Skin (mostly autologous)	Burns
Stem cells (bone marrow, peripheral blood, and cord blood)	Leukaemia, immunodeficiency (e.g., SCID), and thalassemia
Under development	
Pancreas/Islet cells	Diabetes mellitus type I
Small bowel	Cancer and intestinal failure
Neuronal cells	Neurodegenerative conditions, for example, Parkinson's disease

However, there are still many problems associated with transplantation which need to be addressed. These include difficulty in obtaining donor organs and costs involved. Another major problem is the increased susceptibility to cancer and infection associated with the prolonged immunosuppression required in transplant recipients. This has inspired research towards development of strategies to induce graft-specific tolerance. Also, xenografting as an alternative is increasingly being explored.

The immunology of transplantation holds special importance. The focus of this chapter is on the types of grafts, nature of graft antigens, and the effector mechanisms used by the immune system to reject the foreign graft. The different procedures for tissue matching and some immunosuppressive therapies are described. An important future goal in transplantation which is to induce donor-specific tolerance is briefly introduced. The chapter also throws light on immunologically privileged sites, islet cell transplantation, and xenotransplantation. It concludes with a description of bone marrow and haematopoietic stem cell (HSC) transplantation.

TYPES OF GRAFTS

The nature of the immune response to a graft is determined by its type. Special terms are used to denote different types of grafts and genetic relationships between donor and recipient.

Autograft

This is a graft from one area to another on the same individual, for example, a skin graft from trunk to the arm as in burn victims. Rejection does not occur and the autograft heals into position in about twelve days.

Isograft

This is a graft from one individual to another genetically identical (*syngeneic*) individual, such as transplantation of a kidney from one monozygotic twin to another. Rejection of a syngeneic graft does not occur as donor and recipient are *histocompatible*.

Allograft

This is a graft within a species, for example, between man and man or between one mouse strain and another. Due to differences in genetic make-up of donor and recipient, referred to as *allogeneic* differences, the graft is rejected. Donor and recipient in this case are *histoincompatible*. Human transplants are usually allogeneic grafts.

Xenograft

This is a graft from a donor to a recipient of a different species (*xenogeneic*), for example, pig/chimpanzee/baboon to man. Donor and recipient are histoincompatible as genetic differences are maximum.

Some *laws (rules) of transplantation* are depicted in Fig. 17.1. It should be noted that a graft, for example, a skin graft, if syngeneic, is tolerated but allogeneic and xenogeneic grafts are not. A graft from a parent to an offspring heals into place. However, a graft from an offspring to either parent fails. This is because recipient (parent) does not share all the donor's (offspring) histocompatibility antigens. The immune response mounted by the host (recipient) against the graft is called *host-versus-graft (h-v-g) response*.

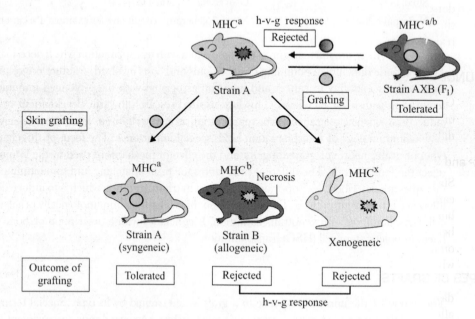

Fig. 17.1 Rules (or laws) of transplantation. Grafting from offspring to only strain A parent is shown. A graft to strain B parent would also be rejected.
Note: As MHC alleles are codominantly expressed, the offspring MHC$^{a/b}$ expresses alleles from both parents and is shown in two colours.

TRANSPLANTATION ANTIGENS

Due to genetic differences, a graft presents a set of foreign proteins or *alloantigens* to the recipient; these can activate an allograft reaction. Besides major and minor histocompatibility antigens described in the following text, the ABO blood group system also provides strong transplantation antigens that can evoke an allograft response.

Major Histocompatibility Antigens

Although the organization of the MHC locus has already been discussed earlier in Chapter 5, a brief revision here will be helpful as it is relevant to transplantation (see Fig. 5.1). The principal regions of the MHC complex that encode transplantation antigens include human leukocyte antigen-A (HLA-A), HLA-C, HLA-B (class I locus), and HLA-D (class II locus). The D region has three subregions: HLA-DP, HLA-DQ, and HLA-DR. The MHC molecules encoded by these genes, as has also been emphasized earlier in Chapter 5, exhibit extreme polymorphism. Considering that each individual inherits two alleles at six different loci from the many variant alleles at each locus, the chance of two people (in a non-inbred population) having identical HLA specificities is very low. Each person, thus, has a unique antigenic profile, just like a fingerprint, which poses a very big barrier to successful transplantation. *It should be noted that a rejection reaction will be mounted by the host if the graft expresses MHC molecules not expressed in the recipient (host).*

Minor Histocompatibility Antigens

Minor histocompatibility antigens are non-MHC antigens that are also important determinants of graft survival. These include non-ABO blood group antigens and antigens on sex chromosomes. Some other proteins, which like MHC proteins exhibit polymorphism and which may be present in donor and recipient in different forms, are also included in this category. Although the response to a single MIH locus is weak, the presence of many MIH loci evokes a response, which though slow, is a reason why certain grafts fail even though they are matched at the MHC locus.

IMMUNOLOGICALLY-MEDIATED GRAFT REJECTION

Graft rejection is an immune phenomenon. The following section focuses on the evidence in support of this, pathways of alloantigen recognition, effector mechanisms that lead to graft rejection, and different patterns of the graft rejection response.

First- and Second-set Rejection Reactions

Sir Peter Medawar inspired the development of the field of transplantation. His research during the early days of the Second World War was motivated by the need to treat aircrew victims suffering from burns. He obtained evidence for the immunological basis of graft rejection from studies in mice on the behaviour of two skin grafts from the same donor to the same recipient (unrelated), the second graft on the animal being placed about one month after the first graft. These experimental observations which established the immunological basis of graft rejection are depicted in Fig. 17.2.

It is seen that a skin graft from a strain X mouse to a strain Y mouse (naïve) is rejected in 7–10 days (*first-set rejection*). A second skin graft from the same donor (X) to the same recipient (Y), placed after some time, is rejected very rapidly (*second-set rejection*). This demonstrates *memory*. If the second graft is derived from donor Z (not shown in the figure), it will be rejected with the kinetics of first-set rejection. This shows the *specificity* of the response. T lymphocytes from a sensitized strain Y mouse can transfer ability to mount a second-set rejection in a naïve strain Y recipient demonstrating that rejection is due to an *adaptive immune response*.

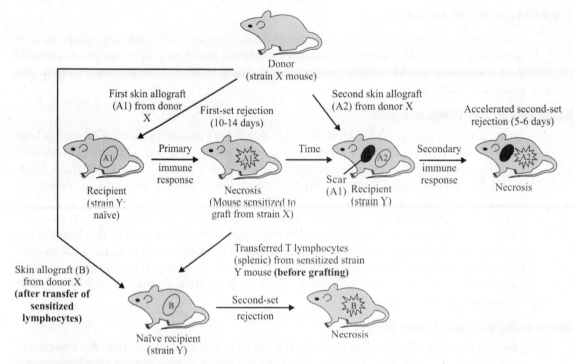

Fig. 17.2 Allograft rejection displays memory and specificity.

There is other evidence also to support the observations that graft rejection is an immune phenomenon:

1. Athymic or nude mice (or even humans with DiGeorge syndrome; see Chapter 16) lack mature T cells and so are unable to reject allografts or xenografts. This shows that T cells have a pivotal role to play in the rejection phenomenon.

2. The process of rejection is slowed considerably or may not occur at all in individuals who are immunosuppressed.

Graft Rejection Occurs in Two Stages

Broadly, graft rejection involves two stages, namely sensitization stage and effector stage. Recognition of graft alloantigens by the recipient's T cells leading to their activation and proliferation, and the effector mechanisms involved in the destruction (rejection) of the allograft are considered in the following text.

Recognition of Alloantigens—Sensitization Stage

There are two main pathways—*direct* and *indirect*—by which T cells (CD4$^+$ and CD8$^+$) of the recipient recognize alloantigens expressed on cells of the foreign graft. The role of TH cells is described here (Fig. 17.3).

Direct allorecognition The recipient's TH cells can recognize donor MHC molecules as such or MHC molecules on the donor cells bound to peptide. The peptide is derived from processing of antigens that occurred in the donor before transplantation. Dendritic cells express high levels of MHC molecules and are the major antigen-presenting cells (APCs) in the graft. They migrate from the graft to the regional lymph nodes where their MHC molecules are recognized as foreign,

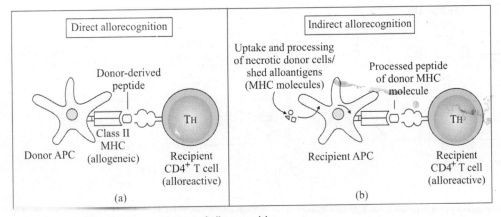

Fig. 17.3   Direct and indirect pathways of allorecognition.
Note: For clarity, signal 2 has not been shown. It should be remembered that the above reactions which lead to T cell activation take place in the local lymph nodes. The endosome in (b) is not shown.

and stimulate activation and proliferation of host T lymphocytes. These activated TH cells play a central role in graft rejection (described in the following text). *Direct activation of T cells by foreign MHC molecules on the graft represents a unique feature of transplantation. This should be compared with the conventional T cell response which requires that foreign protein be processed into peptides and be presented on the surface of APCs in association with self-MHC molecules.* Direct recognition provides a stronger stimulus to rejection than the indirect pathway.

Indirect allorecognition   Host APCs may take up alloantigens (foreign MHC molecules) in the graft, or in the draining lymph nodes to which alloantigens which have been shed from the graft are carried. These alloantigens are processed and presented by host APCs to recipient's own CD4+ TH cells. *Indirect allorecognition bears resemblance to conventional T cell recognition of pathogen-derived antigenic peptides which are processed by host APCs and presented in context of self-MHC molecules.* The indirect pathway is more important in chronic rejection.

Rejection of Allograft—Effector Stage

Alloreactive TH cells which are activated in the regional lymph nodes release cytokines and play a central role in the rejection response. Specific mechanisms, both cell- and antibody-mediated, and non-specific inflammatory reactions, are involved. Migration of effector cells from the lymph nodes to the graft subsequently leads to death of the graft. The effector mechanisms involved are illustrated in Fig. 17.4 and are described in the text that follows.

Cytotoxic T lymphocyte (CTL)-mediated cytotoxicity   Interleukin-2 (IL-2) and interferon-gamma (IFN-γ) are released by TH cells IL-2 stimulates precursor cytotoxic CD8+ T cells to differentiate into effector cells which induce killing of target cells in the graft.

Delayed-type hypersensitivity (DTH) reactions   Activation of macrophages by IFN-γ is critical to the development of a DTH response. Tumour necrosis factor-alpha (TNF-α) released by activated macrophages is an important mediator of inflammatory reactions.

Natural killer cells   Direct killing by NK cells involves ADCC.

Humoral immune response   This is stimulated by TH2 cytokines such as IL-4, IL-5, IL-6, and IL-10. B cells differentiate into plasma cells which produce alloantibodies that mediate antibody-dependent cell-mediated cytotoxicity (ADCC)/complement activation.

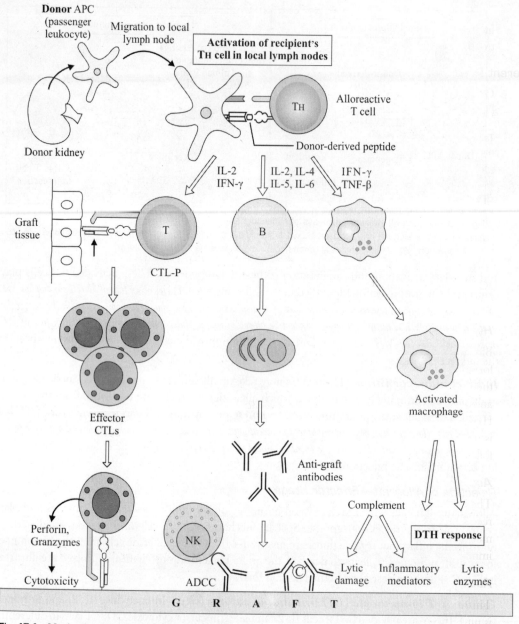

Fig. 17.4 Mechanisms involved in allograft rejection. Donor APCs can activate recipient's CD4+ TH cells to reject the graft. Cytokines from T helper cells play an important role. Although recipient APCs can also process alloantigens and activate TH cells (indirect pathway), this route of allograft rejection is not as efficient as the direct pathway depicted in the figure.

The locally produced IFN-γ induces expression of class I MHC molecules on graft parenchymal cells and vascular endothelial cells which renders these cells targets of CTL-mediated attack. The resultant damage to the vascular endothelium causes haemorrhage, platelet aggregation within the vessels, and formation of microthrombi. Transforming growth factor-beta (TGF-β), a growth factor released by endothelium that is activated by immune attack, causes fibrosis of the graft and results in arteriosclerosis (narrowing of the graft vessels). Loss of blood supply to the graft eventually leads to loss in graft function.

Different Patterns of Graft Rejection Reactions

Graft rejection reactions have various time courses depending on the effector mechanism involved (Table 17.2).

Table 17.2 Different patterns of graft rejection. The time taken for rejection of the graft can vary and ranges from minutes–hours to months–years. The causes for the different types of rejection are indicated here.

Classification of rejection reactions		
Type of rejection	**Time taken**	**Cause**
Hyperacute	Minutes–hours	Preformed anti-donor antibodies and complement
Acute	Days–weeks	Primary activation of alloreactive T cells
Accelerated	Days	Re-activation of sensitized T cells
Chronic	Months–years	Antibodies; immune complex deposition; low-grade T cell response; fibrosis; arteriosclerosis; recurrence of disease

Hyperacute Rejection

Blood transfusions, grafts, or pregnancies in a recipient prior to transplantation may induce antibody formation against alloantigens on the foreign cells, some of which may be specific for antigens on the grafted organ/tissue. These preformed anti-donor antibodies in host bind to cells in the graft and activate complement. There is thrombosis of graft vessels, occlusion, and necrosis of the graft. Hyperacute rejection is typically observed with xenogeneic grafts. A *cross-match test* prior to allografting is used to detect the presence of any anti-donor HLA antibodies in the recipient (described in the following text).

Acute Rejection

There is primary activation of alloreactive T cells in an unsensitized recipient and is due to direct recognition of alloantigens expressed on the graft. Both cell-mediated and antibody-mediated effector mechanisms are involved. Acute rejection occurs when the transplanted tissue is a mismatch or immunosuppressive regimens are not adequate.

Accelerated Rejection

This is a second-set rejection and is due to re-activation of sensitized T cells. Accelerated rejection is mediated by immediate production of cytokines, activation of monocytes and macrophages, and induction of cytotoxic lymphocytes.

Chronic Rejection

This is a slow process taking months to years after the transplanted tissue has assumed normal function. Some causes involved include

- deposition of antibodies and immune complexes in the grafted tissue and consequent inflammation,
- recurrence of the disease process, and
- drug-related toxicities.

Chronic rejection is characterized by fibrosis of the graft and arteriosclerosis.

Before grafting, recipient and potential graft donors need to be matched for blood group antigens and class I and class II MHC antigens. The chapter now proceeds to a description of some of the methods that are employed to avoid graft rejection.

TYPING FOR RBC AND MHC ANTIGENS

Various procedures for typing blood group and MHC antigens are outlined in the following sections.

ABO Blood Group Matching

The ABO blood group system provides strong transplantation antigens which if not matched properly can lead to hyperacute rejection. Red blood cells of a patient (and also donor) are mixed with sera containing anti-A and anti-B antibodies and then observed for the presence of agglutination.

Cross-match Test

This is used to check whether there are preformed antibodies to donor HLA in the recipient (Fig. 17.5). The role of these antibodies in mediating hyperacute rejection has been described in the foregoing discussion. Serum of a recipient is mixed with lymphocytes from a prospective donor in presence of complement. Lysis of donor lymphocytes indicates presence of anti-donor HLA antibodies in recipient's serum. This contraindicates use of the donor organ as these antibodies would result in hyperacute rejection of the graft. A different donor/recipient combination is then tried. Lysed cells take up the dye trypan blue.

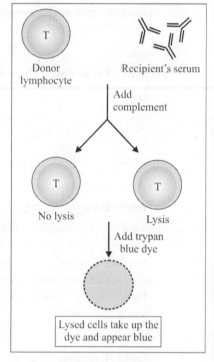

Fig. 17.5   Cross-match test.

Lymphocytotoxicity Assay

Purified B lymphocytes (express both class I and class II MHC molecules) are obtained from donor blood and placed in different wells of a microplate (Fig. 17.6). Antibodies specific for various class II MHC alleles are added to the different wells. Incubation is followed by addition of complement and then a viability dye, for example, trypan blue. Lysis of B cells (these take up the stain) occurs in those wells where antibodies have attached to B cells. These cells express the antigen specificity that caused antibody binding and cell damage. In practice, a battery of monoclonal antibodies is used as numerous HLA antigens are expressed and many allelic forms exist. The test by using the relevant antibodies can also be used to indicate the presence or absence of various class I MHC alleles. Recipient B cells are treated similarly. Matching for HLA class I, especially HLA-A and HLA-B, and HLA class II, particularly HLA-DR, results in better graft survival.

Mixed Lymphocyte Reaction

The mixed lymphocyte reaction (MLR) is an in vitro model of direct T cell recognition of allogeneic MHC molecules. It is used to ascertain how recipient lymphocytes respond to histocompatibility antigens expressed on donor cells (Fig. 17.7). Donor cells are irradiated or treated with mitomycin C

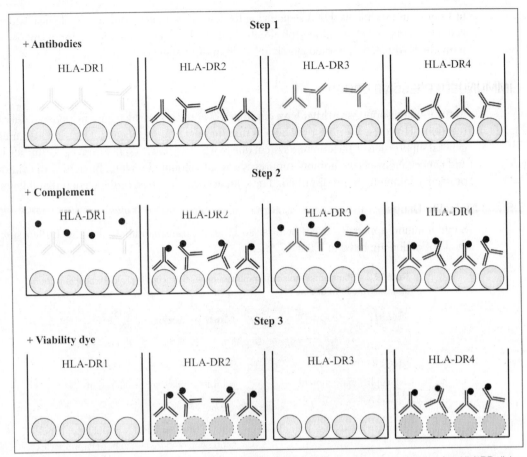

Fig. 17.6 Lymphocytotoxicity assay. The reaction of donor B cells with four antibodies directed against HLA-DR alleles is depicted. Lysis is seen to occur in the second and the fourth panel. So the donor B cells would be typed as HLA-DR2 and HLA-DR4 positive. For convenience, binding of complement to only one Fc region is shown.

to prevent proliferation. Only recipient's T cells proliferate (one-way MLR) when stimulated with foreign class II MHC molecules on donor cells. Synthesis of DNA quantified by the incorporation of tritiated thymidine (^{3}H-T) into cells is a measure of cell proliferation. Greater the class II MHC difference between donor and recipient, more is the proliferation and more uptake of ^{3}H-T is observed. This indicates poor chance of graft survival. A drawback is that it takes about six days to run the MLR.

DNA Analysis

More sensitive and accurate molecular techniques using the polymerase chain reaction (PCR) are now being used to identify HLA genes in the DNA

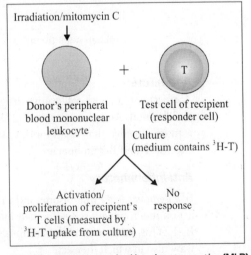

Fig. 17.7 The one-way mixed lymphocyte reaction (MLR).

of donors and recipients. DNA sequencing has shown that alleles that are serologically identical are actually comprised of a number of closely related alleles. DNA analysis is important for unrelated individuals who have inherited closely related but distinct genes.

IMMUNOSUPPRESSIVE DRUGS

Many immunosuppressive drugs have developed over the years which have helped to reduce rejection reactions. However, a serious drawback is that they act non-specifically. Their long-term use causes general suppression of the immune system due to which recipients suffer from opportunistic infections and cancer. Non-specific immunosuppressive agents should, therefore, be used with caution so that protective immunity is not disturbed. These aspects are discussed in the section that follows.

Small Molecule Drugs

Some immunosuppressive drugs being used in organ transplantation along with their summarized mode of action are listed in Table 17.3.

Table 17.3   Some small molecule immunosuppressive drugs in clinical transplantation and their mode of action.

Agent	Mode of action
Antimitotic	
Azathioprine	
Mycophenolate mofetil	Inhibit lymphocyte proliferation
Anti-inflammatory	
Corticosteroids, e.g., prednisone	Alter T cell and PMN trafficking; block expression of cytokines in both lymphocytes and macrophages
Immunophilin-binding drugs	
Cyclosporin	
Tacrolimus (FK 506)	Block T cell IL-2 synthesis
Sirolimus (rapamycin)	Inhibits lymphocyte proliferation by blocking IL-2/IL-2R signal

Antimitotic

Azathioprine is an antiproliferative drug. Its incorporation into DNA of dividing cells prevents further proliferation. *Mycophenolate mofetil (MMF)* was introduced into clinical transplantation in 1995 and is more effective than azathioprine. It limits clonal expansion and reduces the number of specific effector T and B lymphocytes.

Anti-inflammatory

Glucocorticoids (e.g., prednisone and prednisolone) are very potent anti-inflammatory agents. They act on macrophages reducing their effector functions and inhibit secretion of cytokines TNF-α and IL-1. This, in turn, inhibits recruitment of inflammatory cells from blood vessels. There are other ways also in which they act.

Immunophilin-binding Drugs

Cyclosporin is a cyclic 11 amino acid lipophilic peptide derived from a soil fungus. It inhibits the production of IL-2 (the major T cell growth factor) by activated TH cells. *Cyclosporin is currently the most important immunosuppressive agent in clinical use.* Although the benefits of cyclosporin are evident, it is not without its side effects. Acute and chronic nephrotoxicity are severe drawbacks. *Tacrolimus*, earlier known as FK-506, suppresses IL-2 production by TH cells in a way similar to cyclosporin. *Rapamycin (sirolimus)* inhibits IL-2-driven T cell proliferation and, thus, acts distal to IL-2 production.

Immunophilins are intracellular proteins to which cyclosporin, tacrolimus, and rapamycin bind when they cross the T cell membrane. Although the targets for cyclosporin- and tacrolimus-immunophilin complexes are similar, that of rapamycin complex is different. The mode of action of these drugs is a complex one, the overall process interfering in clonal expansion of T cells through inhibition of both DNA and protein biosynthesis.

Some serious side effects associated with the use of the above immunosuppressive agents can be avoided by using *combination therapy*. In this therapy, smaller amounts of each drug are used compared with the high dose required for treatment with a single agent. This minimizes side effects associated with the drug. For instance, MMF can be used in a triple immunosuppression protocol with cyclosporin and prednisone. Corticosteroids are also used in low doses in modern triple therapy. This helps to reduce side effects such as osteoporosis, myopathy, peptic ulceration, and diabetes which occur when higher doses are used.

Protein Drugs

This category includes *polyclonal* and *monoclonal antibodies*, and *fusion proteins*. These are listed in Table 17.4 along with their mode of action. Polyclonal anti-thymocyte globulin is an immunoglobulin preparation from horses or rabbits immunized with human thymocytes. Its drawback is that being foreign, it can cause serum sickness. The safety and efficacy of many monoclonal antibodies are being evaluated in clinical trials.

Table 17.4 Some protein immunosuppressive drugs in clinical transplantation and their mode of action.

Agent	Mode of action
Polyclonal anti-thymocyte globulin	Blocks T cell membrane proteins, e.g., CD2, CD3, and others, altering function and causing lysis
Alemtuzumab†	Binds to membrane protein CD52 on B and T cells (and also on monocytes, macrophages, and NK cells) to cause lysis and depletion
Rituximab ↕	Binds to CD20 on B cells and causes lysis
Basiliximab ↕	Binds CD25 (IL-2Rα chain) on activated T cells; inhibits IL-2-induced T cell activation
Daclizumab†	Action similar to that of basiliximab
CTLA-4–Ig#	Blocks CD28 signalling (signal 2) by binding to B7 on APCs

Note: Humanized monoclonal antibodies (†) are approximately 90 per cent human and 10 per cent murine; chimerized monoclonals (↕) are approximately 75 per cent human and 25 per cent murine. All humanized antibodies contain 'zu', whereas all chimeric antibodies contain 'xi' within their names. #CTLA-4–Ig, cytotoxic T lymphocyte antigen-4–Ig.

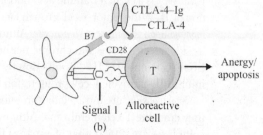

Fig. 17.8 **Costimulatory B7 blockade with CTLA-4–Ig.** (a) T cells require two signals for full activation. (b) Without signal 2, an alloreactive T cell is either anergized or undergoes apoptosis. In experimental settings, signal 2 can be blocked with the soluble fusion protein CTLA-4–Ig.

A soluble *CTLA-4–Ig fusion protein* formed by fusion of the extracellular portion of CTLA-4 and the Fc region of an immunoglobulin molecule (which prolongs half-life in the circulation) blocks costimulatory B7 signals resulting in anergy/apoptosis in alloreactive T cells (Fig. 17.8). Cytotoxic T lymphocyte antigen-4 (CTLA-4), like CD28, is also a ligand for B7 molecules; hence, it can block the interaction with CD28.

Chapter 8 should be referred where the role of CTLA-4 in downregulating T cell responses has been discussed. Use of CTLA-4–Ig in experimental/clinical settings has been shown to suppress graft rejection. The aim is to render the immune system non-responsive to donor antigens while retaining protective immunity. Enhancement of apoptosis of alloantigen-reactive T cells by costimulatory B7 blockade is a means of inducing donor-specific tolerance. There is additional information on donor-specific tolerance and the advantages it offers over blanket immunosuppression in Box 17.1.

IMMUNOLOGICALLY PRIVILEGED SITES

Tissues transplanted at certain sites are protected from the immune response and survive indefinitely. Such sites known as *immunologically privileged sites* include the anterior chamber of the eye, uterus, testes, brain, and others.

Corneal Transplants

These show a high frequency of success and are usually accepted permanently without having to use immunosuppressive therapy or HLA matching. Some factors that contribute to the privileged protection include

- poor lymphatic drainage and lack of vascularization in the anterior chamber of the eye;
- failure of alloantigens to sensitize lymphocytes of the recipient as dendritic cells are few in number;
- local production of the anti-inflammatory cytokine TGF-β which induces mainly TH2 responses rather than TH1;
- expression of Fas L by epithelial cells lining the anterior chamber induces apoptosis of infiltrating Fas-bearing cells such as T cells.

Foetus

This is a natural allograft as paternal MHC molecules and MIH antigens of the foetus differ from those of the mother. The foetus represents a unique example of a foreign tissue that is repeatedly grafted

Box 17.1   Donor-specific tolerance a future goal

Due to various adverse effects of immunosuppressive drugs and increased frequency of malignancy and infection associated with their long-term use, there has been continuing interest in strategies that will promote specific tolerance to graft alloantigens (donor-specific tolerance). *Tolerance in transplantation implies that even in the absence or withdrawal of immunosuppressive and anti-inflammatory agents, the host's immune system does not damage the graft. It is highly desirable because, besides being alloantigen-specific, the immune system's ability to respond to other antigens is left intact.*

Sir Peter Medawar and his colleagues, in early experiments using rodent models, demonstrated that exposure to alloantigens in the neonatal period (when the peripheral T cell system is functionally immature) can induce specific tolerance (Fig. 17.9). However, similar experimental data demonstrating creation of specific tolerance in humans is lacking, though some evidence for the existence of tolerance in humans does exist.

Tolerance to self and tolerance to an allogeneic graft share many common features. Hence, experimental approaches in animal models aim to exploit natural tolerance mechanisms to achieve donor-specific graft tolerance. Induction of anergy/apoptosis in alloreactive T cells using CTLA-4-Ig fusion protein has already been discussed in the preceding section. Besides this, use of donor bone marrow to establish *mixed haematopoietic chimerism* (a state in which cells both lymphoid and myeloid from genetically different individuals coexist) and manipulation of *CD4$^+$ CD25$^+$ T regulatory* (T_{reg}) *cells* to maintain donor-specific tolerance are being extensively explored. *Tregs which are now emerging as central regulators of peripheral tolerance have a crucial role to play in graft protection.* Additional information on regulatory T cells is included in Chapter 15.

Although the approaches discussed in the preceding text are the focus of considerable research in animal models and some encouraging results have been obtained, their feasibility in graft-specific tolerance induction in human transplantation needs to be intensively evaluated.

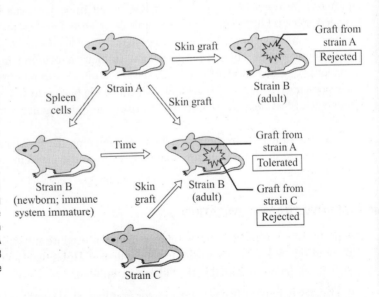

Fig. 17.9 Immunological tolerance is readily demonstrated in mice. A strain B mouse, when newborn, is injected with cells (allogeneic) from strain A. Strain B mouse, when it grows into an adult, is tolerant to skin grafts from strain A (without the need for immunosuppression). But a graft from another strain (strain C) is rejected, revealing the specificity of the tolerance. Note that a graft from a strain A mouse to a strain B mouse would normally be rejected as is shown.

and tolerated. In spite of development of an immune response in a minority of cases and detection of anti-HLA antibodies and cytotoxic T lymphocytes, the foetus avoids rejection. It appears that many factors contribute to survival of the foetus and various explanations have been offered. Of particular importance is the absence of the classical class I and class II MHC molecules on foetal trophoblast cells, the outer layer of the placenta that contacts maternal tissue. An allogeneic response is thereby avoided. Besides, expression of non-classical HLA-G and HLA-E molecules confer protection by preventing cytotoxic attack by maternal NK cells in uterine endometrium. Other defence mechanisms that protect against allogeneic reactions also exist.

ISLET CELL TRANSPLANTATION

Type I diabetes is the result of autoimmune destruction of insulin-secreting β cells in the pancreatic islets. Patients require daily treatment with exogenous insulin to support life, but complications still occur. An alternative to insulin treatment is islet cell transplantation. This is a heterotropic graft—a graft that is located at a site other than its natural location and, hence, differs from other tissue and organ transplants which are generally homotropic. As any injury to the pancreas can lead to severe pancreatitis with pain and tissue destruction, islets are not transplanted homotropically in the pancreas of the recipient.

The β islet cells are isolated and purified from a healthy pancreas obtained from a brain-dead donor (whose heart is beating). After being evaluated for purity and viability, the cells are infused into an ABO compatible recipient through the hepatic portal vein in the liver. The islets engraft in the liver sinusoids and mimic normal insulin secretion in response to blood sugar. Immunosuppressive therapy is needed for as long as the islets work.

XENOTRANSPLANTATION

A major problem being faced in transplantation is the difficulty in finding organs for patients who require them. Hence, an alternative source of donor organs is needed. For ethical reasons, and due to limited availability, species closely related to humans, such as chimpanzee and baboons (non-human primates) have not been widely used. Rather, attention has been focused on the pig, a distantly related species. Physiological and anatomical similarity between pigs and humans and their ability to breed rapidly in large numbers makes pigs a suitable choice. However, there is a major problem in using pig organs. Human recipients have in their circulation natural antibodies to carbohydrate epitopes expressed on graft endothelial cells. As antibodies rapidly activate the complement cascade, a hyperacute rejection reaction ensues which is a big barrier to xenogeneic transplantation. Besides, another very serious safety concern is the risk of introducing new viruses into humans which can be fatal.

Various strategies are being explored to overcome the problem of hyperacute rejection of a xenogeneic graft. This, in future, may help to solve the problems faced due to acute shortage of donor organs.

BONE MARROW TRANSPLANTATION

Bone marrow transplantation is a common clinical procedure and is the most frequent transplantation after the kidney. It provides a self-renewing source of HSCs that can differentiate into all the formed elements of blood. It is used in the following conditions:

- Primary immunodeficiency diseases, for example, SCID and CGD
- Tumours derived from bone marrow precursors, for example, leukaemias and lymphomas
- Haemoglobinopathies, for example, thalassemia and sickle-cell anaemia
- Marrow deficiency, for example, aplasia and agranulocytosis

Chemotherapy in patients suffering from malignant disease of the bone marrow destroys not only cancer cells but also normal elements in the bone marrow. In such cases, bone marrow transplantation is used to 'rescue' patients from side effects of chemotherapy. Another approach, an alternative to allogeneic bone marrow transplantation, is to harvest and store the patient's own marrow before the patient is given radiation and/or chemotherapy. The stored marrow can then be re-infused into

Box 17.2 Use of stem cells to restore the haematopoietic system

Stem cells can be obtained not only from bone marrow but also from umbilical cord blood (obtained from placental tissue which is normally discarded after birth) and peripheral blood. These alternative sources have an advantage over bone marrow extraction as the donor does not have to undergo an invasive procedure or anaesthesia. As HSCs have distinctive surface antigens such as *CD34*, a monoclonal antibody specific for CD34 can be used to select these cells to give a population enriched in $CD34^+$ stem cells. Haematopoietic stem cells can be injected into a vein from where they find their way to the bone marrow where they engraft. Transplantation of HSCs has least complications when genetic disparity between donor and recipient is minimum. Haematopoietic stem cells can even be cryopreserved for later use.

The cytokine *granulocyte-colony stimulating factor* (*G-CSF*) has an important application. It mobilizes donor stem cells out of the bone marrow and increases their number in peripheral blood. Transplantation of peripheral blood stem cells (PBSCs) results in more rapid recovery in neutrophils and platelet numbers than that seen after bone marrow transplantation. In many centres, this is rapidly replacing bone marrow as a source of stem cells.

Today, many centres in India offer the facility of bone marrow/HSC transplantation. The first successful bone marrow transplant was done on 20th March 1983 at Tata Memorial Hospital, Mumbai on a 9-year-old girl suffering from acute myeloid leukaemia. Since 1983, facilities have steadily undergone expansion and the centre is at the forefront of HSCT in India. Cord blood transplants and allogeneic stem cell transplants are being performed successfully. As fewer mature T cells are present in cord blood, the problem of graft-versus-host disease may not be as frequent as in marrow grafts. Also, there is wider use of PBSCs. Moreover, costs involved have also been brought down.

the patient (autologous bone marrow transplantation). The advantage is that it avoids an allogeneic response which is discussed in the following text. Haematopoietic stem cells and stem cells from other sources can also be used in place of bone marrow (Box 17.2).

Graft-versus-host Disease

Bone marrow transplantation differs from solid organ transplantation in that the bone marrow contains immunocompetent T cells. In the routine procedure, the recipient (host) is immunologically suppressed prior to grafting. This makes h-v-g reaction rare allowing donor stem cells to establish themselves in the bone marrow. But the immunocompetent T cells present in donor marrow may react against alloantigens on cells of an immunocompromised host if they are seen as foreign. They proliferate in response and produce cytokines including TNF-β and IFN-γ. These generate an inflammatory reaction called *graft-versus-host (g-v-h) reaction* which can cause severe damage to the host resulting in *graft-versus-host disease* (*GVHD*) (Fig. 17.10). The principal

Graft versus host response

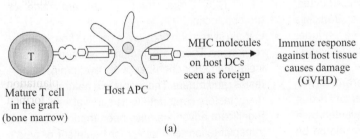

(a)

Use of HSCs avoids GVHD

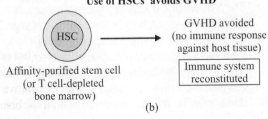

(b)

Fig. 17.10 Problems in bone marrow transplantation. (a) The g-v-h reaction is a problem in bone marrow transplantation. (b) The g-v-h reaction can be avoided by using stem cells/T cell-depleted marrow. Monoclonal antibodies using isotypes that activate the complement system can be used to deplete mature T cells from the bone marrow before transplantation.

targets include skin, gastrointestinal tract, and liver. Pre-treatment of donor bone marrow with a cocktail of monoclonal anti-T cell antibodies can be of benefit. These antibody-coated cells can be removed by complement-mediated lysis or by the use of antibody-coated paramagnetic beads. This technique, known as *purging*, results in depletion of mature T cells including alloreactive T cells. An allogeneic response is thereby avoided.

Graft-versus-host disease is a serious problem, sometimes fatal, and is best prevented by proper HLA matching. DNA typing methods which show greater accuracy are preferred. Most marrow grafts are performed between siblings, or parents and their offspring, as it is rare to find a match that is satisfactory amongst unrelated donors. The ideal situation of course is an identical twin.

SUMMARY

- A variety of organs are transplanted routinely in clinical practice.
- Grafts can be of different types: autograft, isograft, allograft, and xenograft. Human transplants are usually allografts.
- Major histocompatibility molecules on the allograft provoke vigorous graft rejection. Minor histocompatibility antigens can also provoke a rejection reaction which is slower.
- Graft rejection is an immunological reaction and its hallmarks are memory and specificity.
- Graft alloantigens can be presented to recipient T lymphocytes in two ways. They are either directly presented to host T cells by donor APCs (direct pathway) or allogeneic peptides are presented by MHC on host APCs to recipient's own T cells (indirect pathway). Indirect pathway is important in chronic rejection.
- Graft rejection is mediated by T lymphocytes. Cytotoxic T lymphocytes are cytotoxic to graft cells and induce killing whereas T helper cells trigger a DTH response. Antibodies are also involved in rejection.
- Rejection reactions may take different forms. Hyperacute rejection occurs in minutes and is due to preformed antibodies. It can be prevented by a cross-match test. Acute rejection is mediated by primary activation of alloreactive T cells. Accelerated rejection is a second-set rejection reaction in which sensitized T cells are re-activated. Chronic organ rejection involves both cellular and humoral immune components. It is associated with immune complex deposition and vascular injury due to inflammation.
- Matching recipient and donor improves the outcome of transplantation. This can be assessed by typing ABO antigens and by MHC typing.
- Most transplants require generalized immunosuppression of the recipient but its drawbacks include increased risk of cancer and infections. Some agents used include azathioprine/MMF (antimitotic drugs), corticosteroids (anti-inflammatory), and cyclosporin/tacrolimus/sirolimus (T cell-specific drugs).
- Monoclonal antibodies against cell surface molecules may be used to remove alloreactive T cells and other immune cells.
- To avoid drawbacks of blanket immunosuppression, novel methods for inducing tolerance to the graft are being explored. A promising strategy is costimulatory B7 blockade using CTLA-4–Ig fusion protein leading to anergy/apoptosis in alloreactive T cells.
- $CD4^+CD25^+$ T regulatory(T_{reg}) cells are critical for graft protection.
- Certain sites in the body are protected from immune responses. These are immunoprivileged sites and include anterior chamber of the eye, brain, uterus, testes, and others. The foetus is a natural allograft; many factors contribute to its survival.
- Significant advances have been made in islet cell transplantation technology for treatment of type I diabetes.
- The problem of shortage of organs for transplantation may be solved in future by xenotransplantation.
- Bone marrow and HSC transplantation are used to treat various conditions. A special problem of bone marrow transplantation is graft-versus-host disease (GVHD) mediated by mature T lymphocytes in the donor marrow. It is the converse of graft rejection.

REVIEW QUESTIONS

1. Indicate whether the following statements are true or false. If false, explain why.
   - (a) A graft between members of the same species is termed an isograft.
   - (b) Knockout mice lacking CD8$^+$ CTLs still show acute rejection of allografts.
   - (c) A host-versus-graft reaction is common in immunosuppressed individuals.
   - (d) An allograft from a donor to a recipient and which is matched at the MHC locus can still be rejected
   - (e) A second-set rejection reaction occurs only if the first and second skin grafts are derived from different donors.
   - (f) Corneal transplants are often rejected.

2. Self-assessment questions
   - (a) Can you explain why a child suffering from SCID is unable to reject a graft? What problem could arise in SCID children from a bone marrow transplant? Suggest ways that help to overcome problems that may arise.
   - (b) Why is an allograft rejected by a recipient? Explain the immune mechanisms involved in the rejection phenomenon.
   - (c) An allograft was transplanted into normal mice and also knockout mice lacking costimulatory B7 molecules. What in your opinion would be the effect on allograft survival in the two?
   - (d) In a one-way MLR, responder cells proliferated profusely when cultured with stimulator cells that have been treated so that they are incapable of proliferation. Explain the aim of the MLR and the conclusions that can be drawn from the above observation.
   - (e) Describe an experimental approach using skin grafting in mice that suggests that allograft-specific tolerance is possible. What advantage would this offer over non-specific immuno-suppression?

3. For each question, choose the *best* answer.
   - (a) Daclizumab, a monoclonal antibody, suppresses allograft rejection by targeting
     - (i) CD4
     - (ii) IL-2
     - (iii) IL-2 Rα chain
     - (iv) CD3
   - (b) Which is an immunologically privileged site?
     - (i) Uterus
     - (ii) Liver
     - (iii) Pancreas
     - (iv) Lung
   - (c) What is true about cyclosporin?
     - (i) It inhibits transcription of the IL-2 gene.
     - (ii) It is anti-inflammatory.
     - (iii) It is a mitotic inhibitor.
     - (iv) It triggers T cell lysis.
   - (d) Hyperacute graft rejection involves
     - (i) preformed antibodies
     - (ii) cytotoxic T lymphocytes
     - (iii) T helper cells
     - (iv) macrophages

Tumour Immunology

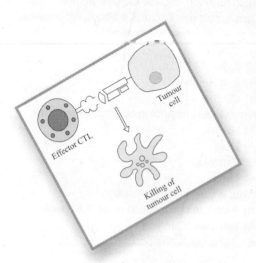

Effector CTL

Tumour cell

Killing of tumour cell

LEARNING OBJECTIVES

Having studied this chapter, you should be able to understand the following:

♦ How the immune system recognizes and reacts to tumours
♦ The nature of antigens on tumours induced by chemical/physical carcinogens and viruses
♦ The importance of cross-presentation and CD8+ CTLs in anti-tumour immunity
♦ Some evasive strategies of tumours that enable them to escape detection by the immune system
♦ Immunotherapeutic approaches in cancer which rely on mAbs and their conjugates, and use of LAK cells and TILs
♦ Therapeutic cancer vaccines which are based on use of tumour antigens/tumour cells transfected with genes encoding costimulatory molecules and/or cytokines/dendritic cells pulsed with tumour antigens, and others

Cancer is a major cause of death worldwide, in both children and adults. Normally, production of new cells in the body is regulated and under control. But sometimes malignant transformation (change to the cancerous state) causes cells to escape from normal growth control mechanisms and proliferate unchecked, producing a tumour. Cancerous cells have the property of invasiveness, that is, they can spread into surrounding tissues unlike cells in a benign tumour. They can enter the blood stream/lymphatic vessels which carry them to distant sites where they form secondary deposits called *metastases*. This property of cancer cells enables them to spread to different parts of the body and initiate new tumour formation. Conventional cancer therapy involves surgical removal (if the tumour is a solid tumour), radiotherapy, or chemotherapy. The aim is to destroy malignant cells without harming normal cells as far as possible. However, side effects occur and some are really nasty, such as loss of hair.

Experiments in animals have demonstrated that tumours express antigens that activate immune responses in a tumour-bearing host. But cancer is a commonly occurring disease which indicates that though immune responses exist, they are generally weak and ineffective. A big challenge for immunologists is to identify potential tumour antigens and to find out ways by which these antigens can be used to enhance host immune responses to specifically destroy cancer cells. Many immunotherapeutic approaches to fight cancer are being investigated and clinical trials are under way for many of them.

This chapter starts with a discussion of the types of antigens expressed on cancer cells and then focuses on major immune effector mechanisms in anti-tumour immunity. Some strategies that tumours have evolved to escape detection by the immune system are described. The final part of the chapter considers some immunotherapeutic approaches in cancer treatment and cancer vaccines which, unlike conventional vaccines, are likely to be (for most cancers) therapeutic rather than prophylactic.

IMMUNOGENICITY OF TUMOURS AND TUMOUR ANTIGENS

Early experiments conducted by Klein et al. and later by Prehn, established the immunogenicity of tumours (Fig. 18.1). Tumour X, a sarcoma induced chemically in a mouse using methylcholanthrene (MCA), was surgically removed and cultured. When a naïve syngeneic mouse and the immunized (cured) mouse were challenged with the cultured tumour cells, the tumour grew in the naïve mouse

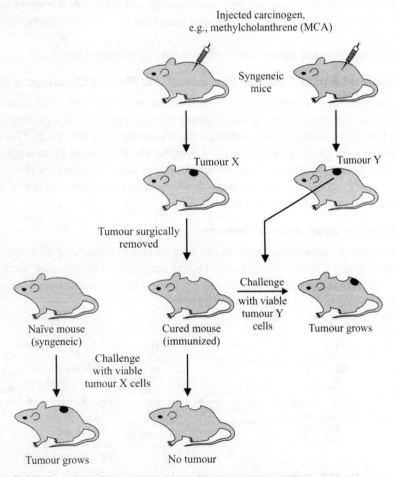

Fig. 18.1 **Immunogenicity of tumours.** Antigens expressed in different tumours induced by the same chemical are distinct and induce immunity that is tumour-specific.

but not in the cured mouse. If the cured mouse was challenged with cells from tumour Y, induced in a different animal with MCA or even in the same animal, a tumour was seen to grow. This provided evidence for the immunogenicity of tumours and demonstrated that two tumours induced by the same chemical in different animals or even the same animal express distinct antigens. As tumours X and Y were not cross-reactive, immunity induced was individually tumour-specific.

Tumour Antigens and Their Classification

Early experiments outlined in the preceding text established that tumours express antigens that are recognized as non-self by the immune system. These antigens were referred to as *tumour-specific transplantation antigens (TSTAs)* or *tumour-specific antigens (TSAs)*. They are unique to tumour cells, that is, they do not occur in normal cells of the body and are rare. *Tumour-associated antigens (TAAs)* are another category of tumour antigens which are not unique to the tumour and are also found in normal cells. Unlike TSAs, these are more common. Tumour antigens may be surface proteins or tumour antigen-derived peptides that are bound in the groove of class I major histocompatibility complex (MHC) molecules. Identifying tumour-specific antigens holds importance because these could be used to vaccinate cancer patients against their own tumours, just as microbial antigens are used to vaccinate against infectious disease though, as we shall learn later in the chapter, an important difference exists (Box 18.1).

The major types of tumour antigens are listed in the following sections.

Antigens on Tumours Induced by Chemical and Physical Carcinogens

Chemical carcinogens and radiations induce mutations in genes encoding normal cellular proteins. Processing of a mutated protein may generate a novel peptide which is displayed in association with class I MHC molecules on the surface of the transformed cell (Fig. 18.2). This may be recognized as foreign by a specific $CD8^+$ cytotoxic T lymphocyte (CTL) resulting in triggering of an immune response. Due to random mutations, different tumours induced by the same chemical express antigens unique to the tumour, that is, they do not show cross-reactivity. These antigens which represent TSAs have limited potential for use as tumour vaccines.

Antigens on Virally-induced Tumours

Unlike tumours induced by chemical carcinogens and radiations, virally-induced tumours express antigens common to all tumours induced by the same virus. This is because virally-encoded proteins act as antigens in the tumour and the same proteins will be expressed in all tumours induced by the same virus (Fig. 18.3).

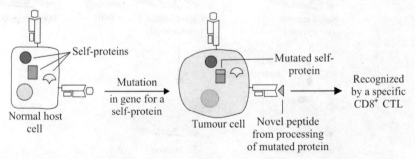

Fig. 18.2 Antigens on tumours induced by chemical carcinogens. Processing of mutated self-proteins generates unique peptides (TSAs) which are specific for individual tumours. These peptides bind to class I MHC molecules and stimulate $CD8^+$ CTL responses.

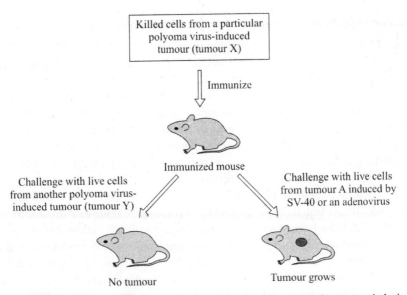

Fig. 18.3   Virally- induced tumours express antigens of the particular tumour-inducing virus. Antigens on killed tumour X cells protect against live cells from tumour Y, another tumour induced by polyoma virus, but not against tumour A induced by SV-40 or other viruses. SV-40, simian virus-40

Therefore, viral antigens have more potential in design of vaccines, unlike antigens on chemically-induced tumours. Two non-structural proteins of *human papilloma virus (HPV)*, namely *E6* and *E7*, and structural capsid proteins *L1* and *L2* of the virion are closely associated with the development of cervical cancer and represent TSAs. As these are foreign proteins, they induce an immune response (CTL-mediated). They are vaccine candidates as preventing HPV infection would help to prevent cervical cancer.

Oncofoetal Antigens

These are found on both cancerous cells and foetal cells, but are absent or expressed at very low levels in normal adult cells. They represent TAAs as they are not specific for the tumour. Two antigens in this category have been well characterized: *α-fetoprotein (AFP)* and *carcinoembryonic antigen (CEA)*. Alpha-fetoprotein increases in serum of patients with liver cancer and sometimes in gastric and pancreatic cancer. It can also be detected in some non-malignant conditions, such as liver cirrhosis. Carcinoembryonic antigen is increased in serum in about 90 per cent of patients with advanced colorectal cancer. It is also detected in serum in cancer of pancreas, stomach, and breast, and in some inflammatory diseases of the gastrointestinal tract and liver. Both CEA and AFP have importance in monitoring tumour growth and response to treatment. Their usefulness as diagnostic markers is limited due to their non-specific expression.

Overexpression of Normal Proteins

Many tumours including breast and ovarian cancers express increased levels of growth factor receptors such as *HER-2/Neu* which is related to epidermal growth factor receptor. It is weakly expressed on epithelial cells of normal tissues. A humanized monoclonal antibody—*anti-HER-2 (herceptin)*—has been approved by US FDA for the treatment of breast cancer.

Tumour-associated Antigens on Human Melanomas

Many TAAs have been identified in human melanoma, a highly malignant tumour of melanocytes (melanin-forming cells in skin) which, besides skin, may also affect the eyes and mucous membranes. These include *MAGE-1*, *MAGE-2*, and *MAGE-3*. These antigens are also expressed in germline cells of testes but are not expressed in other normal differentiated tissues, the reason why they are called *cancer-testis antigens*. As these are shared antigens, being expressed in some other tumours such as of breast, head, and neck, they are candidates for tumour vaccines and are being investigated for clinical purposes. Some other antigens expressed on normal melanocytes and overexpressed in melanoma cells include melanocyte lineage proteins such as *tyrosinase, gp 100, gp 75*, and *MART-1/Melan-A*.

In addition to those mentioned in the preceding text, other categories of tumour antigens also exist. *MUC-1*, a transmembrane molecule, is expressed on breast, ovarian, lung, and pancreatic cancer. Targeting MUC-1 with monoclonal antibodies is an attractive immunotherapeutic approach. Products of mutated cellular oncogenes and tumour-suppressor genes such as *Ras* and *p53*, respectively, also represent tumour antigens. An oncogene is a gene whose protein product is capable of transforming the cell (a change to a malignant state). On the other hand, tumour-suppressor genes encode products that block uncontrolled or excessive proliferation. Peptides derived from these tumour antigens are recognized by tumour-specific CTLs. Identification of many potential tumour antigens is encouraging and a big step forward towards devising ways by which the immune system can be activated against the tumour. It remains to be seen how these antigens can be used effectively to boost the immune system to fight cancer.

IMMUNE RESPONSES TO TUMOURS

According to the concept of *immune surveillance*, proposed by M. Burnet in the 1950s, a major role of the immune system is to eliminate malignant cells as soon as they are recognized, before they grow into an established tumour. The fact that immune surveillance is important in preventing tumour growth is supported by several lines of evidence. For instance, tumour incidence is increased in immunodeficiencies (e.g., acquired immunodeficiency syndrome, AIDS), in transplantation patients on immunosuppressive therapy, and in the neonatal period and old age. In spite of controversies regarding the validity of the concept of immune surveillance, it is clear that an immune response is mounted against tumours. The way these immune responses can be exploited to destroy tumours is an area that is being actively pursued.

Both cell-mediated and humoral immunity have been shown to be involved in destruction of tumour cells. Cell-mediated immune reactions play a major role and are similar to immune responses mounted by a host against pathogens. How various immune components contribute to anti-tumour immunity is discussed in the following text.

CD8+ cytotoxic T lymphocytes The major mechanism in tumour cell killing is mediated by CD8+ CTLs (Fig. 18.4).

Cross-priming or cross-presentation Antigen-presenting cells (APCs) particularly dendritic cells (DCs) near the tumour site and TH cells are critical for induction of CTL responses. The mechanism involved is called *cross-priming* or *cross-presentation* in which exogenous antigens enter the class I MHC pathway of antigen processing and presentation (see Fig. 5.10). As is described again in a later section, peptides derived from tumour antigens are presented on the DC surface associated with class I MHC molecules which are recognized by tumour-specific CTL-precursors. CD4+ TH cells are activated by DCs to release interleukin-2 (IL-2) and interferon-gamma (IFN-γ). Interleukin-2 provides signals for

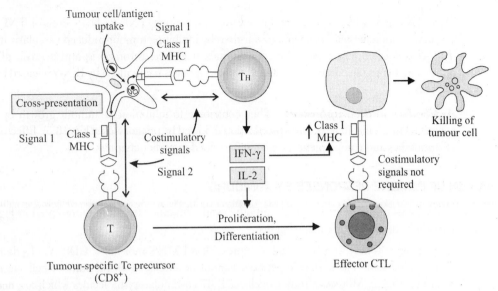

Fig. 18.4 Role of cytotoxic T lymphocytes (CTLs) in tumour cell killing. Interaction of B7 molecules on dendritic cells with CD28 on T cells provides the costimulatory signal.

proliferation and differentiation of precursor CTLs while IFN-γ increases class I MHC expression on tumour cells. This enhances recognition and killing of tumour cells by effector CTLs.

Cross-presentation has an important practical application. Dendritic cells from a cancer patient are grown and then incubated with antigens from the patient's own tumour. There is uptake of tumour antigens by DCs. These antigen-pulsed (loaded) DCs can be used as vaccines to actively stimulate T cell responses against the tumour. A lot of interest is focused on developing DC-based vaccines (described in a later section).

Natural killer cells These cells play an important role in host defence during early stages of tumour growth before development of CTLs and activated macrophages. With the help of their Fc receptors (CD16), natural killer (NK) cells bind to antibody-coated tumour cells and mediate antibody-dependent cell-mediated cytotoxicity (ADCC; Fig. 18.5).

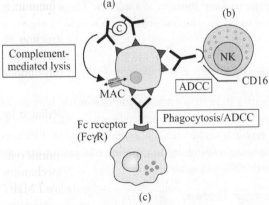

Fig. 18.5 Immune response to tumours. Different ways by which the immune system of a tumour-bearing host targets tumour cells are shown.
Note: The role of CTLs has been omitted here.

There are other mechanisms also by which NK cells kill target cells. Tumour cells which have lost expression of class I MHC molecules fail to be recognized by CTLs but are potential targets for NK cells. By releasing granule contents, NK cells induce apoptosis in their cellular targets similar to mechanisms used by CTLs (see Chapter 9). The ability of NK cells to kill tumour cells is enhanced by cytokines, for example, IL-2. Natural killer cells activated in vitro by IL-2 are called *lymphokine-activated killer (LAK) cells.* These are important in cancer immunotherapy and are described in a later part of the chapter.

Macrophages They have a significant role in anti-tumour immunity and mediate phagocytosis/ADCC (Fig. 18.5). Macrophages release lytic enzymes, reactive

O_2 and N_2 intermediates, and tumour necrosis factor-alpha (TNF-α). High levels of TNF-α damage vascular endothelial cells near the tumour thereby inhibiting tumour-induced vascularization. When TNF-α is injected into tumour-bearing animals, it induces thrombosis, and necrosis of tumours/ regression, hence the name. Cytotoxicity of macrophages is enhanced by IFN-γ released by activated TH cells.

Antibodies and complement They contribute to inhibition of tumour growth by mediating complement-mediated lysis, and opsonization followed by phagocytosis (Fig. 18.5). Effector functions of antibodies and complement have been described in earlier chapters.

EVASION OF IMMUNE RESPONSES BY TUMOURS

The various mechanisms by which tumours evade immune attack are represented in Fig. 18.6 and are briefly outlined in the following text.

1. Tumour cells may sometimes fail to express class I MHC molecules. CD8$^+$ CTLs do not receive activation signals as antigenic peptides cannot be displayed on the tumour cell surface as seen in Fig. 18.6(a). Moreover, tumour cells lack B7 costimulatory molecules which are necessary for providing the second signal for naïve T cell activation.
2. Tumour cells secrete the immunosuppressive cytokine *transforming growth factor-beta (TGF-β)*. It derives its name from the fact that it was first identified in culture supernatants of tumours. It directly inhibits antigen-specific T cell activation. It should be recalled that TH1 cells are important for development of inflammatory T cell responses/cell-mediated immunity (CMI) which are critical for controlling tumour growth. Transforming growth factor-beta also recruits CD4$^+$ CD25$^+$ T regulatory (Treg) cells which block local T cell effector responses as seen in Fig. 18.6(b). These cells and also their crucial role are described in Chapter 15.
3. Some antigens expressed on tumour cells, and which are recognized by the immune system, may gradually be lost from the surface due to antibody-induced internalization. Also, due to rapid mitotic rate and genetic instability of tumours (Fig. 18.6c), mutations/deletion of genes that encode tumour antigens are frequent. This gives rise to *antigen-loss* variants which go unrecognized by tumour-specific CTLs (or serum antibody).
4. Antibodies interact with shed tumour antigens to form immune complexes. These bind to Fc receptors (CD16) on NK cells but are unable to bridge tumour cells and NK cells. This blocks ADCC as seen in Fig. 18.6(d).

VARIOUS APPROACHES TO CANCER IMMUNOTHERAPY

Although immunotherapy is still in its experimental stage, it is encouraging that it has become an important part of therapy in some forms of cancer. It is likely to be more effective after the tumour mass has been reduced in size and when used in combination with other conventional forms of therapy. Various immunotherapeutic strategies which are being investigated in experimental animals and are undergoing clinical trials in humans are discussed in the following sections.

Monoclonal Antibodies and Their Conjugates in Tumour Therapy

Use of monoclonal antibodies, a form of passive immunization, allows the immune response to be directed specifically against the tumour. But, there are some serious problems associated with the use of murine monoclonals for therapy such as the following.

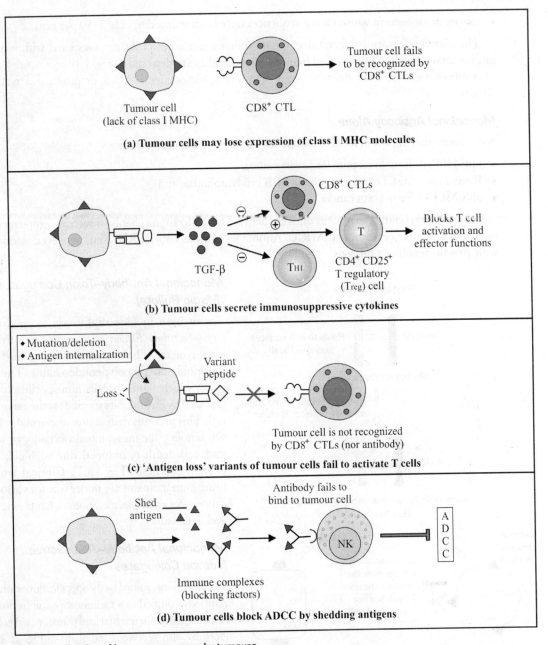

Fig. 18.6 Evasion of immune responses by tumours.

1. Being foreign, they evoke a *human anti-mouse antibody (HAMA) response*; the immune complexes formed have damaging effects on the kidney and half-life of the antibody is shortened.
2. Murine antibodies do not efface well with human effector cells such as NK cells; in other words, Fc region of murine antibodies are poor activators of human Fc receptor-bearing cells.

Technological advances in protein engineering have made available

◆ *hybrid* or *chimeric antibodies* which have approximately 25 per cent mouse sequences; and

- *humanized antibodies* in which mouse sequences have been reduced to only 5–10 per cent.

These antibodies are less immunogenic in humans and avoid problems associated with use of murine monoclonals. Chimeric and humanized antibodies are depicted in Fig. 4.19.

Antibodies can be used alone or coupled to toxins, radioactive isotopes, or prodrug-activating enzymes.

Monoclonal Antibody Alone

Some antibodies approved for therapeutic use for selected cancers include

- anti-HER-2/Neu (herceptin) for breast cancer,
- Rituximab (anti-CD20) for treatment of B cell lymphoma, and
- anti-MUC-1 for ovarian cancer.

Antibodies on binding to tumour antigens activate host effector mechanisms such as complement-mediated lysis, phagocytosis, and ADCC. Antibodies, such as anti-HER-2/Neu, may even interfere with growth-signalling functions.

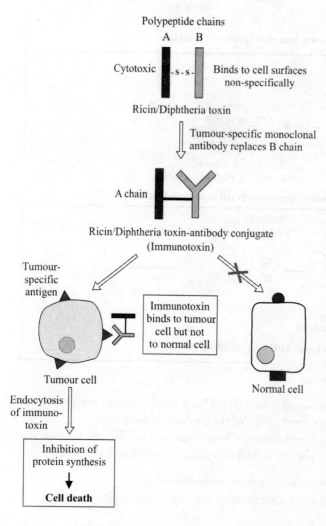

Monoclonal Antibody–Toxin Conjugates (Magic Bullets)

Toxins used include diphtheria toxin from *Corynebacterium diphtheriae* or ricin toxin from castor-bean. These toxins have A and B disulphide-linked polypeptide chains. The B chain which binds to cells non-specifically is replaced by an antibody specific for the tumour cell. This prevents destruction of normal cells. On binding, the immunotoxin is endocytosed and cell death is induced due to block in protein synthesis (Fig. 18.7). Clinical trials using immunotoxins are under way for various cancers, for example, melanomas, lymphomas, and leukaemias.

Monoclonal Antibody–Radioactive Isotope Conjugates

The radiations emitted by the specific monoclonal antibody coupled to a radioisotope kill tumour cells, though both normal and transformed cells close by also receive a lethal dose (Fig. 18.8). Antibody–Radioisotope conjugates specific for CD20 on B cells are in use for treatment of lymphoma patients.

Fig. 18.7 Immunotoxins in cancer therapy. When injected into patients, the immunotoxin seeks out the tumour and binds specifically to it. It exerts its cytotoxic effect without involvement of host effector mechanisms. Some immunotoxins are undergoing clinical trials.

Monoclonal Antibody–Enzyme Conjugates

A prodrug-activating enzyme conjugated to a specific monoclonal antibody is administered and is given time to gather at the tumour surface. Then the prodrug (non-toxic) is given which is converted by the enzyme to a cytotoxic agent at the tumour site. This strategy is referred to as *ADEPT* (*antibody-directed enzyme prodrug therapy*).

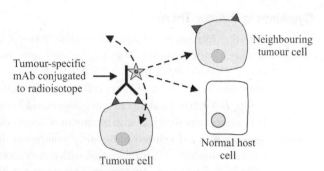

Fig. 18.8 Tumour therapy by monoclonal antibodyradioactive isotope conjugates.

Adoptive Cellular Immunotherapy

This involves first culturing the patient's immune cells having anti-tumour activity with IL-2 and then transferring them back into the patient. Cells used include *LAK cells* and *tumour-infiltrating lymphocytes* (*TILs*). Lymphokine-activated killer cells are mostly NK cells obtained from the peripheral blood of cancer patients. They are expanded in vitro with IL-2 and then re-infused into the patient with IL-2. Encouraging results have been obtained in advanced melanoma and kidney cancers. Tumour-infiltrating lymphocytes are obtained from the actual tumour mass of a cancer patient by biopsy and are mostly CD8$^+$ T cells specific for the tumour (Fig. 18.9). Tumour-infiltrating lymphocytes were obtained from melanoma patients and expanded in vitro with IL-2. Re-infusion with IL-2 into patients has shown a good response.

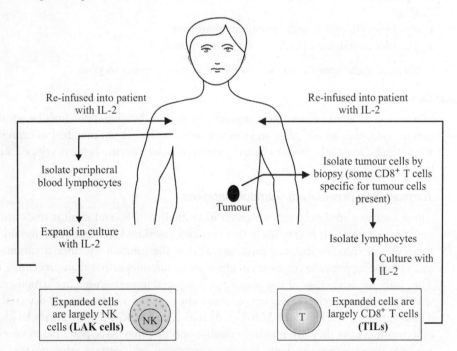

Fig. 18.9 LAK cells and TILs in cancer immunotherapy. LAK cells are mostly NK cells obtained from peripheral blood. TILs are largely CD8$^+$ T cells obtained from the actual tumour mass.

Cytokines in Tumour Therapy

With the isolation and cloning of cytokine genes, it is possible to produce large amounts of cytokines for therapeutic purposes. They can be used alone or along with chemotherapy. Some cytokines have shown a positive response in animal models and in clinical settings. The most positive response has been seen in treatment of hairy cell leukaemia with *IFN-α*. Besides its antiproliferative and antiviral effects, *IFN-α* has the ability to upregulate class I MHC molecule expression. An encouraging response has been obtained with *IL-2* in treatment of renal cell carcinoma and advanced melanoma. It induces tumour-specific T cell activation and proliferation and also NK cell activation. Many tumour vaccine trials are conducted in combination with this cytokine. *Granulocyte monocyte-colony stimulating factor (GM-CSF)* is used to reconstitute the haematopoietic system destroyed by radiotherapy or chemotherapy. Additionally, it enhances differentiation of immature DCs to mature DCs. Some other cytokines being evaluated include *IFN-β*, *IFN-γ*, *IL-12*, and *TNF*.

In spite of obstacles in the use of cytokines, such as their short half-life, undesirable side effects, and complexity of the cytokine network, cytokines hold promise in cancer therapy.

CANCER VACCINES

The aim of cancer vaccines is to stimulate the patient's own immune response against the tumour (active immunization). This can be achieved by vaccinating cancer patients with

- irradiated tumour cells (autologous),
- tumour antigens,
- tumour cells transfected with genes encoding costimulatory molecules and/or cytokines (e.g., IL-2),
- dendritic cells pulsed with tumour antigens, and
- plasmids containing cDNA encoding tumour antigens.

Some of these approaches are considered in the following sections.

Tumour Cell-based Vaccines

Stimulation of active anti-tumour immunity in tumour-bearing individuals by administering killed tumour cells, tumour antigens, and tumour cells that have been modified to express costimulatory B7 molecules and/or to secrete cytokines are approaches that are being developed and are described here.

Tumour Cells (Irradiated)/Tumour Antigens

These vaccines are being experimented in animal models, and clinical trials are in progress in melanoma patients. It is very likely that vaccines based on killed tumour cells and shared tumour antigens will enhance immune responses against the tumour. Melanoma vaccines, for instance, aim at boosting immune responses to pre-existing tumours rather than preventing the melanoma. They have the advantage of low toxicity as compared to agents used in chemotherapy. Focus is on shared tumour antigens such as cancer-testes antigens which were initially detected in melanomas. These antigens, which include *MAGE-1*, *MAGE-2*, and *MAGE-3*, have also been identified in some other tumours. As they are relatively tumour-specific, they have potential as vaccine candidates, not only for melanoma patients, but also for patients with certain other types of cancer (e.g., of breast, head, and neck).

Tumour Cells Transfected with Genes Encoding Costimulators and/or Cytokines

In this approach, the patient's own tumour cells are isolated, propagated, and transfected with the relevant gene. The transfected tumour cells are re-infused into the patient after irradiation (Fig. 18.10). Genes used to transfect tumour cells include those encoding

- *Costimulatory molecules (e.g., B7)* This would help to convert tumour cells which lack costimulatory molecules into efficient APCs. These could then directly activate CTL-precursors (CTL-Ps). It is reminded here that lack of B7 molecules on tumour cells is an escape mechanism of the tumour as it results in anergy in T cells. Transfection of tumour cells with genes for B7 molecules would prevent T cells from becoming anergic.
- *Cytokines* Proliferation and differentiation of tumour-specific CTL-Ps is enhanced by IL-2. CTL-Ps on receiving both signal 1 and 2 from the tumour cell, and activating signals from IL-2, differentiate into effector CTLs which would lead to tumour cell destruction.

The approach has the advantage that tumour antigens need not be identified.

Dendritic Cell-based Vaccines

The role of DCs in stimulating CTL responses against the tumour has been highlighted in the preceding text. A potential approach for enhancing host immunity to tumours using the patient's own dendritic cells is briefly discussed here.

Dendritic cells are purified from patients, expanded in vitro, and pulsed with antigens from the patient's own tumour. These antigen-pulsed DCs are re-introduced into the patient. Dendritic cell-based vaccines stimulate cytotoxic T cell responses to the tumour. This approach exploits the unique ability of DCs to present exogenous antigens via the class I MHC pathway to CD8$^+$ cytotoxic T lymphocytes (cross-presentation), thereby boosting immune responses against the tumour by CTLs. Due to the immense potential of this approach, DC-based vaccines are being extensively explored for cancer therapy in patients with metastatic melanoma, renal carcinoma, and prostate cancer.

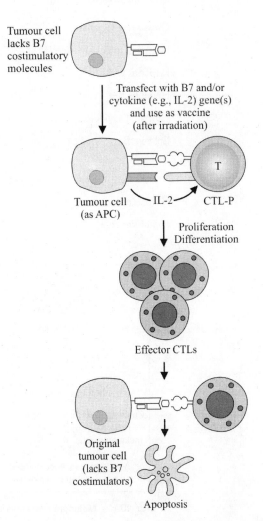

Fig. 18.10 Tumour cell-based vaccines. Tumour cells are transfected with B7 and/or cytokine gene(s), irradiated and then used as a vaccine. This converts B7-transfected tumour cells into APCs which may activate CTL-Ps into effector CTLs which are likely to kill tumour cells.
CTL-P, CTL-precursor

Box 18.1   Cancer vaccines versus traditional vaccines

Prophylactic vaccines which are generally used to protect against infectious disease may also be used to prevent cancers induced by viruses. It is very likely that preventing viral infection will prevent development of the associated cancer. Using this approach, some successes have been met with in veterinary medicine. These include reduction in incidence of

*   haematologic malignant tumours in cats induced by feline leukaemia virus, and
*   Marek's disease (a lymphoma) in chickens induced by a herpes virus.

Vaccines based on HPV proteins have yielded promising results in prevention of cervical cancer in humans. Besides, it is anticipated, and there have been some positive results, that the vaccination programme to prevent Hepatitis B virus infection will help to reduce the incidence of hepatocellular carcinoma in humans. But vaccine development for other types of cancers faces many challenges. While only 15–20 per cent of cancers are caused by infectious agents particularly viruses (Table 18.1), most cancers (chemical carcinogens/radiation

Table 18.1   Cancers associated with infectious agents. About 15–20% of all cancers are known to be associated with infectious organisms. It is likely that vaccinating against the causative agent will prevent the associated cancer

Causative agent	Cancer
Human papilloma virus (HPV)	Cervical cancer
Hepatitis C	Liver cancer
Hepatitis B	Liver cancer
Human T cell leukaemia virus -1 (HTLV-1)	Adult T cell leukaemia
Epstein–Barr virus (EBV)	B cell lymphoma
	Nasopharyngeal carcinoma
	Hodgkin's disease
Human herpes virus (HHV) 8	Kaposi's sarcoma
Helicobacter pylori	Stomach cancer

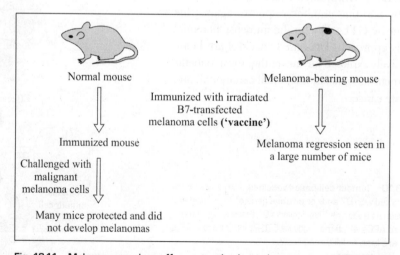

Fig. 18.11   **Melanoma vaccines offer protection in murine tumour models.**

induced) are caused by defects in cellular proteins. Though these mutated proteins represent antigens that are unique to the tumour, there are many obstacles in the way of using them to develop vaccines that would target cancer cells specifically while sparing normal cells. A major obstacle is that very few tumour-specific antigens have been identified. Moreover, as discussed in the main text, cancers induced by chemicals express antigens novel to each tumour. A prophylactic vaccine for such cancers is thus not possible. However, a vaccine that will boost immune responses against an already established tumour (*therapeutic vaccine*) using shared antigens, or even tumour cells/dendritic cells transfected with relevant genes, is a more feasible approach that is being pursued. From the encouraging results obtained with melanoma 'vaccines' in murine tumour models, it is hoped that similar vaccines may help to prevent metastases after surgical removal of a primary melanoma in human patients (Fig. 18.11). This has led to initiation of clinical trials in patients with advanced melanoma using transfected tumour cell-based vaccines.

SUMMARY

- Tumour cells express antigens which are of two types. These include tumour-specific transplantation antigens (TSTAs) and tumour-associated antigens (TAAs).
- Tumour immunity can be induced by immunization. For chemically-induced tumours, immunity induced is individually tumour-specific. So antigens on chemically- induced tumours have limited potential as tumour vaccines.
- For virally-induced tumours, all tumours induced by the same virus have shared antigens. Shared tumour antigens have more potential in design of vaccines.
- Principal mechanism of tumour rejection is mediated by CTLs. T$_H$ cells primed by APCs provide help for effective CD8$^+$ T cell functioning. Natural killer cells, macrophages, and antibodies are also involved in anti-tumour immunity.
- Tumours evolve various mechanisms to escape host immune responses such as downregulation of class I MHC molecules, secretion of immunosuppressive cytokines (TGF-β) besides others.
- Passive immunotherapy involves use of mAbs specific for tumour antigens (these can be coupled

to toxins, drugs, or radioactive isotopes), and TILs and LAK cells obtained from cancer patients. These are expanded in vitro and re-infused into patients (adoptive cellular immunotherapy).
- Administration of some cytokines systemically enhances the immune response against tumours. These cytokines have shown a positive response in clinical settings.
- Active immunotherapy is based on vaccination with: purified tumour antigens, tumour cells transfected with genes encoding cytokines and/or costimulatory B7 molecules, and dendritic cells pulsed with antigens from the patient's tumour.
- Most vaccines against cancer are likely to be therapeutic, that is, will be used for patients who already have cancer. Prophylactic (preventive) vaccines may be used for prevention of virally-induced cancers such as cervical cancer.
- Most immunotherapeutic strategies are in the experimental stage. They are likely to be effective after the tumour mass has been reduced in size and when used in combination with other conventional forms of therapy.

REVIEW QUESTIONS

1. Indicate whether the following statements are true or false. If false, explain why.
   (a) Alpha-fetoprotein is used to monitor growth and progression of tumours of the colon.
   (b) Immunotoxins are toxic substances released by phagocytic cells.
   (c) T cell-mediated cytotoxicity is important in tumour rejection.
   (d) Herceptin has been approved by FDA (USA) for treatment of cancer of the liver.
   (e) T regulatory (T$_{reg}$) CD4$^+$ CD25$^+$ cells down-regulate anti-tumour immunity.

(f) Like CTLs, recognition of tumour cells by NK cells is MHC restricted.

2. Self-assessment questions
   (a) Why is it that unlike methylcholanthrene (MCA)-induced tumour antigens, virally-encoded tumour antigens have more potential in design of vaccines?
   (b) What are the different ways in which monoclonal antibodies can be used against cancer? Why are murine monoclonals avoided? Are there any alternatives available?
   (c) Explain mechanisms by which tumours down-regulate host anti-tumour immune responses and evade the immune system.
   (d) Explain why infusion of melanoma cells transfected with B7 and IL-2 genes are of benefit in melanoma patients? Can vaccines based on melanoma antigens be used for treating patients with other types of cancer?
   (e) An animal is immunized with adenovirus. What is the type of protective immunity induced? How do you think that an APC presents internalized tumour antigens associated with class I MHC molecules?

3. For each question, choose the *best* answer.
   (a) The virus involved in cervical cancer aetiology is:
      (i) Epstein–Barr virus (EBV)
      (ii) Human papilloma virus (HPV)
      (iii) Human T cell leukaemia virus (HTLV-1)
      (iv) Human immunodeficiency virus (HIV)
   (b) Anti-tumour activity of IFN-α involves:
      (i) increase in class I MHC expression
      (ii) damage to vascular endothelial cells
      (iii) decrease in blood flow
      (iv) inhibition of vascularization of tumours
   (c) The cytokine that stimulates differentiation of immature dendritic cells is
      (i) IFN-γ
      (ii) IFN-α
      (iii) GM-CSF
      (iv) TGF-β
   (d) Anti-tumour immunity is downregulated by
      (i) TGF-β
      (ii) IFN-γ + IL-2
      (iii) IL-12
      (iv) GM-CSF

Immunological Techniques—Principles and Applications

We have seen how antibodies represent an important defence mechanism by which our bodies stay protected from various infectious microbes present in the environment. In addition to this role, antibodies are amazingly useful reagents that find use in many laboratory techniques. As seen in Chapter 4, the interaction between an antigen and antibody is a bimolecular reaction comparable to the reaction between an enzyme and its substrate, but with the important difference that both reactants remain unchanged. It is the exquisite specificity of the interaction that makes antibodies very handy and indispensable reagents. Development of a method for generating monoclonal antibodies (mAbs) has greatly enhanced our ability to generate antibodies of an enormously wide range of specificities. Many immunoassays have been developed that are used in research and which rely on antibodies. Besides being exploited for therapeutic purposes, antibodies are also important tools for clinicians as they help in disease diagnosis.

Included in the appendix are some commonly used immunological techniques and assays that make use of antibodies for detection, purification, and quantitation of antigens. The principles that underlie the techniques along with a brief methodology, and applications are described.

PRODUCTION OF POLYCLONAL ANTISERUM

A suitable polyclonal antiserum or monoclonal antibodies against the antigen of interest is essential for all immunochemical procedures. The choice of animal for production of polyclonal antiserum depends on the volume of antiserum that is required, though other considerations such as the amount of antigen available are also important. The rabbit is a popular animal for immunization and production of most conventional polyclonal antisera (Fig. A.1). Sheep, goats, and horses are used when a greater volume of antiserum is required. Rats and mice are used for recovery of spleen cells.

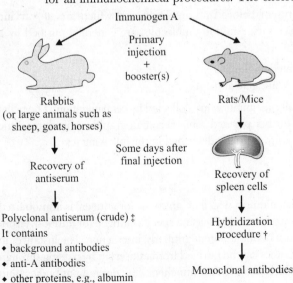

Fig. A.1 Production of polyclonal antiserum and monoclonal antibodies. The polyclonal antiserum contains antibodies arising from many B cell clones. It is *antigen-specific*. Monoclonal antibodies originate from a single clone and are *epitope-specific*.

‡ The crude polyclonal antiserum can be purified to give a preparation specific for immunogen A.

† The hybridization procedure for monoclonal antibodies is depicted in Fig. A.3.

It is to be remembered that splenic lymphocytes from immunized animals are the key starting cells for production of hybridomas and mAbs.

Immunization Procedure

Polyclonal antibodies are raised by injecting an immunogen into an animal and then collecting the blood containing the desired antibodies after a suitable time. The immunizing dose range varies. It is generally between 50–1000 µg in rabbits and other large animals and about 10–100 µg in mouse or a rat. The route of immunization affects immunogenicity and can be intradermal, intramuscular, intraperitoneal, intravascular, or subcutaneous. Antigens given subcutaneously are carried to the regional lymph nodes whereas those administered by the intravenous route (generally used for final boosting for hybridoma generation) are carried to the spleen. Particulate antigens (e.g., bacterial cells and red blood cells) being good immunogens can be injected alone, but soluble molecules, such as proteins require the use of adjuvants in order to improve or enhance the immune response mounted by the animal. Freund's complete adjuvant (FCA) is the most commonly employed adjuvant and is used in the first immunization. Subsequent immunizations make use of Freund's incomplete adjuvant (FIA) which lacks killed mycobacteria (see Chapter 13).

The animal is given a priming injection followed by booster doses administered at intervals of several weeks or months. Delivering booster doses increases the effectiveness of the immune response activated and helps to maintain it. It is important to collect blood from the animals before the first injection is given. This serves as control for subsequent tests. Also, it is necessary to collect blood after each injection to test the sera of animals for the presence of antibodies and to assess the antibody titre. If there is indication of good antibody formation, further booster injections are not required.

To obtain serum/antiserum, blood is allowed to stand at room temperature to clot. Antibodies remain in the exuded fluid called serum. Serum that contains antibodies specific for a particular antigen is called *antiserum*. Decomplement antiserum by heating at 56°C for 30 minutes.

Production of antisera having high-affinity antibodies usually takes a minimum of about 3 months. Aliquots of antisera can be stored in tubes at 4°C for up to 6 months. They can also be placed in deep -freeze for long term storage Addition of sodium azide prevents bacterial contamination.

Purification of Antibody

As background antibodies (antibodies present before immunization and which are of varying specificities) are present, purification is necessary. Antibody molecules are generally purified by a two-step procedure:

♦ Precipitation with 40–50 per cent saturated $(NH_4)_2SO_4$
♦ Affinity chromatography using protein A/antigen/anti-IgG

The partially purified antibodies after salt precipitation are collected by centrifugation. The pellet is redissolved in buffer and antibodies are further purified using chromatographic procedures. One such procedure, called affinity chromatography, is briefly described in the following text.

AFFINITY CHROMATOGRAPHY

Affinity chromatography is a purification technique in which an antibody (or antigen) is immobilized on a solid support, such as sepharose beads and is used to select a specific antigen (or antibody) from a mixture. It exploits the exquisite specificity of the antigen–antibody interaction. For instance, in the example shown in Fig. A.2, anti-A antibodies can be purified from antiserum by passing through a column containing sepharose beads to which antigen A is attached. The desired antibodies bind to the antigen while unwanted antibodies and other serum proteins which remain unbound are removed by washing. The bound anti-A antibodies can be eluted by a change in pH which disrupts the antigen–antibody interaction. *Protein A* is present in the cell wall of *S. aureus* and is available as a recombinant product. It binds to the Fc region of IgG of several species and so is useful for affinity purification of IgG from antiserum.

HYBRIDOMA TECHNOLOGY FOR MONOCLONAL ANTIBODY PRODUCTION

A polyclonal antibody preparation besides containing the desired antibody against the immunizing antigen contains background antibodies (Fig. A.1). This may yield misleading results in a particular immunological test as some of the antibodies may cross-react with the test antigens. Another limitation is that it is very difficult to produce the same polyclonal preparation once it has been used up. These limitations of polyclonal antibodies were overcome when G. Kohler and C. Milstein in 1975 developed a remarkable technique for producing mAbs, a major achievement in immunology which has greatly benefited the field of medicine.

The technology for mAb production starts traditionally with injection of antigen (antigen A) into a mouse. The sequential steps are represented schematically in Fig. A.3.

When the mouse is making a good antibody response, the spleen is removed and a cell suspension prepared. This is a source of plasma cells, some of which are secreting antibody of the desired specificity (anti-A) while others are secreting background antibodies. Spleen cells are fused with immortal myeloma cells (lymphoid tumour cells) using polyethylene glycol (PEG) which promotes membrane fusion. Only some cells fuse successfully to produce hybrid cells which secrete antibodies. The hybrid cell proliferates into a clone called a *hybridoma*. Like myeloma cells, these cells are immortal.

By culturing in a selective medium called *HAT*, unfused myeloma cells die whereas hybrid cells survive. HAT medium which contains hypoxanthine (a purine), aminopterin (a folic acid antagonist), and

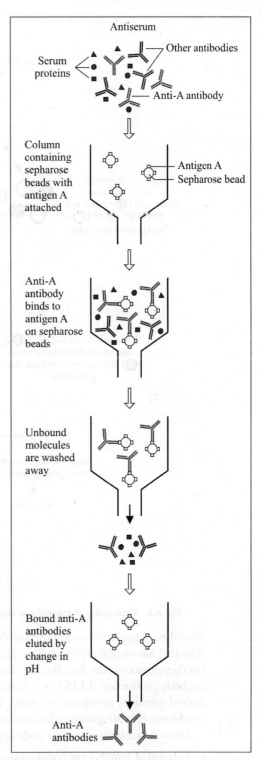

Fig. A.2 Affinity chromatography.

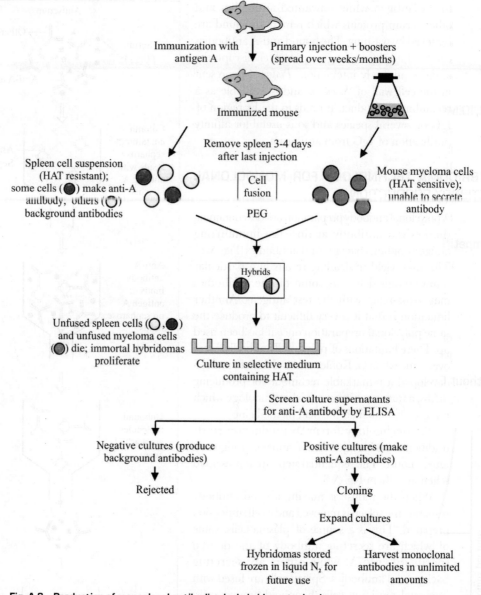

Fig. A.3   Production of monoclonal antibodies by hybridoma technology.

thymidine (a nucleoside composed of deoxyribose, a pentose sugar, linked to the pyrimidine base thymine) allows only hybrid cells to grow. Unfused spleen cells are able to grow in HAT medium but they do not survive in culture for more than a few days. Individual hybridomas are screened for antibody production (ELISA is commonly used for this purpose). Cells secreting antibody of the desired specificity are cloned by plating them out so that each well contains a single cell. The cloned hybridoma cells are grown in bulk culture to produce large amounts of homogeneous antibody.

Monoclonal antibodies have wide applications some of which include:

- isolation of lymphocyte populations and subpopulations,
- tissue typing,

- immunoassays,
- diagnosis of malignancy,
- as therapeutic agents,
- 'magic bullet' therapy in cancer, and
- affinity chromatography for protein purification.

RADIOIMMUNOASSAY

Radioimmunoassay (RIA) is a competitive binding assay which was introduced by Berson and Yalow for determination of human insulin. Yalow was awarded the Nobel Prize in 1977, a few years after Berson's death.

In a RIA, a fixed amount of radiolabelled antigen and the corresponding unlabelled antigen compete for binding to a limited number of antigen-combining sites on a high-affinity antibody. The components react as shown in the following text:

Competition

$$\underset{\substack{\text{unlabelled} \\ \text{antigen}}}{X} + \underset{\substack{\text{radiolabelled} \\ \text{antigen}}}{X^*} + \underset{\text{anti-X}}{Y} \rightleftharpoons \underset{\text{bound fraction}}{X-Y+X^*-Y} + \underset{\text{free fraction}}{X+X^*}$$

Due to competition the amount of label in the bound fraction decreases with increase in concentration of the unlabelled antigen. This decrease is measured to determine the amount of antigen present in a test sample. It is to be noted that without unlabelled antigen there would be no competition.

Without Competition

$$X^* + Y \rightleftharpoons X^*-Y + X^*$$

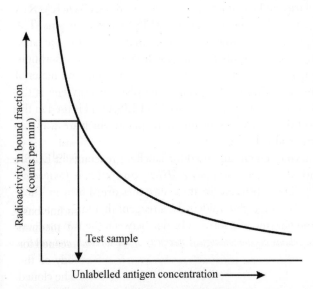

Fig. A.4 **Competitive radioimmunoassay.** The dose-response curve is obtained by adding increasing concentrations of unlabelled antigen to a fixed concentration of labelled antigen and its antibody. The linear part of the curve can be used to determine the concentration of antigen in the test sample.

Predetermined amounts of labelled antigen (X^*) and anti-X antibody are taken in a series of tubes. The concentration of labelled antigen should be such that the number of epitopes presented by it should be in excess of binding sites on the antibody. Normally, concentrations selected are such that 50–70 per cent of labelled antigen is bound. Added known increasing amounts of unlabelled antigen (X) and incubated. The soluble antigen–antibody complexes formed can be separated from the free antigen (free fraction) by various separation methods. A commonly used method is precipitation by *antiglobulin* which is an anti-isotype antibody (Fig. A.8). This leaves the unbound antigen (X and X^*) in the supernatant. The radioactivity of the immune complexes is determined and plotted against amounts of X added. It is inversely proportional to the concentration of unlabelled antigen. The concentration of antigen in a test sample can be determined from the dose-response curve (Fig. A.4).

Choice of radioisotopes for labelling antigen usually lies between ^{125}I (γ-emitting) and ^3H (β-emitting). Phenolic groups of the aromatic ring of protein tyrosine residues facilitate direct iodination with ^{125}I in presence of a mild oxidizing agent. *The labelling procedure should be such that there is least alteration in immunological reactivity of the molecule.*

Radioimmunoassays are accurate and sensitive. Some compounds can even be measured in the pg ml^{-1} range. However, they have many limitations:

- Hazards of radioactive reagents; thyroid gland is a major target for ^{125}I which can be incorporated into the thyroid hormones T_3/T_4
- High cost of equipment and its maintenance
- Short half-life of reagents; ^{125}I and ^{131}I have a half-life of 60 days and 8 days, respectively
- Need for trained technical staff
- Prompt disposal of radioactive waste

Radioimmunoassays have been most widely used in endocrinology for measurement of hormones in serum/plasma. They can also be used to measure drugs, vitamins, antibodies, and various other substances found in low levels in biological fluids.

However, due to its limitations and with ELISA's growing popularity there has been a dramatic reduction in the use of RIA technology.

ENZYME-LINKED IMMUNOSORBENT ASSAY

Enzyme-linked immunosorbent assay (ELISA) was devised by two Swedish scientists Eva Engvall and Peter Perlman in 1971. It is a useful analytical tool for antigens and antibodies in human serum and other biological fluids and is widely used in clinical diagnostics today. This powerful tool has grown both in importance and popularity and has almost entirely replaced RIA. Whereas RIA makes use of a radioactive label, ELISA uses an enzyme. The solid phase is the immunosorbent on which one of the reactants, either antigen or antibody, is immobilized by passive adsorbtion. This makes it easy to separate bound from unbound material during assay by simply washing the plate. Polystyrene is the most popular solid phase material in ELISA and is used in the form of disposable 96-well microtitre plates which are available commercially (Fig. A.5).

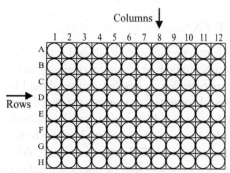

96 - well microtitre plate
(showing numbering and lettering)

Fig. A.5   A microtitre plate.

Enzymes commonly used for labelling reactants in ELISA include *horse radish peroxidase* (*HRP*) and *alkaline phosphatase* (*ALP*). The substrates for these enzymes are shown in Table A.1. The enzymes can be coupled to antibodies using glutaraldehyde, a reagent that targets the free amino group of lysine on both antibody and enzyme and forms a bridge between the two proteins. *It is important that the antibody–enzyme conjugate retains the immunological specificity of the antibody and catalytic activity of the enzyme.*

ELISA can be used in various ways:

Sandwich ELISA

The sandwich assay is so named because the antigen to be measured is bound (sandwiched) between two antibodies. The steps in sandwich ELISA are described in Fig. A.6. The *second (detection) antibody*

Table A.1 Enzymes and their substrates commonly used in immunoassays and other related colour reactions. In enzyme immunoassays, the OD of the coloured product is measured. Hence, the product needs to be soluble. In immunoblotting the product must be insoluble to allow precise localization of the antigen–antibody interaction. Chemiluminescent substrates are also available for HRP which increase detection limit.

Enzymes and substrates	Product solubility	Applications
Horse radish peroxidase (HRP) †		
◆ Tetramethyl benzidine (TMB)	soluble yellow (450nm)	enzyme immunoassays
◆ Diaminobenzidine (DAB)	insoluble brown	immunoblots
◆ Chloronaphthol	insoluble blue-black	immunoblots
Alkaline phosphatase (ALP)		
◆ Nitrophenyl phosphate	soluble yellow (405 nm)	enzyme immunoassays
◆ BCIP-NBT combination	insoluble dark purple	immunoblots

BCIP-NBT, bromochloroindolyl phosphate-nitro blue tetrazolium

† H_2O_2 is always required along with a chromogen

which carries the enzyme label binds to an epitope (binding site for antibody) on the antigen distinct from the epitope recognized by the *first (capture) antibody*. *Blocking* is an essential step in ELISA. It is used to block unreacted protein-binding sites in the plastic plate by incubating with an inert protein such as bovine serum albumin (BSA), gelatin, or casein. This prevents proteins added in later steps from binding non-specifically to the plastic. Sandwich ELISA can be used to estimate cytokines and other molecules in an unknown sample.

Indirect ELISA

This variant of ELISA can be used to detect or quantitate antibody in serum or other samples (Fig. A.7). The *primary antibody*, the antibody to be quantitated, binds to antigen coating the wells. The binding can be detected with an enzyme-conjugated *secondary antibody* (antiglobulin; Fig. A.8). No binding occurs if primary antibody is absent in the test sample. Indirect ELISA is useful for detecting presence of anti-HIV antibodies in HIV-infected individuals.

The indirect system is particularly useful in in vitro diagnostics. Any number of antisera can be screened by binding to a given antigen using the universal antiglobulin reagent. This reagent is both economical and convenient. Use of antiglobulin overcomes a limitation of the sandwich assay in which each antigen-specific antibody has to be labelled.

Protein A introduced earlier in the chapter, like antiglobulin, binds to Fc regions of immunoglobulin molecules, particularly IgG of several species. It can be covalently coupled to any of the enzymes used in ELISA. The resultant conjugate can then be used as a substitute for the enzyme-conjugated secondary antibody in the indirect ELISA system.

Competitive ELISA

Competitive assays are generally used when the antigen is small (such as a drug or steroid hormone) and has a single epitope. Instead of antibody, it is the antigen that is often labelled with enzyme. Labelled and unlabelled (test) antigens compete for binding to the capture antibody immobilized on the plastic well. Labelled antigen is kept constant in all the wells. A calibration graph is drawn using known increasing concentrations of unlabelled antigen taken in different wells. The concentration of test antigen is determined with reference to the standard curve. It is inversely proportional to colour

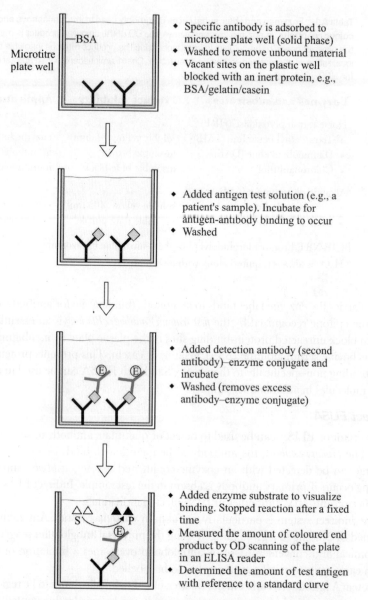

Microtitre
plate well

—BSA

- Specific antibody is adsorbed to microtitre plate well (solid phase)
- Washed to remove unbound material
- Vacant sites on the plastic well blocked with an inert protein, e.g., BSA/gelatin/casein

- Added antigen test solution (e.g., a patient's sample). Incubate for antigen-antibody binding to occur
- Washed

- Added detection antibody (second antibody)–enzyme conjugate and incubate
- Washed (removes excess antibody–enzyme conjugate)

- Added enzyme substrate to visualize binding. Stopped reaction after a fixed time
- Measured the amount of coloured end product by OD scanning of the plate in an ELISA reader
- Determined the amount of test antigen with reference to a standard curve

Fig. A.6 The two-antibody sandwich assay for estimation of an unknown antigen.

intensity (Fig. A.9). A limitation of this method is that different methods have to be used to couple antigens, which chemically are very diverse, to an enzyme.

Advantages of ELISA

- It is economical and suitable for use in small laboratories.
- As a solid phase is used, bound antigen–antibody complex can be separated from free reactants by simply washing the plate.

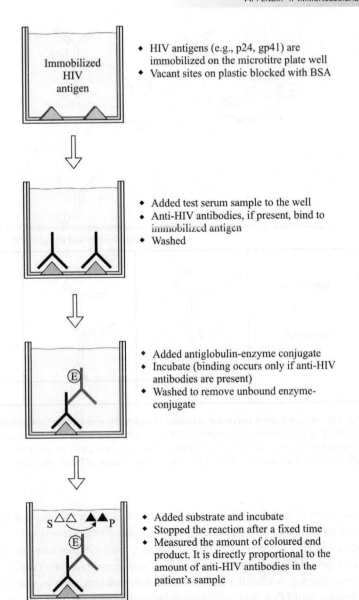

- HIV antigens (e.g., p24, gp41) are immobilized on the microtitre plate well
- Vacant sites on plastic blocked with BSA

- Added test serum sample to the well
- Anti-HIV antibodies, if present, bind to immobilized antigen
- Washed

- Added antiglobulin-enzyme conjugate
- Incubate (binding occurs only if anti-HIV antibodies are present)
- Washed to remove unbound enzyme-conjugate

- Added substrate and incubate
- Stopped the reaction after a fixed time
- Measured the amount of coloured end product. It is directly proportional to the amount of anti-HIV antibodies in the patient's sample

Fig. A.7 An indirect ELISA system for detecting anti-HIV antibodies in serum. Anti-HIV antibodies cannot be detected in the window-period (about 6–7 weeks) that exists just after infection.

- It is rapid and sensitive.
- Disposable polystyrene microtitre plates or tubes as solid phase carriers are readily available.
- The shelf-life of reagents is more favourable than RIA.
- ELISA plate readers are commercially available which can measure absorbance of 96 wells in less than a minute.
- It lacks radiological hazards that are associated with RIA.

The many advantages of ELISA account for its growing popularity.

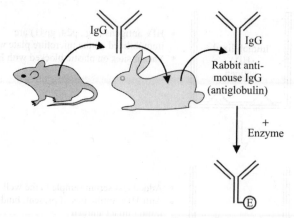

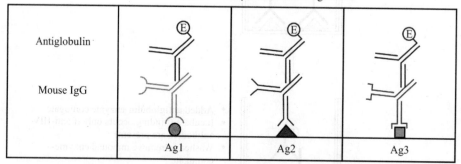

Fig. A.8   Antiglobulin-a universal indicator reagent. Enzyme-labelled antiglobulin raised in rabbit to mouse IgG antibody can bind to any mouse IgG molecule irrespective of its specificity. Similarly, antibodies to human IgG can be raised in rabbits or other species (in this case the antiglobulin is rabbit anti-human IgG). The figure, an over simplification, depicts the practical utility of antiglobulin.

Applications

ELISA can be used in clinical laboratories for assay of almost any antigen, hapten, or antibody. Some compounds measured are: HBsAg, α-fetoprotein (an oncofoetal protein used to monitor tumour growth; see Chapter 18), HIV antigens, anti-HIV antibodies, cytokines in serum, and hormones, for example, insulin, estrogens, HCG, thyroxine, and TSH. It can be used to detect antibacterial and antiparasite antibodies in disease. Antibodies in hybridoma supernatants, such as anti-cytokine antibodies, and autoantibodies (anti-DNA and anti-thyroglobulin) can also be detected. Besides, therapeutic drug levels can be monitored. ELISA-based kits are widespread and successful.

Sandwich Immunoassay in a Home Pregnancy-detection Kit

Human chorionic gonadotropin (HCG) is a glycoprotein hormone produced by the developing placenta shortly after fertilization. Its early detection in the urine 7–10 days after conception confirms pregnancy. The device used in detection is shown in Fig. A.10.

The test urine is added to the sample well. As it flows through the device, HCG, if present in the sample, reacts with the anti-HCG– gold conjugate. The coloured complex moves up the membrane to the test region where it is immobilized by a polyclonal anti-HCG antibody coated on the membrane forming a pink-coloured band. Absence of this pink band in the test region indicates a negative result. The unreacted anti-HCG–gold conjugate (with no HCG bound) and any unbound complex

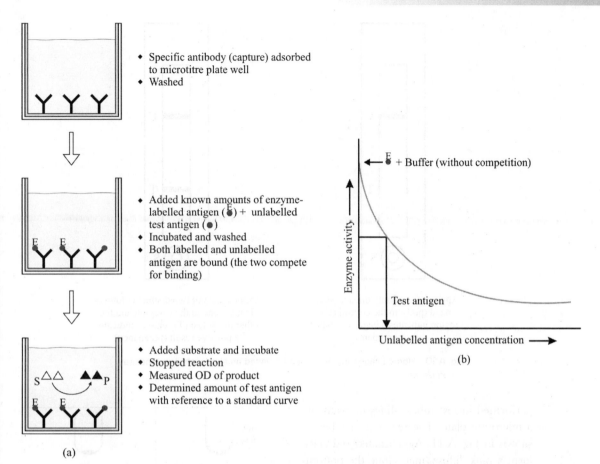

- Specific antibody (capture) adsorbed to microtitre plate well
- Washed

- Added known amounts of enzyme-labelled antigen (E) + unlabelled test antigen (●)
- Incubated and washed
- Both labelled and unlabelled antigen are bound (the two compete for binding)

- Added substrate and incubate
- Stopped reaction
- Measured OD of product
- Determined amount of test antigen with reference to a standard curve

(a)

E + Buffer (without competition)

Enzyme activity

Test antigen

Unlabelled antigen concentration ⟶

(b)

Fig. A.9 Competitive ELISA. (a) There are many variants of competitive ELISA. In the form shown, antibody is adsorbed to the microtitre well. Some variants make use of antigen adsorbed on the solid phase. (b) Concentration of antigen is inversely proportional to the colour produced. Note that the labelled antigen is kept constant throughout.

move further up the membrane and are immobilized in the control region of the strip. This region has anti-mouse antibodies coated on the membrane. Appearance of two distinct coloured bands indicates a positive result.

Many commercial diagnostic kits, such as the kit for HCG detection in urine described in the preceding text and others make use of antibodies bound to minute colloidal *gold particles* (usually 2–40 nm in diameter). Depending on the size of the gold particles used for labelling, a red or blue colour is imparted to sites where binding to antibody occurs. Colloidal gold bound to antibody finds wide use in immunoblotting and in immunoelectron microscopy. Its use allows more than one antigen to be simultaneously localized in the same tissue.

AGGLUTINATION REACTIONS

Interaction between an antibody and a particulate antigen results in visible clumping or agglutination. Microbial cells, RBCs and even inert particles, such as latex and gelatin can be agglutinated. IgM due to its multiple antigen-binding sites and higher avidity is able to agglutinate cells more efficiently than IgG (see Chapter 4). Agglutination reactions are simple, rapid, and sensitive. They can be

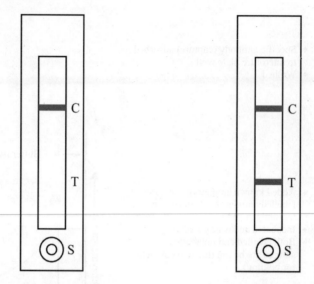

Appearance of only one coloured band (pink) in the control (C) region indicates a negative result (not pregnant)

Appearance of two distinct coloured bands - one in the C region and the other in the test (T) region - indicates a positive result (pregnancy)

Fig. A.10 **Home pregnancy-detection kit based on sandwich immunoassay.**
S, sample well

performed in test tubes, slides or wells of a microtitre plate. The reaction in tubes is shown in Fig. A.11. Agglutinated red cells form a pink diffuse 'mat' along the bottom and sides of the tube while non-agglutinated cells settle at the bottom forming a small compact 'button'. Agglutination reactions can be *direct* or *indirect*.

Direct Agglutination

This results when antibodies are directed to antigens that are part of the cell surface. If the cells are RBCs, the term *direct haemagglutination* is used. Some clinical applications of direct agglutination reactions include the following:

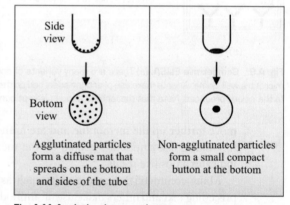

Agglutinated particles form a diffuse mat that spreads on the bottom and sides of the tube

Non-agglutinated particles form a small compact button at the bottom

Fig. A.11 Agglutination reactions.

- ◆ Red cell typing
- ◆ Detection of anti-Rh (D antigen) antibodies in an Rh negative mother who has delivered an Rh positive child (Fig. A.12); a positive test indicates chances of haemolytic disease of the newborn (HDN) in the next childbirth. If the memory response is stimulated, anti-D antibodies bind to foetal RBCs leading to their destruction (see Fig. 14.8).
- ◆ Detection of autoantibodies to RBCs in autoimmune haemolytic anaemia (*Coomb's test*)
- ◆ Detection of antibodies specific for surface antigens on a bacterial cell; a rising titre is used to confirm infection

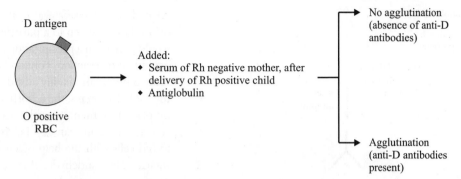

Fig. A.12 Detection of anti-D antibodies in serum of an Rh negative mother.

Titre is defined as the highest dilution of antiserum which gives a visible agglutination reaction. It is a semi-quantitative expression of the antibodies present in serum. A good example is the *Widal test* for typhoid which is performed by mixing gradually increasing dilutions of the patient's serum with a suspension of *Salmonella typhi*, incubating, and looking for agglutination.

Determination of Titre

A bacterial suspension (for instance *S. typhi)* is titrated with specific antisera (anti-X). The steps described are shown in Fig. A.13 in the following text.

Saline, 0.1 ml, is added to a series of wells in a microtitre plate. An equal volume of test antiserum (anti-X) which has been diluted (1:5 dilution) is added to the first well and mixed with the saline. A 0.1 ml sample from the first well is transferred to saline in the second well, mixed and transferred 0.1 ml to the third well and so on. This method doubles the dilution in each consecutive well and is called *serial dilution.* In the next step, 0.1 ml bacterial suspension is added to each well with gentle mixing and kept at room temperature for 1 hour. A clear red button (or cell pellet) at the bottom of the well indicates non-agglutinated cells. Agglutinated cells, on the other hand, settle as a pink diffuse mat. The last well identified showing agglutination gives the *titre value.* The first few tubes which contain the most concentrated antiserum sometimes fail to agglutinate cells. This is called *prozone effect* and is due to excess antibodies which bind to single cells and do not link them together.

Indirect/Passive Agglutination

Inert particles (and even RBCs) can be made to serve as carriers for an antigen which can be covalently or non-covalently attached to the surface. Agglutination of such particles by antibodies is

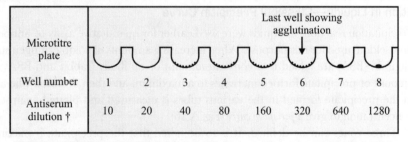

Fig. A.13 Determination of titre. Well no. 6 is the last well showing a visible agglutination reaction. Hence the titre of the antiserum is 320.

† Figures are arbitrary .

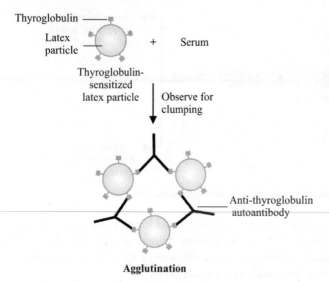

Agglutination

Fig. A.14 Detection of autoantibodies to thyroglobulin in serum of a suspected thyroid patient.

termed *indirect/passive agglutination*. Attachment of a soluble antigen to a particle converts what would have been a precipitation reaction into an agglutination reaction. Polysaccharides and also some proteins are readily adsorbed to RBCs. In the case of proteins, the adsorbtion is facilitated by prior treatment of red cells with chromic chloride. Proteins can also be covalently linked to red cells with the help of coupling reagents such as glutaraldehyde. Passive agglutination reactions can be used to detect:

♦ *Autoantibodies to thyroglobulin in the serum of a patient with thyroid disease* Serum of a suspected patient is added to a drop of sensitized latex particles on a slide and observed for clumping. A positive agglutination reaction indicates presence of anti-thyroglobulin autoantibodies in the serum (Fig. A.14).

♦ *Rheumatoid factors (RFs) in serum of rheumatoid arthritis patients* The patient's serum is added to a drop of IgG-sensitized latex particles on a glass slide and observed for agglutination.

Commercial kits are available for the above purposes and are widely used.

Haemagglutination Inhibition Assay

The assay is based on the principle that soluble antigen (in test sample such as urine/serum) competes with antigen coating the indicator cells for binding to a limiting amount of antibody. The assay can be used to determine presence/absence of Factor VIII in the sera of patients suspected to be suffering from haemophilia (Fig. A.15).

PRECIPITATION REACTIONS

Precipitation reactions can be performed in liquids or in semi-solid media such as agar. Although the reactions performed in liquids have only historical significance, precipitation reactions in gels are in common use.

Precipitation in Liquids—Classical Precipitin Curve

Precipitation reactions in liquids were used earlier for quantitative assay of antibody/antigen but are now seldom used for this purpose. When increasing amounts of soluble antigen such as bovine serum albumin (BSA) are added to a constant amount of antibody (rabbit anti-BSA) and incubated, the amount of precipitate formed increases to a maximum and then declines. The amount of antibody in the precipitate formed in the various tubes is measured and plotted against increasing antigen concentration to give a *precipitin curve* (Fig. A.16).

Three zones can be defined. It is to be noted that the precipitate is maximum in the *zone of equivalence*. Here, the ratio of antigen and antibody is optimal and large lattices form. Some soluble immune complexes which are too small to precipitate out are present in the *zone of antigen excess* and

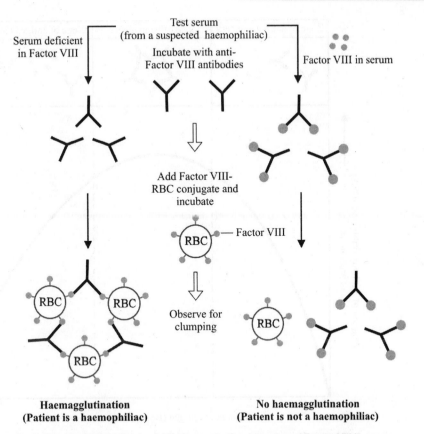

Fig. A.15 Haemagglutination inhibition assay for detection of Factor VIII in serum.

also in the *zone of antibody excess*. The precipitin reaction, though not in use now, holds importance as all quantitative studies of antigen–antibody interactions are based on it.

Immune responses in vivo are continually generating immune complexes. Small immune complexes persist in the circulation and can lead to undesirable consequences due to their effect in small blood vessels.

Precipitation in Gels

Precipitation reactions in gels are routinely performed in semi-solid media such as agar which is allowed to solidify on a microscopic glass slide or a petri-dish. They are cheap, easy to perform, and satisfactory, and can be used for both qualitative and quantitative work. Some techniques based on precipitation reaction in gels are described here.

Single Radial Immunodiffusion (SRID)

Buffered agar into which antiserum (raised against the antigen to be determined) has been incorporated is allowed to solidify on a glass slide. When an antigen solution is placed in a well punched in the agar, it diffuses radially into the surrounding gel and complexes with the antibody. A ring of precipitation forms around the well and moves outwards. When the entire antigen has entered the well (end point), the ring becomes stationary. At this point, the diameter/area of the ring is related to antigen concentration (Fig. A.17).

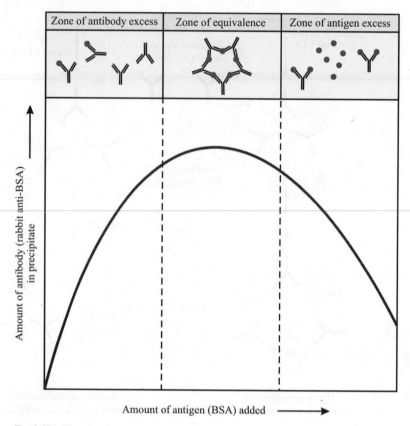

Zone of antibody excess	Zone of equivalence	Zone of antigen excess

Amount of antibody (rabbit anti-BSA) in precipitate

Amount of antigen (BSA) added →

Fig. A.16   The classical precipitin curve.

SRID is a simple and sensitive quantitative technique that can be used to determine IgG levels and also other plasma proteins in human serum. A calibration curve can be constructed using an antigen of known concentrations and plotted against ring diameter. An unknown concentration of the same antigen can be determined with reference to the standard curve (Fig. A.18). If a voltage is applied, SRID becomes *rocket immunoelectrophoresis*.

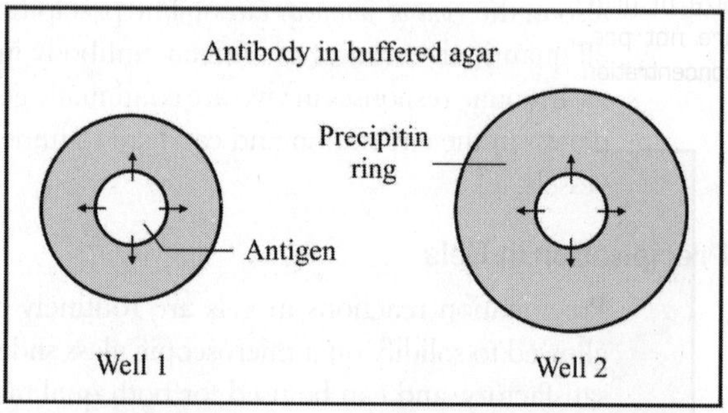

Double Immunodiffusion (Ouchterlony's Technique)

Antibody in buffered agar

Precipitin ring

Antigen

Well 1   Well 2

Fig. A.17   Single radial immunodiffusion (SRID). Antigen in well 2 diffuses further from the well than antigen in well 1 as concentration of antigen in well 2 is higher than in well 1.

Buffered agar is allowed to solidify on a glass slide. Wells are then cut in the agar at a suitable distance from each other according to the pattern diagrammed in Fig. A.19. Antigen and antibody solutions are placed in wells and the plate is incubated in a moist chamber. Both the reactants diffuse radially into the agar (double immunodiffusion) to form a visible precipitin line at equivalence. Three major patterns are depicted in the figure: *reactions of identity, partial identity*, and *non-identity*. The technique

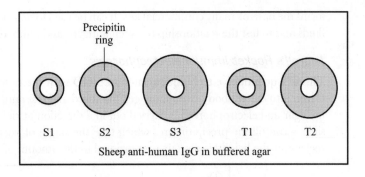

(a)

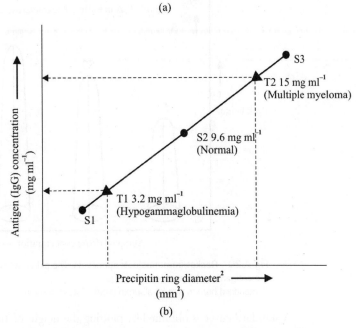

Fig. A.18 Measurement of IgG concentration in serum by SRID. (a) Standard (S) concentrations of IgG and test (T) serum samples from two patients are subjected to SRID. Diameter of the precipitin rings are measured when they become stable. (b) A calibration graph is constructed to determine IgG levels in test samples. The precipitin ring diameter squared (at equivalence) is a function of antigen concentration. The sample T2 is from a myeloma patient while the level of IgG in T1 indicates hypogammaglobulinemia. Size of precipitin rings shown here are not precisely related to antigen concentration.

(b)

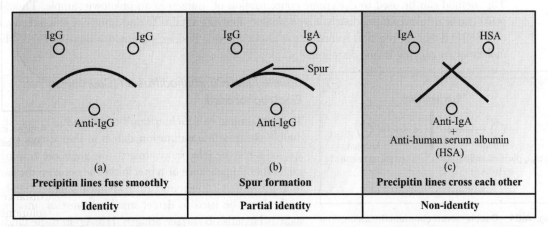

Fig. A.19 Ouchterlony's technique. The figure depicts reactions of (a) identity (b) partial identity and (c) non-identity. It is to be noted that in (b) the spur points to the well containing IgA which lacks some epitopes present in IgG, the isotype against which the antiserum is raised.

forms the basis of many commercial kits. It can be used to detect the presence of antigens in biological fluids and to test the relationship between antigens and antibodies.

Laurell's Rocket Immunoelectrophoresis

This is a quantitative technique related to SRID with the difference that the antigen is electrically driven into the antibody-containing gel. Standard and test antigen samples are placed in wells cut in the agar and electrophoresis is carried out in a direction at right angles to the wells (Fig. A.20). The slide is run till the precipitin arcs which take the shape of rockets become stable. The area of the rockets (or the height) is directly proportional to the amount of antigen in the well.

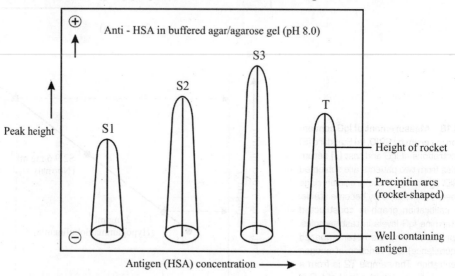

Fig. A.20 Rocket immunoelectrophoresis. The pH of gel is such that the antibody is immobile while the antigen carries a negative charge.
S, standard human serum albumin (HSA); T, test sample

A standard curve is obtained by plotting the height of the rocket against antigen concentration. The method can be used to determine concentration of antigen in an unknown sample. Though peaks can be measured immediately, it is easier after applying a stain. The advantage of this technique over SRID is that the reaction is complete in about 2 hours. Besides, sensitivity is increased as all the molecules are moving in one direction.

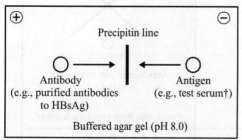

Fig. A.21 Double electroimmunodiffusion. The precipitin line confirms infection with Hepatitis B virus. † Serum of suspected Hepatitis B virus-infected patient

Double Electroimmunodiffusion (Counter-current Electrophoresis)

Though similar to Ouchterlony's technique in principle, double electroimmunodiffusion differs in that a voltage is applied across the gel to move antigens and antibodies towards each other. Appearance of a precipitin line between the two wells shows that antigen and antibody have interacted. The method can be used to detect small amounts of antigens such as Hepatitis B surface antigen (HBsAg) in tissue fluids. This helps in rapid diagnosis of Hepatitis B virus infection (Fig. A.21).

The technique takes advantage of the cathodic migration of the γ-globulins (due to electro-endoosmotic flow) and migration of antigens to the anode.

The advantages of this technique include the following:

- Precipitin bands appear fast (15-20 min) while Ouchterlony's technique (unassisted) may take days to produce a clear result
- Sensitivity is increased as the reactants migrate towards each other rather than diffusing radially

IMMUNOELECTROPHORESIS

This technique is used for qualitative analysis of complex antigens (proteins) in biological fluids. It is a combination of electrophoretic separation of antigens on basis of charge and immunodiffusion against an antiserum (Fig. A.22). The two stages include:

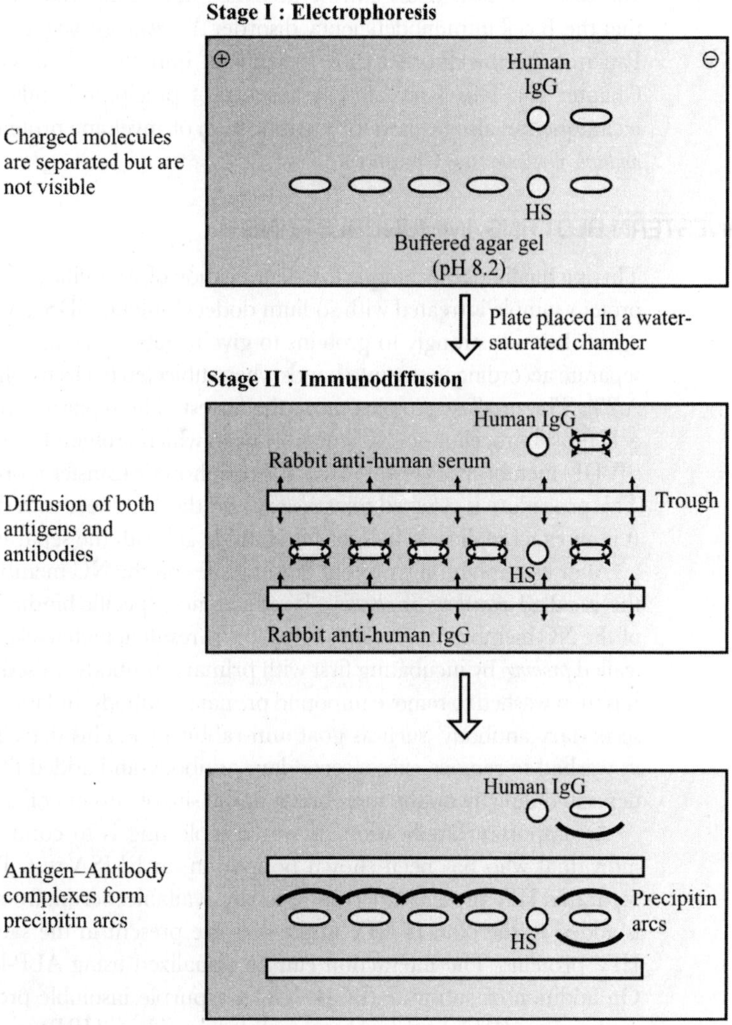

Fig. A.22 Principle of immunoelectrophoresis. The results shown are of a human serum sample. Precipitin arcs can be identified using purified antigens, e.g., pure IgG. For clarity, many precipitin arcs have not been shown.
HS, human serum

Stage I—Electrophoresis

The antigen sample is placed in a small well in the agar gel layer on a glass slide or plate. When an electric current is applied through the gel, antigens separate on the basis of charge and move to different positions in the gel depending on their electrophoretic mobility. The current is stopped at the end of 1–2 hours when the antigens are sufficiently separated.

Stage II—Immunodiffusion

A trough is cut in the agar, parallel to the direction of electrophoresis, and filled with antiserum (rabbit anti-human serum). The slide is placed in a water-saturated chamber for diffusion of antigen and antibody to occur. A precipitin arc forms at equivalence when antibody recognizes its specific protein. Each antigen–antibody complex forms an arc of precipitate which can be stained with a protein stain such as Coomassie Brilliant Blue.

This qualitative technique has major applications in disease diagnosis. Serum samples from normal and diseased individuals can be analyzed and compared. It was through immunoelectrophoresis that the B cell immunodeficiency disorder *X-linked agammaglobulinemia* (*X-LA*) was identified in 1952. Patients with this disorder show absence of immunoglobulins of several isotypes in their serum (see Chapter 16). This is revealed by absence of precipitin bands for IgM, IgA, and IgG isotypes. The technique can also be used for identification of myeloma proteins in serum of patients suffering from *multiple myeloma* (see Chapter 4).

WESTERN BLOTTING/IMMUNOBLOTTING

This is a qualitative technique for identification of a specific protein in a complex protein mixture. The protein sample is treated with sodium dodecyl sulfate (SDS) , an anionic detergent and a dissociating agent. It binds strongly to proteins to give negatively charged linear SDS-protein complexes which separate according to size into bands when subjected to electrophoresis in SDS-polyacrylamide gel (Fig. A.23). The smallest proteins move the fastest. The separated proteins are then transferred from the gel onto a nitrocellulose (NC) membrane to which proteins bind irreversibly. Polyvinylidene difluoride (PVDF) membranes are also used. Electrophoretic transfer is preferred due to its speed and efficiency. This procedure is referred to as *blotting* and the NC sheet with the transferred proteins is called a *blot*. It is an exact replica of the polyacrylamide gel with the separated proteins.

After electroblotting, protein binding sites on the NC membrane are blocked with BSA or casein; this is called *quenching* or *blocking*. It reduces non-specific binding of antibodies to the charged surface of the NC membrane. A failure to do so will result in high background signals. The blot is then probed (called *probing*) by incubating first with primary antibody (raised say in rabbit) specific for the antigen. It is then washed to remove unbound primary antibody and incubated with enzyme (ALP)-conjugated secondary antibody (such as goat anti-rabbit IgG).This detects the primary antibody and binds to it; washed to remove excess secondary antibody and added the substrate. A coloured precipitate is deposited directly on the membrane at the site of protein of interest.

An important application of western blotting is to confirm presence of HIV infection in an individual who has been shown positive in an ELISA test. Pre-blotted NC strips containing the separated HIV proteins are commercially available. Serum from a suspected HIV-infected individual is added to the blot. If HIV antibodies are present in the sample, they will bind to the separated HIV proteins. The interaction can be visualized using ALP-labelled goat anti-human antibodies. On addition of substrate (BCIP-NBT), a purple insoluble product is deposited on the membrane confirming HIV infection. Horse radish peroxidase (HRP)-conjugated secondary antibody, too, can be used with a suitable substrate.

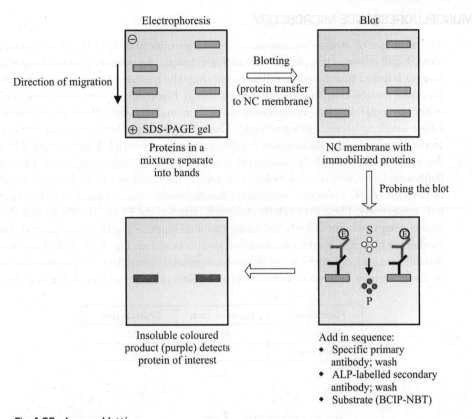

Fig. A.23   Immunoblotting.

IMMUNOPRECIPITATION

An antigen can be isolated from a mixture of proteins using a monoclonal antibody immobilized on sepharose beads by a technique called *immunoprecipitation* (Fig. A.24). The antibody-coated beads are incubated with the antigen mixture allowing the antibody to bind to its specific antigen. Unbound molecules are centrifuged and removed from the complex by washing. The antigen of interest is released from the antibody by a change in pH or ionic strength which lowers the affinity of antigen–antibody binding. Antigens purified by immunoprecipitation can be characterized by SDS–polyacrylamide gel electrophoresis.

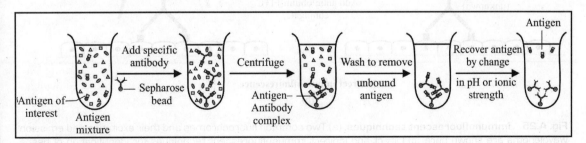

Fig. A.24   Immunoprecipitation.

IMMUNOFLUORESCENCE MICROSCOPY

The technique of *immunofluorescence microscopy* was introduced in 1941 by Albert Coons who used it to identify antibody-secreting plasma cells. In this technique, the primary antibody/universal antiglobulin reagent is linked to a *fluorochrome* (fluorescent dye) which is used as a probe to identify and locate a particular antigen in a tissue, cell, or biological fluid. Fluorochromes are molecules which absorb light at one particular wavelength (excitation wavelength) and emit light (fluoresce) at another specific and longer wavelength (emission wavelength). The site of binding of antibody to antigen in a tissue section can be visualized with a fluorescence microscope equipped with a UV light source. The site is revealed due to the bright glow of the fluorescent antibody against a dark background. The commonly used fluorescent labels *fluorescein* and *rhodamine* are used as their isothiocyanate derivatives, namely, *fluorescein isothiocyanate* (*FITC*; fluoresces green) and *tetramethyl rhodamine isothiocyanate* (*TRITC*; fluoresces orange-red), respectively. These dyes can be covalently linked to the Fc region of a specific antibody (to free amino groups on lysine side chains) taking care that immune reactivity is unaltered. Fluorescein and rhodamine have non-overlapping emission spectra as seen in Fig. A.25 (a) and so can be attached to two different antibodies which can be used simultaneously to detect two proteins within the same cell or tissue. Immunofluorescent techniques can be *direct* or *indirect* as seen in Fig. A.25 (b).

Fluorochrome	Excitation (nm)	Emission (nm)
Fluorescein	495	525
Rhodamine	550	573

(a)

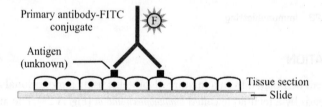

Direct immunofluorescence

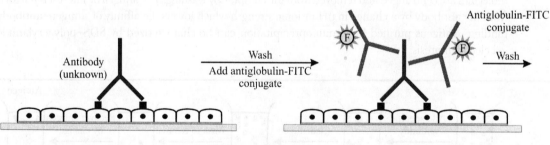

Indirect immunofluorescence

(b)

Fig. A.25 **Immunofluorescent techniques.** (a) Two common fluorochromes and their excitation and emission wavelengths are shown here. (b) Direct and indirect immunofluorescent techniques for identification of tissue antigens or their antibodies. *Cells are visualized for staining with a fluorescence microscope.*

Direct Immunofluorescence

This is a one-step procedure. The antibody-FITC conjugate is directly applied to the tissue section, incubated, and washed. The washing removes antibody that is unbound. The bound antibody is revealed by viewing under a fluorescence microscope; it is seen to fluoresce green in a dark background. The procedure requires a separate antibody-FITC conjugate specific for each antigen. This is a limitation considering the lengthy conjugation process involved. The technique is widely used for examining solid tissue biopsies of skin, kidney, lymphoid tissue, and gut from patients.

Indirect Immunofluorescence

This is a two-step procedure in which an antiglobulin bears the fluorochrome. The initial step involves applying the test sample (suspected to contain antibody specific for a known antigen), as a solution, to the sectioned tissue. In the next step, antiglobulin-FITC conjugate is added which reacts with the primary antibody if it is present in the test sample. Washings are necessary after each incubation.

As several antiglobulin-FITC conjugates bind to each of the primary antibody molecules present in the first layer, fluorescence is brighter than with direct tests and sensitivity is increased. The technique can be used to detect presence of anti-nuclear and anti-thyroglobulin autoantibodies in sera of systemic lupus erythematosus (SLE) and thyroid patients, respectively. Some other applications of immunofluorescence microscopy include identification/detection of

- B and T cells and their subsets in blood;
- transplantation and tumour-specific antigens;
- microorganisms in tissues or culture and, conversely, antibodies specific for pathogens in sera of patients(this has diagnostic importance);
- immune complexes in a pathological sample; and
- complement components in tissues.

FLOW CYTOMETRY—FLUORESCENCE-ACTIVATED CELL SORTER

Identification and counting of immune cells in peripheral blood is often necessary for clinicians and for research also. Traditionally, fluorescence microscopy using fluorescent mAbs to label cells of interest was used for this purpose but this is laborious and time-consuming. With the development of flow cytometry, a very sophisticated alternative is now available and quantitative measurements have been made easy.

A flow cytometer can identify fluorochrome-labelled cells by measuring the fluorescence that they emit and the light that they scatter as they flow though a laser beam. The number of cells of a particular type in a mixed population can also be determined. A *fluorescence-activated cell sorter* (*FACS*), an instrument based on flow cytometry, is shown in its most basic form in Fig. A.26. It can, in addition, select the desired cells from a mixture of cells and sort them into separate containers. The figure depicts the separation of T cells in a mixed population by tagging with monoclonal fluorescein-labelled anti-CD3 (CD3 is a pan T cell marker).

The following steps are involved:

- Cells are introduced into the flow chamber of the machine.
- The cell stream passes through a vibrating nozzle under pressure and breaks into tiny droplets which contain at the most a single cell.
- The machine moves the cells in single file through a laser beam.
- Fluorescent light emitted by a labelled cell is measured by sensitive detectors and the cell is given an electric charge.

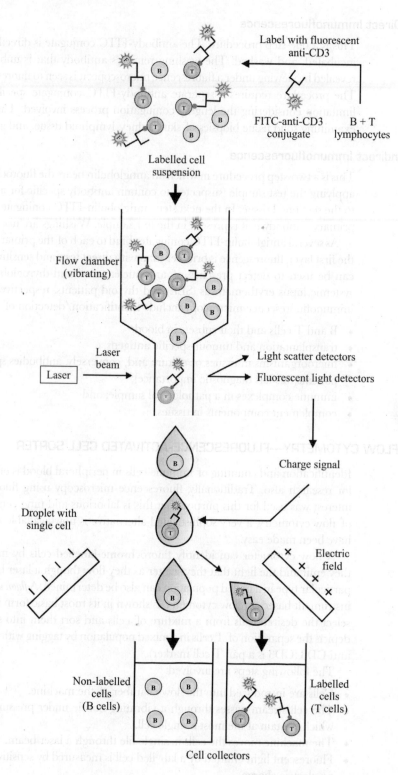

Label with fluorescent anti-CD3

FITC-anti-CD3 conjugate

B + T lymphocytes

Labelled cell suspension

Flow chamber (vibrating)

Laser

Laser beam

Light scatter detectors

Fluorescent light detectors

Charge signal

Droplet with single cell

Electric field

Non-labelled cells (B cells)

Labelled cells (T cells)

Cell collectors

Fig. A.26 Separation of B and T lymphocytes using FACS. The figure shows the separation of T lymphocytes from a mixed (B+T) lymphocyte suspension using anti-CD3. Quantitative analysis can also be done.

♦ Uncharged droplets and those with varying electric charge are separated in an electric field and collected in separate vessels.

Computer analysis of data gives the number of cells expressing the molecule (in this case CD3) to which the fluorescent antibody binds. The FACS machine also measures the way the laser light is scattered when it strikes a cell. This helps to measure each cell for:

♦ Size (forward or low-angle light scatter).

♦ Granularity (side or 90° light scatter).

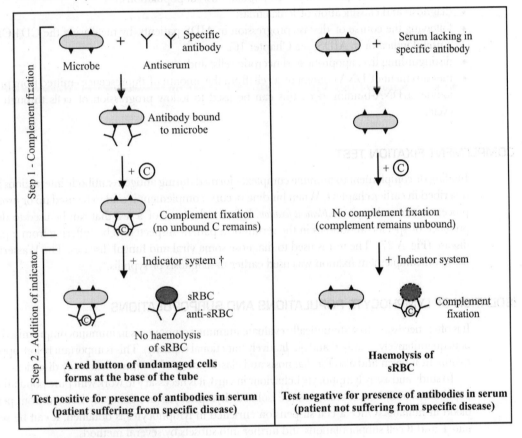

Fig. A.27   Complement fixation test.
† Sheep RBC (sRBC) and anti-sheep RBC

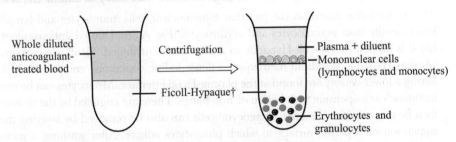

Fig. A.28   Separation of mononuclear cells by density gradient centrifugation. Mononuclear cells can be recovered from the interface of the medium and Ficoll.
† Specific gravity of Ficoll-Hypaque=1.078

Such data helps to distinguish different cell populations. For instance, neutrophils cause more 90° light scatter than lymphocytes due to presence of granules in their cytoplasm.

With modern instruments, it is possible to label cell populations to be analyzed with two, three, or more differently labelled monoclonal antibodies (each specific for a particular marker) in a single test, provided emission spectra of the fluorochromes do not overlap. Some applications of FACS include

- enumeration and separation of cell populations/subpopulations;
- diagnosis and classification of leukaemias;
- following the course of disease progression in AIDS patients (by measuring the CD4:CD8 ratio, a useful indicator in AIDS; see Chapter 16);
- distinguishing live, apoptotic and necrotic cells; and
- measurement of DNA content of a cell (from the amount of fluorescence emitted from propidium iodide, a DNA-binding dye); this can be used to follow progression of cells through the cell-cycle.

COMPLEMENT FIXATION TEST

Binding of complement to immune complexes formed during antigen–antibody interactions has been described in earlier chapters. When binding occurs, complement is said to be used up or *fixed* and the process is referred to as *complement fixation*. It forms the basis of a test that can be used to detect the presence of specific antibodies in the serum of a patient suspected to be suffering from a particular disease (Fig. A.27). The test is used to diagnose some viral and fungal diseases. The Wasserman test based on complement fixation was used earlier in diagnosis of syphilis.

ISOLATION OF LYMPHOCYTE POPULATIONS AND SUBPOPULATIONS

It is often necessary to systematically evaluate immune components in immunocompromised patients both quantitatively (number) and qualitatively (functional capacity). This is important before appropriate treatment is given and also for diagnosis and classification of immunodeficiency disorders.

To study and assay lymphocyte behaviour in vitro, it is necessary to work with pure populations/sub-populations and, hence, cells must be isolated. Lymphocytes are generally isolated from peripheral blood in humans. Once a cell suspension enriched in lymphocytes is obtained, it can be separated into T and B cell subpopulations and further into subsets by several methods.

Separation of Mononuclear Cells from Peripheral Blood—Density Gradient Centrifugation

The separation is based on the fact that mononuclear cells (monocytes and lymphocytes) have a lower density than granulocytes and erythrocytes (Fig. A.28). Diluted anticoagulant treated whole blood is layered over Ficoll-Hypaque in a tube and centrifuged. Ficoll is a carbohydrate polymer whereas Hypaque is sodium metrizoate, a dense iodine containing compound. Mononuclear cells having a lower density are found at the plasma-Ficoll interface. Monocytes can be removed from the mononuclear suspension by addition of iron filings. These are engulfed by the monocytes which can then be drawn with a magnet. Phagocytic cells can also be removed by layering the mononuclear suspension on a plastic surface to which phagocytes adhere. After washing, a monocyte-depleted lymphocyte population is obtained.

Separation of T and B Lymphocytes

Expression of characteristic surface molecules on T and B cells permits the two subpopulations to be separated from each other using antibodies specific for surface markers. Separation by FACS has already been described earlier Some other commonly used procedures (bulk techniques) for separation are outlined here.

Panning The lymphocyte suspension is applied to an antibody-sensitized polystyrene plate (a plate to which antibody is non-covalently bound). T cells bind to anti-CD3 antibodies through their membrane CD3. B cells do not adhere and can be separated by carefully washing the plate. It is possible to recover adherent cells by changing culture conditions such as pH and ionic strength (Fig. A.29). Panning can also be used to separate TH and TC cell subpopulations using anti-CD4 and anti-CD8 antibodies, respectively.

Immunomagnetic separation The method is simple and can handle a large number of cells. Magnetic beads coated with anti-CD3 monoclonal antibody can be used to positively select T cells (Fig. A.30).

The above bulk separation techniques are fast and purified populations can be obtained. Once T and B cell subpopulations have been isolated, they can be analyzed quantitatively and also for functional competence. Various in vitro assays are available for functional assessment of lymphocytes. One such assay called the *chromium (^{51}Cr) release assay* tests effector function of cytotoxic T lymphocytes (CTLs).

EXPERIMENTAL ANIMAL MODELS

Studies on various aspects of the immune system require a suitable animal model and mice generally are preferred by researchers. Some animal models useful for immunological research—the inbred mouse strain, and transgenic and knockout mice—are described here.

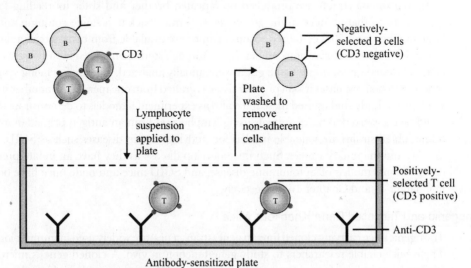

Antibody-sensitized plate

Fig. A.29 Panning for isolation of lymphocyte subpopulations. The procedure shown here can be modified for non-immobilized (negatively-selected) T cells. For this, the microtitre plate requires sensitization with anti-IgM antibodies.

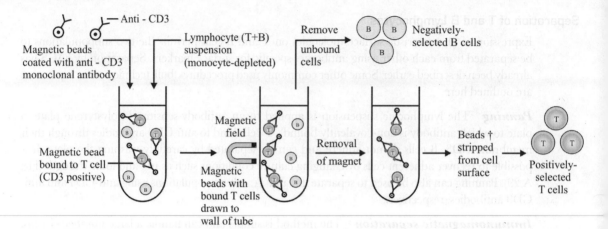

Fig. A.30 Separation of T and B lymphocytes using immunomagnetic beads.
† By sudden reapplication of high magnetic field or slight warming

Inbred Mouse Strain

A major drawback of conducting studies on mice from the outbred population is that variables are introduced due to genetic differences and, hence, results obtained by different groups cannot be compared. In contrast, inbred strains of mice are essentially *syngeneic*, that is, genetically identical. As this reduces variables, they are preferred as experimental models. Other reasons which make inbred strains of mice a popular model system include

- easy handling,
- rapid breeding, and
- easy maintenance in the laboratory environment.

Inbred mouse strains are produced by repeated brother and sister inbreeding for at least 20 generations so that all mice in the last generation trace back to a single common ancestor. A very large number (over 500) of inbred strains of mice are available from commercial animal dealers or research laboratories for various studies. It was through studies on inbred mouse strains that rejection of transplanted tumours and tissue grafts were initially analyzed. These mice being syngeneic do not mount rejection responses if skin or other tissue is grafted from one member to another member of the same strain. Early studies used these mice also as experimental models to demonstrate that immunity could be transferred to naïve animals using lymphocytes from an antigen-primed (immune) animal. Some inbred strains are valuable models for studying certain diseases such as SCID, autoimmune disease, and mammary cancer. Such mice develop disease as they have an innate predisposition to do so. Animal models of autoimmune disease, and SCID mice and nude mice have been described in Chapter 15 and Chapter 16, respectively.

Transgenic and Targeted Gene Knockout Mice

Transgenic mice carrying cloned foreign genes (transgenes) are widely used in immunological research. These mice enable researchers to study gene function in vivo. A cloned gene is microinjected into fertilized eggs isolated from a pregnant female mouse. The eggs are implanted into the uterus of foster mice and the offsprings are screened for expression of the transgene. The success rate is somewhat low with the transgene being incorporated into chromosomal DNA of about 10–30 per cent of the offspring. These animals are then bred to generate the transgenic strain (Fig. A.31).

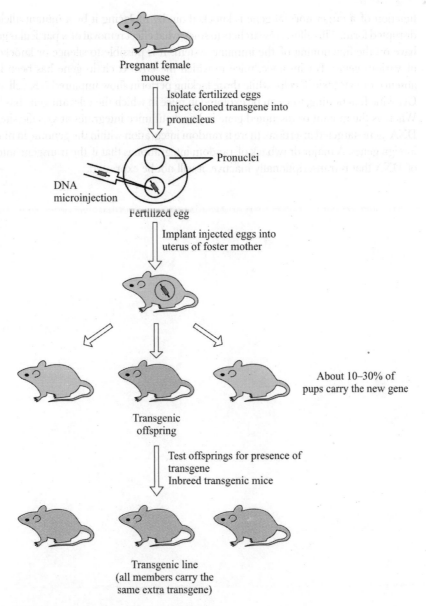

Pregnant female mouse

Isolate fertilized eggs
Inject cloned transgene into
pronucleus

Pronuclei

DNA
microinjection

Fertilized egg

Implant injected eggs into
uterus of foster mother

About 10–30% of
pups carry the new gene

Transgenic
offspring

Test offsprings for presence of
transgene
Inbreed transgenic mice

Transgenic line
(all members carry the
same extra transgene)

Fig. A.31 Production of transgenic mice.

The expression of the transgene can be confined to a particular tissue if it is constructed with a particular tissue-specific promoter. For instance, a transgene linked to the insulin promoter would be expressed in the pancreas while one linked to the thyroglobulin promoter would be expressed in the thyroid. Availability of transgenic lines has greatly facilitated immunological research. Transgenic mice have provided valuable information regarding functional role of cytokines, various cell surface molecules such as T cell receptor and class I and class II MHC molecules, and signalling molecules.

Often, it is necessary for immunologists to understand what effect removal of a particular gene product would have on the immune system. This is possible with the use of *knockout mice* in which the function of a target normal gene is knocked out by replacing it by a mutant allele or the gene in a disrupted form. This allows researchers to study what effect removal of a particular gene product would have on the functioning of the immune system. It is possible to silence or knockout the expression of various genes. For instance, mice in which the CD8 α chain gene has been knocked out show absence of cytotoxic T cells, while those lacking perforin show impaired NK cell and CTL function. Cytokine functioning, too, can be explored in mice in which the relevant gene has been knocked out. Whereas the mutant or disrupted gene in knockout mice integrates at specific sites in chromosomal DNA (gene-targeted insertion), there is random integration within the genome in mice carrying cloned foreign genes. A major drawback of random integration is that if the transgene integrates in a region of DNA that is transcriptionally inactive, it will not be expressed.

Cumulative Glossary

Acquired immune deficiency Immunodeficiency of the immune system that is acquired after birth and is not due to genetic defects. Some causes include cytotoxic therapy, malnutrition, and infections.

Acquired immunodeficiency syndrome An immunodeficiency disorder caused by infection of $CD4^+$ T helper cells with human immunodeficiency virus (HIV). There is $CD4^+$ T cell depletion leading to defects in cell-mediated immunity (CMI) and other aspects of immune functioning.

Acute-phase proteins Proteins whose concentration increases in serum during infection and inflammation and which are involved in the early phase of innate immune response to infection, for example, C-reactive protein (CRP) and mannose-binding lectin (MBL).

Adaptive immunity Immunity mediated by lymphocytes following exposure to antigen. Its key features include specificity and memory.

Adjuvant A substance which non-specifically enhances immune responses to an antigen when injected along with that antigen.

Affinity A measure of the binding strength between a single antigen-binding site of an antibody and an antigenic determinant.

Affinity chromatography Purification of a substance based on its affinity for another substance that has been immobilized on a solid support.

Affinity maturation The events that lead to increase in affinity of antibodies for a specific protein antigen during the course of a humoral immune response. It is due to somatic hypermutation in Ig V region genes and selection of B cells bearing high-affinity receptors for the antigen. The process of affinity maturation improves during a secondary immune response, and with further booster injections.

Agglutination The clumping of particulate antigens by antibodies.

Allele One form (variant) of a polymorphic gene present at a particular genetic locus.

Allergen An antigen (e.g., pollen, dust) that produces an allergic type I hypersensitivity reaction in atopic individuals by inducing synthesis of IgE and mast cell/basophil activation.

Allergy An immediate hypersensitivity type I reaction in atopic individuals triggered by allergen which induces synthesis of IgE and mast cell/basophil activation.

Alloantigens Antigens expressed in cells and tissues which differ in genetically non-identical members of a species. Alloantigens in a graft when seen as foreign stimulate a graft rejection response.

Allogeneic graft An organ or a tissue graft from a donor to a recipient of the same species who is genetically dissimilar.

Allotypes The protein product of an allele that is seen as foreign by a different member of the same species. The term with reference to antibodies refers to antigenic determinants (allotopes) in C domains of antibodies of the same class present in some individuals but not in others.

Alternative complement pathway A pathway of complement activation that is triggered by microbial surfaces and not by antibodies. It is initiated by C3 activation and C3b deposition on the microbial surface.

Anaphylactic shock An allergic reaction that causes cardiovascular collapse and suffocation. It is due to binding of an antigen to IgE on mast cells throughout the body.

Anaphylatoxins Small fragments (C5a, C3a, and C4a) formed by cleavage of complement proteins when they undergo activation. They bind to receptors on mast cells/basophils and stimulate them to release histamine and other mediators which promote inflammation. They also promote chemotaxis of defensive cells from blood vessels to infected sites.

Antibody A glycoprotein molecule (also called immunoglobulin) secreted by B lymphocytes that binds with high specificity to an antigen that induced its production. Membrane-bound antibodies on the B cell surface serve as receptor for antigens.

Antibody-dependent cell-mediated cytotoxicity (ADCC) A cytotoxic mechanism for inducing target cell killing. It is triggered when an antibody coating a target cell binds to Fc receptor-bearing killer cells, such as NK cells, eosinophils, and macrophages.

Antibody repertoire The entire collection of antibody molecules of varying specificities expressed in an individual.

Antigen A molecule (generally foreign) that binds specifically to a secreted antibody or lymphocyte receptors (BCR/TCR). While B cells recognize antigens in their native state, TCR on T cells recognizes only short peptide fragments derived from native proteins, and which are bound to MHC molecules.

Antigen-binding site The site on an antibody molecule which physically contacts an antigenic determinant (epitope). It is made up of six hypervariable domains or complimentarity determining regions (CDRs), three from V_L and three from V_H.

Antigen presentation This is the display of peptide fragments (derived from proteolysis of antigen by one of two different pathways) associated with MHC molecules on the surface of an antigen-presenting cell (APC), or other cells such as altered cells. Recognition of specific peptide-MHC complexes by TCR activates the T cell.

Antigen-presenting cells These are specialized cells including B cells, dendritic cells, and macrophages. They process protein antigens and present small peptide fragments on the cell surface associated with MHC molecules to antigen-specific T cells. Besides, they express costimulatory B7 molecules and are also known as professional antigen-presenting cells .

Antigen processing Degradation of protein antigens (extracellular or cytosolic) into peptides that bind to the peptide-binding groove of MHC molecules for display to T cells.

Antigenic determinant *See* Epitope

Antiserum Serum from an immunized individual that contains antibodies specific for the antigen used for immunization.

Antitoxin An antibody that neutralizes the exotoxins produced by some microbes, such as those that cause tetanus and diphtheria.

Apoptosis *See* Programmed cell death

Atopy This refers to the genetic predisposition of some individuals to mount IgE-mediated type I or immediate hypersensitivity reactions against various environmental antigens (allergens), such as dust and pollen.

Autoantibody An antibody specific for a self-antigen which may injure cells and tissues.

Autocrine This refers to the ability of a cytokine to act on the same cell that produced it.

Autograft A graft from one area to another on the same individual such as a skin graft in burn victims.

Autoimmunity An adaptive immune response mounted against self-components due to failure in self-tolerance mechanisms. When such immune responses cause damage to cells and tissues, it leads to autoimmune disease.

Autoreactivity This describes immune responses directed at self-antigens.

Avidity The overall strength of binding between a bivalent/multivalent antibody with a multideterminant antigen. Avidity of IgM (pentameric) for a multideterminant antigen far exceeds the avidity of IgG (dimeric) for the same antigen.

Basophils A circulating polymorphonuclear leukocyte with granules that stain with basic dyes and which resemble mast cells in tissues.

B cells The central cells of humoral immunity that arise and develop in the bone marrow. The antigen receptor on their surface is membrane-bound Ig. On stimulation by antigens, they differentiate into antibody-secreting plasma cells.

B cell receptor (BCR) This is the receptor for antigen expressed on the B cell surface. It is composed of a transmembrane Ig molecule (which binds to antigens) and invariant Ig-α and Ig-β proteins (which are signalling molecules).

β_2 microglobulin A protein that is part of the structure of class I MHC molecules but which, unlike MHC molecules, is not encoded within the MHC.

Bone marrow The site in adult humans where all cellular elements of blood are generated including erythrocytes, platelets, polymorphonuclear leukocytes, and immature lymphocytes. It is also the site of B cell maturation in mammals.

Bone marrow transplantation A clinical procedure which restores all cellular elements of blood including lymphocytes and is used to treat immunodeficiency, such as SCID, and malignant conditions such as leukaemia besides others.

Bradykinin A vasoactive peptide produced by the kinin system, an enzyme system in the plasma triggered when tissues are damaged and which mediates inflammation.

Bronchus-associated lymphoid tissue (BALT) The secondary lymphoid tissue located in the respiratory tract which is the site of induction of immune responses to inhaled antigens.

Burkitt's lymphoma A malignant tumour affecting B cells and which is caused by the Epstein–Barr virus (EBV).

Bursa of Fabricius A primary lymphoid organ in birds and the site of B cell development.

Carcinoembryonic antigen (CEA) A membrane glycoprotein expressed during foetal life in many tissues but not in adults. Its expression is increased in cancer of colon, pancreas, and breast resulting in elevated levels of CEA in serum.

Cell adhesion molecules Cell surface molecules (e.g., selectins and integrins) that mediate binding to other cells or to the extracellular matrix. They play a major role in migration of leukocytes from the bloodstream, and cellular activation in both innate and adaptive immunity.

Cell-mediated cytotoxicity This refers to lysis of a target cell by effector cytotoxic T lymphocytes (CTLs), and NK cells. It defends against intracellular pathogens such as viruses and some bacteria. Tumour cells are also targeted by cytotoxic cells. Myeloid cells can also mediate destruction of their targets but in a different way.

Cell-mediated immunity A type of adaptive immunity mediated by CD4$^+$ TH1 lymphocytes which defends against intracellular microbes within phagocytic- or non-phagocytic cells. It also includes the immunity mediated by CD8$^+$ cytotoxic T cells against virally-infected cells.

Central lymphoid organs These include the bone marrow and thymus and are the sites where lymphocytes undergo development and acquire antigen-specific receptors. Development of B lymphocytes in mammals occurs in the bone marrow while T lymphocyte development takes place in the thymus.

Central tolerance This refers to self-tolerance induced in lymphocytes in central lymphoid organs—in bone marrow for B cells and in thymus for T cells. It is a consequence of immature self-reactive lymphocytes recognizing self-antigens leading to death by apoptosis (clonal deletion), or functional inactivation (clonal anergy).

Chemokines These are low molecular weight chemoattractant cytokines that stimulate migration and activation of cells, especially phagocytic cells and lymphocytes. They play important roles in inflammation and influence cell compartmentalization within lymphoid tissues.

Chemotaxis This is the migration of leukocytes up a concentration gradient of chemotactic molecules which guide movement of defensive cells into tissues to sites of infection.

Class I MHC molecules These are one of two types of heterodimeric surface glycoproteins and are expressed on almost all nucleated cells. They display peptide fragments generally derived from intracellular protein antigens on the cell surface for T cell recognition.

Class II-associated invariant chain peptide (CLIP) It is a peptide formed when the invariant chain is cleaved by proteases during processing of an antigen by the exogenous pathway. It remains bound to the peptide-binding cleft of class II MHC molecules and when removed by HLA-DM, allows antigen-derived peptides to bind to the cleft.

Classical pathway of complement activation The pathway of complement activation involving complement components C1, C4, C2, and C3. It is initiated by binding of antigen–antibody complex to C1 component of the complement cascade.

Clonal anergy This is the failure of a self-reactive T or B lymphocyte to mount an immune response on stimulation by self-antigen in the periphery due to absence of the costimulatory second signal. It is one of the mechanisms that maintains immunologic tolerance to self. Lack of a DTH response to common antigens such as *Candida* antigens is a sign of T cell dysfunction, also referred to as anergy. It is to be distinguished from clonal anergy.

Clonal deletion The process by which lymphocytes during early stages of differentiation undergo cell death by apoptosis on contact with self-antigen.

Clonal selection The selection of a specific lymphocyte by antigen (pathogen). It is followed by proliferation of the selected lymphocyte to form an expanded clone. Lymphocytes in the expanded clone bear receptors of identical specificity. They effectively fight the pathogen which initiated the immune response.

Clone An identical cell population derived from a single progenitor cell.

Cluster of differentiation (CD) A set of monoclonal antibodies that identify a particular cell surface molecule. The surface molecule is designated CD and is assigned a number, for example, CD1, CD2, and so on.

Colony stimulating factors (CSFs) Cytokines that stimulate proliferation and differentiation of progenitor cells in the bone marrow to various cell types in blood including red blood cells, platelets, granulocytes, monocytes, and lymphocytes.

Combinatorial diversity Mechanism for generating a large number of diverse antigen receptors from a limited number of gene segments. First, gene segments join in different ways to generate diverse receptor chains (heavy and light chains for immunoglobulins; α and β or γ and δ chains for T cell receptors). Two different chains of the receptor then combine to make the complete receptor capable of recognizing antigen.

Complement A set of serum proteins that are activated by three different pathways—classical pathway, alternative pathway, and the lectin pathway. These proteins interact with each other in an enzymatic cascade to produce various effector molecules.

Complimentarity-determining regions (CDRs) *See* Hypervariable regions.

Complement receptors (CRs) Receptors on various cells that recognize and bind complement proteins, e.g., CR1 on red blood cells that binds to complement component C3b.

Co-receptor A lymphocyte cell surface protein that binds to antigen at the same time that the antigen is bound by antigen receptor (membrane-bound Ig or TCR) and which delivers the signals for activation. The T cell co-receptors CD4 and CD8 bind to non-polymorphic regions of MHC molecules at the same time that the TCR recognizes a specific peptide-MHC complex.

Corticosteroids A group of drugs related to steroid hormones of the adrenal cortex. Corticosteroids are potent anti-inflammatory and immunosuppressive agents. They induce apoptosis in developing lymphocytes.

Costimulatory molecules Molecules present on the surface of specialized antigen-presenting cells which provide second signals needed to fully activate a naïve T cell. They include B7-1 and B7-2 molecules which on binding to the T cell surface molecule CD28 transduce activating signals to the T cell. The costimulatory CD40 molecule on B cells and macrophages interacts with CD40 L on activated Tн cells delivering similar activating signals to B cells and macrophages.

CTLA-4 A cell surface molecule on activated T cells which binds to B7 costimulatory molecules on antigen-presenting cells delivering inhibitory signals which are important for homeostasis.

Cyclophosphamide A DNA alkylating agent that is cytotoxic and is used as an immunosuppressive drug. It acts by killing rapidly dividing cells, including proliferating lymphocytes.

Cyclosporin A widely used immunosuppressive drug which acts by blocking transcription of T cell cytokine genes, for example, IL-2, thereby inhibiting T cell activation and effector function.

Cytokines Secreted proteins of low molecular weight that promote or inhibit differentiation, proliferation, and functioning of various cells of the immune system. They are produced by macrophages and NK cells during innate immune responses and largely by T lymphocytes in adaptive immunity.

Cytotoxic T lymphocyte (CTL) A type of T cell expressing CD8 and which recognizes microbial peptides displayed by class I MHC molecules. When activated to effector cells, it induces apoptosis in target cells infected with intracellular microbes such as viruses.

Defensins A group of cysteine-rich antimicrobial basic proteins present in neutrophil granules and also in skin.

Delayed-type hypersensitivity (DTH) A type IV hypersensitivity reaction which occurs within 48–72 hours and is mediated by cytokines released by CD4$^+$ TH1 cells. Macrophage activation and inflammation cause damage to tissues.

Dendritic cells These are cells found in tissues and are so called because of their long dendrite-like processes. They are very efficient at capturing antigens after which they migrate to lymph nodes where they function as APCs for naïve T lymphocytes.

Desensitization A treatment which aims to inhibit allergic reactions in individuals and involves exposing the individual to increasing doses of allergen.

Diapedesis A process by which blood cells mainly leukocytes move out from the blood vessels into tissues to sites of infection.

Diversity This refers to the structural variations in the antigen-binding site of lymphocyte receptors for antigen, namely BCR and TCR, which allows the immune system to respond to diverse antigens entering the body.

Diversity (D) gene segments These are short DNA sequences found between the V and J gene segments in immunoglobulin heavy chain genes, and T cell receptor β and δ chain genes. D gene segments together with J gene segments are somatically recombined with V segments during lymphocyte development. The recombined V-D-J DNA codes for the V region of the antigen receptor.

DNA vaccination A vaccination approach in which bacterial plasmids containing cDNA encoding a protein antigen (from an infectious microbe) is injected intramuscularly. The DNA is expressed and the encoded protein initiates both CTL-mediated and antibody responses.

Double-negative thymocytes Immature T cells (thymocytes) in the thymus that lack expression of T cell co-receptors CD4 and CD8 (and also CD3 and TCR). This stage progresses to an intermediate double-positive (DP) stage in which both CD4 and CD8 co-receptors (and also CD3 and TCR) are expressed on thymocytes.

Double-positive thymocytes Cells (thymocytes) in an intermediate stage of T cell development in the thymus expressing both CD4 and CD8 co-receptor proteins, CD3 and also the TCR. After undergoing selection processes, surviving cells mature into single-positive mature T cells expressing either CD4 or CD8.

Endogenous pyrogen Substances produced in the body, such as some cytokines that can elevate body temperature. These are distinct from endotoxin, a bacterial toxin from Gram-negative bacteria.

Endosome Intracellular membrane-bound vesicles containing endocytosed material. Here, protein antigens are partially degraded by proteolytic enzymes to generate peptides, some of which can bind to class II MHC molecules, a necessary step before antigen presentation by the class II MHC pathway.

Endotoxin This is a bacterial toxin released only when there is damage to a bacterial cell, unlike bacterial exotoxins which are secreted. Lipopolysaccharide (LPS) is a potent endotoxin from Gram-negative bacteria that induces fever by triggering synthesis of cytokines (endogenous pyrogens).

Enzyme-linked immunosorbent assay An important assay for detection and quantitation of an antigen or antibody.

A linked enzyme (e.g., to antiglobulin or second antibody) is used to detect a bound antibody or antigen. The enzyme converts a colourless substrate into a coloured product which can be measured spectrophotometrically.

Eosinophils A type of granulocyte that defends against extracellular parasite infections, such as helminths, besides having an important role in allergic responses (atopy). They have cell surface receptors for IgE. Their number shows a marked increase in blood (eosinophilia) both in parasitic infections and atopy.

Epitope A small part of an antigen that is recognized and bound by an antibody or an antigen receptor. A T cell epitope is a short linear sequence, derived from a protein antigen, bound to an MHC molecule. B cell epitopes are generally discontinuous sequences brought together due to folding of the protein.

Epstein–Barr virus A double-stranded DNA virus belonging to the herpes virus family. It specifically infects B cells by binding to complement receptor 2 (CR2) and is the cause of Burkitt's lymphoma.

Exocytosis Release of contents of intracellular vesicles to the exterior on fusion of vesicles with the plasma membrane.

Exotoxin Toxins secreted by bacteria.

Extravasation Movement of cellular components and fluid from inside the blood vessels into tissues.

Fab An antibody fragment with one antigen-binding site formed when an antibody is digested with the enzyme papain. Papain digestion yields two Fab fragments each consisting of an intact light chain and the N-terminal V_H and C_{H1} domains of the heavy chain.

F(ab')$_2$ An antibody fragment with two antigen-binding sites formed when an antibody molecule is cleaved by the enzyme pepsin.

Fas ligand (Fas L) A cell surface protein expressed on activated T cells. Binding of Fas L to Fas , a monomeric protein, initiates a signalling cascade leading to apoptotic death of the Fas-bearing cell.

Fc A crystallizable fragment obtained when an immunoglobulin molecule is digested with papain. It consists of the disulphide-linked carboxyl-terminal parts of the two heavy chains which can bind to Fc receptors on many immune cells, and to C1q component of the complement protein C1.

FcR Receptors on the surface of many cell types which bind to the Fc region of particular immunoglobulin isotypes, for example, Fcγ and Fcε receptors specific for IgG and IgE isotypes, respectively.

FcεRI A receptor expressed on mast cells and basophils that binds with high affinity to the C-terminal constant region of IgE. When antigen binds IgE bound to mast cells/basophils, there is cross-linking of FcεRI which activates the mast cell.

FcγR Specific receptors on the cell surface that bind to the Fc region of IgG molecules. Many different types of Fcγ receptors are known.

Fibroblast A cell of the connective tissue that plays an important role in wound healing by producing collagen.

Fluorescein isothiocyanate (FITC) A dye which emits a green fluorescence and which is used to label antibodies (or other proteins) for use in immunofluorescence.

Follicular dendritic cells Dendritic cells having long branching processes and which are found in lymphoid follicles. They lack class II MHC molecules and carry Fc receptors which bind to immune complexes without undergoing receptor-mediated endocytosis.

Framework regions Segments of antibody V regions that lie between the hypervariable regions.

Freund's complete adjuvant (FCA) An emulsion of aqueous immunogen in oil and containing killed *M. tuberculosis*. It serves to enhance immune responses to the immunogen when injected along with it. Freund's incomplete adjuvant lacks mycobacteria.

Frustrated phagocytosis This refers to events that occur when phagocytes fail in their attempt to phagocytose immune complexes/antigenic particles. Phagocyte granule contents are discharged outside leading to tissue damage.

Germinal centres Secondary lymphoid structures in lymph nodes and spleen which form around follicular dendritic cells after B cells, on receiving activation signals from T helper cells, have migrated into lymphoid follicles. Here, B cells undergo proliferation, selection, and affinity maturation.

Germline The arrangement of the genetic material in germ cells that is passed down to offspring before being altered by somatic recombination or other mechanisms.

Glomerulonephritis Inflammation of renal glomeruli due to deposition of immune complexes or due to binding of antibodies to glomerular antigens. Activation of complement and phagocytes cause injury and lead to renal failure.

Graft An organ (or tissue) that is removed from one site in a particular individual and placed at another site usually in a different individual.

Graft rejection This refers to destruction of the grafted tissue due to an immune response mounted by the host against the graft.

Graft-versus-host disease (GVHD) The reaction mounted by allogeneic donor lymphocytes against tissues of an immunocompromised host.

Granulocytes Cells of the myeloid lineage containing cytoplasmic granules and which include neutrophils, eosinophils, and basophils.

Granuloma A nodule formed in tissues due to chronic inflammation triggered by persistent infection, such as by mycobacteria or due to continued presence of antigen. It is a form of a delayed-type hypersensitivity reaction. Cells inside a granuloma are mostly fused macrophages surrounded by T lymphocytes.

Granzymes Enzymes found in granules in cytotoxic T lymphocytes (CTLs) and natural killer (NK) cells. They enter target cells through perforin channels and trigger apoptosis.

Gut-associated lymphoid tissue (GALT) The lymphoid tissue associated with the gastrointestinal mucosa and submucosa.

H-2 The major histocompatibility complex (MHC) of mouse.

Haematopoiesis The generation of all mature blood cells including red blood cells, leukocytes, and platelets from pluripotent stem cells (haematopoietic stem cells) in bone marrow and foetal liver. The process is regulated by various haematopoietic cytokines/growth factors produced by bone marrow stromal cells and other cell types.

Haematopoietic stem cell A pluripotent stem cell in the bone marrow that is capable of self-renewal, that is, it divides continuously to generate additional stem cells. It gives rise to all formed elements of blood belonging to the myeloid, lymphoid, and erythrocyte lineage.

Haplotype The set of MHC alleles or other genetic determinants inherited from any one parent and located on a single chromosome.

Hapten A small molecule that can bind to an antibody but must be conjugated to an immunogenic carrier protein in order to stimulate an anti-hapten immune response.

HAT A selective cell culture medium (hypoxanthine-aminopterin-thymidine) used when generating hybridomas for production of monoclonal antibodies.

T helper lymphocytes A subclass of T cells most of which express the CD4 molecule. When activated to effector cells, they stimulate macrophages (CMI), and help B cells to make antibody (humoral immunity) against thymus-dependent antigens. They also help in differentiation of cytotoxic T cells.

Heterodimer A molecule such as a protein which is composed of two peptide chains that are non-identical, for example, class I and class II MHC molecules, and the $\alpha\beta$ and $\gamma\delta$ TCR.

Heterozygous Possessing two different alleles for a particular gene on the two homologous chromosomes.

High endothelial venule (HEV) Highly specialized venules found in lymphoid tissues. They are lined with endothelial cells that allow migration of naïve T lymphocytes from blood vessels into lymphoid organs.

Hinge region The region of the immunoglobulin heavy chain between the Fab portion and the Fc tails. It allows flexibility in the molecule and permits the two Fab portions to adopt a wide range of angles and combine with epitopes spaced apart from each other.

Histamine A major vasoactive amine released on degranulation of basophils and mast cells. It causes dilation of local blood vessels and smooth muscle contraction.

HLA-DM A class II MHC-like protein that is non-polymorphic and which participates in the class II MHC pathway of antigen presentation by facilitating removal of CLIP. This allows binding of other antigenic peptides to the cleft of class II MHC molecules.

Homing receptor Adhesion molecules expressed on the surface of leukocytes that direct their movement to specific tissues (homing).

Homodimer A molecule such as a protein having two identical peptide chains.

Homozygous Possessing the same allele for a particular gene on the two homologous chromosomes.

Human immunodeficiency virus (HIV) A retrovirus that causes AIDS. Of the two variants HIV-1 and HIV-2, HIV-1 is more global and causes disease worldwide.

Humanized antibody Non-human monoclonal antibodies (e.g., murine) which are genetically engineered so that all sequences except the antigen-binding CDR sequences are replaced with sequences of a human antibody. They are less likely to induce an immune response and can be used for therapeutic purposes, such as in treatment of tumours.

Humoral immunity The branch of adaptive immunity that is mediated by antibodies (and complement proteins) produced by B lymphocytes. It provides defence against extracellular microbes and their toxins.

Hybridoma A hybrid cell line formed by fusion of a specific antibody producing B cell with a myeloma cell (lymphoid tumour cell). The hybridoma has the immortality of the tumour cell and the ability to secrete antibody, a property of the B cell. Monoclonal antibodies are commonly produced from hybridomas.

Hyperacute rejection Immediate rejection of an allograft or xenograft due to preformed antibodies against foreign antigens on the graft. Binding of antibodies to the graft endothelium triggers activation of the complement and the clotting cascade, resulting in destruction of the organ.

Hypersensitivity Excessive or uncontrolled immune reactivity to antigens that causes tissue or organ damage. The injury is due to the same effector mechanisms that the immune system uses to provide defence against microbes.

Hypervariable regions Short amino acid sequences about 10 amino acids in length within the variable regions of the immunoglobulin and T cell receptor which show the greatest variability in amino acid sequence between different antigen receptors. They form loop structures and contribute to the antigen-binding site. There are three hypervariable loops (also known as complimentarity determining regions or CDRs) present in each antibody heavy chain and light chain, and in each TCR chain.

Idiotope An antigenic determinant in the variable region of an antibody.

Idiotype The collection of idiotopes expressed by an antibody molecule is called its idiotype.

Immediate hypersensitivity Hypersensitivity that occurs within minutes of exposure to antigen. It is mediated by antibody (IgE) and is also known as type I hypersensitivity.

Immune complex The complex formed when antibody reacts with an antigen and which may also contain C3b, a breakdown product of the complement protein C3.

Immunity The ability of the body to resist infection.

Immunoblotting A technique which makes use of antibodies for identifying and characterizing proteins.

Immunodeficiency Absence or functional defect in some component(s) or aspect(s) of the immune system and which leads to immunodeficiency disease.

Immunodiffusion Identification of antigen or antibody by the formation of antigen-antibody precipitate in agar gel.

Immunofluorescence analysis A technique which makes use of antibodies labelled with a fluorescent dye for detecting cell/tissue antigens or other molecules. The fluorescence can be detected using a fluorescence microscope.

Immunogen Any substance that can induce an adaptive immune response on injection and which can react with products of the immune response. All immunogens are antigens but not all antigens are immunogens.

Immunoglobulin All serum antibodies including IgG, IgM, IgA, IgE, and IgD. Membrane-bound immunoglobulin serves as the B cell receptor for antigen.

Immunoglobulin domains A characteristic feature of proteins of the immunoglobulin superfamily. An Ig domain has about 110 amino acid residues and includes two layers of antiparallel β-pleated sheets held together by hydrophobic interactions and a disulphide bond. There are two main types of Ig domains: C domains and V domains.

Immunoglobulin superfamily A family of proteins having domains homologous to those seen in antibody molecules and which include CD2, CD3, CD4, CD8, TCR, class I and class II MHC molecules, and ICAM, besides others.

Immunoprecipitation A technique which makes use of a specific antibody for isolating a molecule from a complex protein mixture such as a cell lysate, and then precipitating the complex with an antiglobulin, or by coupling the primary antibody to an insoluble particle or a bead (agarose).

Immunostimulating complexes (ISCOMs) These consist of antigen held within a lipid matrix. They allow antigen to be taken up into the cytoplasm of APCs after fusion of the lipid with the plasma membrane.

Immunotoxins A reagent consisting of antibody specific for an antigen on a tumour cell and which is conjugated to a cytotoxic molecule such as a toxin (ricin/diphtheria toxin). Such reagents are being investigated in treatment of cancer.

Inflammation A protective response of the innate immune system which is amplified by local adaptive immune responses. Its aim is to control infection and promote tissue repair but it can also cause tissue damage and disease.

Innate immunity The early immune response to infection which depends on mechanisms that are inborn, rapid, and which react in essentially the same way to repeated infections. It relies mainly on phagocytic cells, NK cells, cytokines, and complement.

Integrins A family of heterodimeric cell surface proteins some of which can interact with cell adhesion molecules (CAMs) on vascular endothelium and have a role in leukocyte extravasation. Others interact with extracellular matrix proteins.

Intercellular adhesion molecules (ICAMs) They are members of the Ig superfamily of proteins which function as adhesion molecules. They have a role in binding of lymphocytes (and other leukocytes) to certain cells, such as APCs and endothelial cells and are ligands for integrins.

Interdigitating dendritic cells Dendritic cells found in T cell areas of the lymph nodes and spleen, and which are rich in class II MHC molecules.

Interferons A group of proteins which can induce an antiviral state in cells. They include IFN-α and IFN-β which can be induced in most cell types, and IFN-γ produced by T lymphocytes and also NK cells. Interferon-γ has a more important role in regulation of immune responses.

Interleukins (ILs) A designation for cytokines secreted by various leukocytes that have effects on other leukocytes.

Intron A DNA segment that is transcribed but removed by splicing and so is not present in mRNA.

Isograft Tissue transplanted between two genetically identical individuals. The term syngraft is also used.

Isotypes These are immunoglobulin classes and include IgM, IgG, IgA, IgE, and IgD. Each has a distinct heavy chain constant region. Effector functions of antibodies vary with the isotype.

J (joining) chain A polypeptide produced in mature B cells that is involved in polymerization of IgM and IgA molecules.

Joining (J) gene segments These are immunoglobulin and T cell receptor gene segments which lie 5′ to the C genes. A V and D gene segment must rearrange to a J gene segment during lymphocyte development. The recombined V-D-J DNA codes for the V region of the antigen receptor.

Junctional diversity This is the diversity generated in antigen receptors on lymphocytes due to addition or removal of nucleotide sequences at junctions during joining of V, D, and J gene segments.

Kappa (κ) chain One of the two types (isotypes) of immunoglobulin light chains, the other being the lambda (λ) isotype.

Kinins Plasma proteins that work as an enzymatic cascade and whose activation is triggered during inflammatory reactions. Vasoactive mediators (e.g., bradykinin) are released which serve to increase vascular permeability and smooth muscle contraction.

Knockout mice Mice in which a functional gene (in embryonic stem cells) is replaced with a defective copy of the gene. These mice lacking functional genes are valuable for studying roles of various molecules in the immune system such as cell surface receptors and cytokines.

Kupffer cell A type of macrophage fixed in liver.

Langerhans cells Immature dendritic cells found in skin which function to capture and transport antigen to local lymph nodes. During migration, they transform into mature dendritic cells which are efficient antigen-presenting cells.

Large granular lymphocytes (LGLs) *See* Natural killer cells.

Lectins Proteins that bind specifically to sugars in glycoproteins and glycolipids. Some plant lectins such as ConA and PHA have a mitogenic effect.

Leukocytes All white blood cells including neutrophils, basophils, eosinophils, monocytes/macrophages, and lymphocytes.

Leukaemia Uncontrolled proliferation of bone marrow precursors of blood cells. Most leukaemias are lymphocytic (derived from T or B cell precursors) or myelogenous (derived from myeloid precursor cells). Leukaemic cells are found in the bone marrow and in blood circulation.

Leukotrienes Lipid inflammatory mediators derived from arachidonic acid and produced by many cell types, such as mast cells and basophils. They promote chemotaxis and increase vascular permeability.

Ligand A term used generally for any molecule that is recognized and bound by a receptor.

Lipopolysaccharide (LPS) A component also called endotoxin present in Gram-negative bacterial cell walls. It has inflammatory and mitogenic effects.

Lymph node A secondary lymphoid organ in which adaptive immune responses are initiated. Here, mature naïve B and T lymphocytes respond to antigen—either free or associated with dendritic cells, respectively.

Lymphoma A malignant tumour of lymphocytes which arises in lymphoid tissues and is generally not found in blood.

Lymphotoxin (TNF-β) A T cell cytokine which, like TNF-α, has a proinflammatory role and may be toxic for some tumour cells.

Lysosomes Membrane-bound cytoplasmic granules containing hydrolytic enzymes. On fusion with phagosomes, they help to degrade proteins which have been phagocytosed from the extracellular space.

Lysozyme An enzyme present in tears, saliva, and phagocytic cell granules which has antibacterial effects. It digests peptidoglycans present in cell walls of bacteria.

Major histocompatibility complex A cluster of genes on human chromosome 6 that encodes the highly polymorphic class I and class II MHC molecules. Other proteins (non-polymorphic) encoded in this region include cytokines, complement proteins, and molecules of the antigen processing machinery.

Mannose-binding lectin (MBL) An acute-phase protein and a member of the collectin family. It binds to mannose residues on microbial surfaces and functions as an opsonin. It activates the lectin pathway of complement activation.

Mast cells Cells which reside in connective tissue adjacent to blood vessels. They are rich in granules and resemble blood basophils. Both cell types express high affinity FcεRs and have a role in immediate hypersensitivity reactions.

Membrane attack complex A complex formed from terminal components of the complement cascade which forms a pore in the target cell membrane.

Mitogen A substance that non-specifically causes proliferation in lymphocytes.

Molecular mimicry A proposed mechanism of autoimmunity which is triggered due to similarity of epitopes on microbes and self-molecules.

Monoclonal antibodies Homogenous antibodies that are reactive with a specific epitope. They are produced by a B cell hybridoma (a cell line that is the product of fusion of a specific antibody producing B cell from spleen and a myeloma cell).

Monocyte A type of circulating WBC having a bean-shaped nucleus and which is a precursor of tissue macrophages.

Mucosa-associated lymphoid tissue (MALT) Lymphoid tissue that is associated with mucosal surfaces. The main sites of MALT include the gut-associated lymphoid tissue (GALT) and bronchial-associated lymphoid tissue (BALT).

Multiple myeloma A cancer of the plasma cell which secretes monoclonal Ig called a myeloma protein. Sometimes there is excess synthesis of light chains over heavy chains. These are excreted in the urine of patients and are called Bence Jones proteins.

Murine Pertaining to mice.

Naïve lymphocytes These are mature lymphocytes that have not encountered a specific antigen. On stimulation by antigens, they differentiate into effector cells, such as antibody-secreting B cells or effector T cells.

Natural killer (NK) cells Cells of the lymphoid lineage also known as large granular lymphocytes (LGLs), a name derived from the morphologic appearance of NK cells which contain cytoplasmic granules. They do not express the antigen-specific receptors of T and B lymphocytes. Their granules contain granzymes which enter target cells, such as virally-infected cells through a channel created by perforin resulting in apoptotic death of the target cell. These cells also target certain types of tumour cells. Natural killer cells also mediate ADCC.

Necrosis A form of cell death due to chemical or physical injury as compared to apoptosis which is a programmed form of cell death. Unlike apoptosis, necrosis leaves considerable cellular debris which can trigger inflammatory reactions.

Negative selection A mechanism for maintenance of self-tolerance as it prevents development of autoreactive lymphocytes. T and B lymphocytes undergo apoptotic cell death when they recognize self-antigens in thymus and bone marrow, respectively.

Neutralization A mechanism by which antibodies block or inhibit the effect of a virus.

Neutropenia A reduction in neutrophil count in blood.

Neutrophil A polymorphonuclear granulocyte with phagocytic activity. It is the first cell type to migrate from blood vessels to inflammatory sites.

Nude mice Mice with a homozygous gene defect designated *nu/nu*. They lack a thymus and have no mature T cells. They are so called as they lack fur.

Oncofoetal antigens Proteins expressed on certain types of cancer cells and foetal cells but not in adult tissue. They include carcinoembryonic antigen (CEA) and α-fetoprotein (AFP). Their measurement in serum is used to follow progression of tumour growth in patients.

Opsonins These are substances that coat antigens/pathogens enabling them to be ingested more rapidly by phagocytes. Antibody and C3b (a complement split product) opsonize pathogens which are readily phagocytosed and destroyed by neutrophils and macrophages.

Opsonization The process of coating of antigens/pathogens with opsonins (antibody and C3b) is called opsonization.

Opportunistic pathogens Microbes that cause disease only in immunocompromised individuals such as AIDS patients.

Organ-specific autoimmune disease These are autoimmune diseases that target a particular organ, such as the thyroid (Graves' disease) or pancreas (insulin-dependent diabetes mellitus, type I).

Paracortex The T cell area of a lymph node that lies between the cortex (that has primarily B cells) and medulla.

Pathogen-associated molecular patterns (PAMPs) Molecules such as lipopolysaccharide (LPS), lipoteichoic acid (LTA), and peptidoglycans besides others expressed by pathogens but not by host tissues.

Pattern-recognition receptors (PRRs) Receptors of innate immunity found on many cell types that recognize molecular structures on microbes (PAMPs) and promote innate immune responses against them. Some examples include toll-like receptors and mannose receptor.

Perforin A protein present in granules of NK cells and cytotoxic T cells which, like complement component C9, polymerizes to form a channel with a hydrophilic core in the membrane of a target cell leading to its death.

Periarteriolar lymphoid sheath (PALS) The lymphoid tissue in the spleen that surrounds small arterioles and which forms part of the white pulp. It contains mainly CD1$^+$ T lymphocytes.

Peripheral lymphoid organs These are sites where adaptive immune responses are initiated, for example, lymph nodes and spleen.

Peripheral tolerance This is immunological tolerance to self-antigens acquired by mature lymphocytes outside primary lymphoid organs in peripheral tissues.

Peyer's patches These are part of gut-associated lymphoid tissue (GALT). They are clusters of lymphocytes which form distinct lymphoid nodules along the small intestine, particularly the ileum. Cells present here comprise mostly B cells with smaller numbers of T cells and APCs.

Phagocytosis The uptake and destruction of microbial cells and other particulate matter by phagocytic cells, namely, macrophages and neutrophils. The material is ingested into a vesicle called a phagosome which fuses with lysosomes to form a phagolysosome.

Pluripotent stem cell *See* Haematopoietic stem cell

Polyclonal This refers to many different clones or the product of many clones such as a polyclonal antiserum.

Polyclonal activators These are agents that activate many clones of lymphocytes regardless of their specificity as opposed to specific activation of lymphocytes by antigens. Phytohaemagglutinin (PHA), a plant lectin, is a polyclonal activator for T cells.

Poly-Ig receptor A receptor at the basolateral membrane of epithelia. It binds specifically to dimeric IgA and pentameric IgM, and transports them across the cell to epithelial surfaces (a process called transcytosis).

Polymorphism This refers to variability in structure or sequence and is due to existence of multiple alleles (variants) at a particular genetic locus. The genes that encode the major histocompatibility molecules are the most polymorphic genes in the human genome. An individual may carry two different alleles of a particular gene which are inherited from the two parents.

Polymorphonuclear (PMN) leukocytes These are WBCs having a segmented multilobed nucleus and cytoplasmic granules containing hydrolytic enzymes. There are three types including mostly neutrophils (commonly referred to as PMNs; their granules stain with neutral dyes), eosinophils (have granules that stain with eosin), and basophils (have granules that stain with basic dyes).

Positive selection This is selection in the thymus of those developing T cells carrying receptors that recognize self-MHC molecules. These cells are prevented from undergoing apoptosis while all remaining developing T cells die.

Pre-B cell A B cell developmental stage in which heavy chain genes have rearranged but not light chain genes.

Primary immune response This is the adaptive immune response activated in response to initial exposure to an antigen.

Primary immunodeficiency Deficiency in some component of the innate or adaptive immune system due to a genetic defect and which increases susceptibility to infection.

Pro-B cell The earliest cell of the B lymphocyte lineage in the bone marrow which has not yet completed heavy chain gene rearrangement and does not produce Ig.

Programmed cell death A form of cell death by apoptosis triggered from inside the dying cell and characterized by DNA fragmentation. In contrast to cell death by necrosis, an inflammatory response does not occur. It has an important role in maintaining appropriate lymphocyte numbers.

Properdin A component of the alternative pathway of complement activation that functions as a positive regulator of complement activation. It helps to stabilize $C\overline{3bBb}$.

Prostaglandins Lipid mediators derived from arachidonic acid in many cell types which both facilitate and inhibit immunological responses.

Pro-T cell An early cell that enters the thymic cortex from the bone marrow and is double-negative (CD4⁻ CD8⁻) and also lacks CD3.

Proteasome A multi-subunit proteolytic complex found in the cytoplasm of most cells and which has a role in degradation of cytosolic proteins. Peptides presented by class I MHC molecules are generated in the proteasome.

Protein A A component of cell membrane of *Staphylococcus aureus* which can bind to the Fc region of IgG, thereby blocking effector functions of an antibody. It has practical importance in IgG purification.

Pyrogen A substance that induces fever.

Receptor-mediated endocytosis The internalization of a molecule into endosomes after binding to cell surface receptors (such as antigens bound to B cell receptors).

Recombination activating genes These include RAG-1 and RAG-2 genes which encode the proteins RAG-1 and RAG-2. These proteins have a critical role in receptor gene rearrangement events in lymphocytes.

Respiratory burst The increase in oxygen consumption that occurs in phagocytic cells following activation by foreign matter.

Rheumatoid factors Autoantibodies usually of the IgM class directed against Fc portion of IgG and which are present in serum of rheumatoid arthritis patients.

Scavenger receptors Cell surface receptors expressed on phagocytic cells, such as macrophages, which mediate phagocytosis of any matter (cells/molecules) that needs to be cleared from the body, such as apoptotic cells.

Secondary immune response The immune response activated when primed lymphocytes are re-exposed to the same antigen that initially stimulated them. It is rapid and more intense than the primary immune response.

Secretory component A product of proteolytic cleavage of the poly-Ig receptor which remains associated with secretory IgA molecules. It protects IgA from proteolytic enzymes in the intestinal lumen.

Selectin A family of cell surface adhesion molecules of leukocytes and endothelial cells. They are carbohydrate-binding proteins that allow leukocytes to adhere to endothelial cells.

Self-tolerance This refers to lack of responsiveness of the adaptive immune system to self-antigens. Its failure may lead to autoimmune disease.

Seroconversion The appearance of detectable antibodies in the serum during the course of a microbial infection.

Severe combined immunodeficiency (SCID) Severe immunodeficiency disorders affecting T lymphocytes and which may extend to B cells and also NK cells. Several different genetic defects result in SCID in which both humoral and cell-mediated immunity is affected.

Somatic hypermutation The increased rate of point mutations in the V region genes during B cell response to antigens and which generates variant antibodies some with higher affinity for antigen.

Somatic recombination A process occurring in developing B and T lymphocytes in which a limited set of inherited (germline) DNA sequences, which are separated from each other, are brought together to form complete genes encoding the variable regions of antigen receptors. During this process, there is enzymatic deletion of intervening sequences followed by ligation.

Superantigen An antigen (e.g., staphylococcal enterotoxin) that binds to all T cells in an individual that express a particular set of Vβ TCR genes. Superantigens activate a large number of T cells unlike conventional antigens.

Syngeneic The term denotes genetic identity. Monozygotic twins and inbred strains of mice are syngeneic.

Systemic A term that relates to or affects the body as a whole.

T cells A subset of lymphocytes that matures in the thymus and which is central to development of a cell-mediated immune response. They express antigen receptors (TCRs) of which the more common αβ TCR recognizes short peptide fragments associated with MHC molecules displayed on the cell surface. There are two major subsets which differ functionally, including cytotoxic T cells (Tc) and T helper cells (TH).

T cell receptor (TCR) The heterodimeric T cell antigen receptor which exists in two forms, consisting of α and β chains or γ and δ chains. The αβ TCR is the more common of the two.

TH1 cells A CD4$^+$ T cell subset whose main function is to activate macrophages. Cells in this subset secrete a distinct set of cytokines including IL-2, TNF-β and IFN-γ. They are also known as inflammatory CD4$^+$ T cells.

TH2 cells A CD4$^+$ T cell subset which secretes a distinct set of cytokines including IL-4, IL-5, IL-10, and IL-13. These cells are primarily involved in class-switching to IgE in B cells, and in eosinophil activation.

TH3 cells These are cells involved in the mucosal immune response to orally-presented antigen. They are characterized by production of TGF-β.

Thymocyte Immature T lymphocyte which undergoes development in the thymus.

Thymus-dependent (TD) antigens These are antigens that require both T helper cells and B cells to induce an antibody response.

Thymus-independent (TI) antigens These are antigens that can induce an antibody response independent of T cell help.

Tissue typing Determination of MHC alleles of an individual which is required for matching allograft donors and recipients.

Tolerance A state of immunological unresponsiveness of the adaptive immune system to antigens.

Toll-like receptors (TLRs) Cell surface receptors of innate immunity that recognize molecular patterns on pathogens.

Toxoid A modified toxin that is no longer harmful but retains its immunogenicity.

TR1 cells Regulatory T cells that secrete IL-10 and suppress T cell responses.

Transcytosis The process of transport of molecules such as IgA across intestinal epithelial cells.

Transgenic mouse A mouse in which one or more new genes have been introduced. They are important in immunological research for functional studies on cytokines, cell surface molecules, such as receptors on immune cells, and intracellular molecules that mediate signal transduction, besides others.

Transplantation The process of grafting of organs/tissues/cells from one individual to another, or from one site to another in the same individual.

T regulatory (Treg) cell A CD4$^+$ CD25$^+$ T cell which suppresses functioning of lymphocytes. It has a role in maintenance of tolerance to self-antigens.

Tumour-infiltrating lymphocytes (TILs) These are mononuclear cells infiltrating the tumour mass. They are obtained from cancer patients by biopsy, expanded in vitro with IL-2, and then re-infused into patients (adoptive transfer). TILs are mostly CD8$^+$ T cells specific for the tumour. This is an approach to cancer immunotherapy.

Tumour necrosis factor (TNF)-α A cytokine produced by activated macrophages which has a proinflammatory effect. TNF-β or lymphotoxin is a related cytokine produced by T cells and which has similar effects.

Vaccination Immunization against infectious disease by injecting a vaccine which consists of a killed or attenuated form of the pathogen, or parts derived from it.

V (D) J recombination The process in which V, D, and J gene segments join to generate antigen-specific receptors of T and B cells. The joining of gene segments into a V (D) J unit is mediated by an enzyme complex with various activities called V (D) J recombinase.

Variable (V) gene segments Multiple gene segments in the germline that rearrange together with D(diversity) and J (joining) gene segments to encode the V region of B and T cell receptors.

Vasoactive amines Products such as histamine released by basophils and mast cells which act on local endothelium and smooth muscle.

Wheal and flare Local swelling (oedema) and redness produced in an allergic individual when small amounts of allergen are injected into the dermis. These effects are induced by histamine released from mast cells.

Xenogeneic Interspecies genetic differences.

Xenograft A graft between individuals of different species.

Further Reading

TEXTBOOKS FOR GENERAL READING

- Coico, R., G. Sunshine, and E. Benjamini (2003), *Immunology: A Short Course*, 5th Edn, Wiley, Hoboken, New Jersey.
- Delves, P.J., S.J. Martin, D.R. Burton, and I.M. Roitt (2006), *Roitt's Essential Immunology*, 11th Edn, Blackwell Publishing, Oxford, UK.
- Elgert, K.D. (2009), *Immunology Understanding the Immune System*, 2nd Edn, John Wiley & Sons, Inc., New Jersey.
- Janeway, C.A. Jr, P. Travers, M. Walport, and M.J. Shlomchik (2005), *Immunobiology: The Immune System in Health and Disease*, 6th Edn, Garland Science, Taylor & Francis Group, New York and London.
- Kenneth, M., P. Travers, and M. Walport (2008), *Janeway's Immunobiology*, 7th Edn, Garland Science, Taylor & Francis Group, New York and London.
- Kindt, T.J., R.A. Goldsby, and B.A. Osborne (2007), *Kuby Immunology*, 6th Edn, W.H. Freeman and Company, New York.
- Roitt, I., J. Brostoff, and D. Male (2001), *Immunology*, 6th Edn, Mosby (an imprint of Elsevier Science Ltd), St. Louis, USA.

SELECTED ARTICLES ON SPECIFIC SUBJECTS

The articles listed below provide additional and advanced information for readers interested in a particular subject.

Chapter 1

Burnet, F.M. (1959), *The Clonal Selection Theory of Acquired Immunity*, Cambridge University Press, London.

Burnet, F.M. (1957), 'A modification of Jerne's theory of antibody production using the concept of clonal selection', *Australian Journal of Science*, Vol. 20, Australian National Research Council, Australia, pp. 67–69.

Delves, P.J. and I.M. Roitt (2000), 'The immune system—first of two parts', *The New England Journal of Medicine*, Vol. 343, Massachusetts Medical Society, USA, pp. 37–49.

Jerne, N.K. (1955), 'The natural selection theory of antibody formation', *Proceedings of the National Academy of Sciences*, Vol. 41, National Academy of Sciences, USA, pp. 849–857.

Rajewsky, K. (1996), 'Clonal selection and learning in the antibody system', *Nature*, Vol. 381, Nature Publishing Group, UK, pp. 751–758.

Chapter 2

Aderem, A. and D.M. Underhill (1999), 'Mechanisms of phagocytosis in macrophages', *Annual Review of Immunology*, Vol. 17, Annual Reviews, California, USA, pp. 593–623.

Blanchard, C.M. and E. Rothenberg (2009), 'Biology of the eosinophil', *Advances in Immunology*, Vol. 101, Elsevier Science, Netherlands, pp. 81–121.

Gabay, C. and I. Kushner (1999), 'Acute-phase proteins and other systemic responses to inflammation', *The New England Journal of Medicine*, Vol. 340, Massachusetts Medical Society, USA, pp. 448–454.

Ganz, T. (2003), 'Defensins: Antimicrobial peptides of innate immunity', *Nature Reviews Immunology*, Vol. 3, Nature Publishing Group, USA, pp. 710–720.

Nathan, C. (2006), 'Neutrophils and immunity: Challenges and opportunities', *Nature Reviews Immunology*, Vol. 6, Nature Publishing Group, USA, pp. 173–182.

Ramachandra, L., D. Simmons, and C.V. Harding (2009), 'MHC molecules and microbial antigen processing in phagosomes', *Current Opinion in Immunology*, Vol. 21, No. 1, Elsevier Science, Netherlands, pp. 98–104.

Shaw, M.H., T. Reimer, Y. Kim, and G. Nuñez (2008), 'NOD-like receptors (NLRs): Bona fide intracellular microbial sensors', *Current Opinion in Immunology*, Vol. 20, No. 4, Elsevier Science, Netherlands, pp. 377–382.

Takeda, K. and S. Akira (2005), 'Toll-like receptors in innate immunity', *International Immunology*, Vol. 17, Oxford University Press, UK, pp. 1–14.

Trinchieri, G. (2003), 'Interleukin-12 and the regulation of innate resistance and adaptive immunity', *Nature Reviews Immunology*, Vol. 3, Nature Publishing Group, USA, pp.133–146.

Turner, M.W. (2003), 'The role of mannose-binding lectin in health and disease', *Molecular Immunology*, Vol. 40, Elsevier Science, Netherlands, pp. 423–429.

Chapter 3

Banchereau, J. and R.M. Steinman (1998), 'Dendritic cells and the control of immunity', *Nature*, Vol. 392, Nature Publishing Group, UK, pp. 245–252.

Born, W.K., C.L. Reardon, and R.L. O' Brien (2006), 'The function of γδ T cells in innate immunity', *Current Opinion in Immunology*, Vol. 18, Elsevier Science, Netherlands, pp. 31–38.

Butcher, E. and L.J. Picker (1996), 'Lymphocyte homing and homeostasis', *Science*, Vol. 272, American Association for the Advancement of Science (AAAS), USA, pp. 60–67.

Erwig, Lars-P. and P.M. Henson (2007), 'Immunological consequences of apoptotic cell phagocytosis', *The American Journal of Pathology*, Vol. 171, American Society for Investigative Pathology, USA, pp. 2–8.

Osborne, B.A. (1996), 'Apoptosis and the maintenance of homeostasis in the immune system', *Current Opinion in Immunology*, Vol. 8, Elsevier Science, Netherlands, pp. 245–254.

LaRosa, D.F. and J.S. Orange (2008), Lymphocytes. *Journal of Allergy and Clinical Immunology*, Vol. 121, Elsevier Science, Netherlands, pp. S364–S369.

Chapter 4

Alkan, S.S. (2004), 'Monoclonal antibodies: The story of a discovery that revolutionized science and medicine', *Nature Reviews Immunology*, Vol. 4, Nature Publishing Group, USA, pp. 153–156.

Davies, D.R., E.A. Padlan, and S. Sheriff (1990), 'Antibody–Antigen complexes', *Annual Review of Biochemistry*, Vol. 59, Annual Reviews, California, USA, pp. 439–473.

Groner, B., C. Hartmann, and W. Wels (2004), 'Therapeutic antibodies', *Current Molecular Medicine*, Vol. 4, Bentham Science Publishers Ltd, USA, pp. 539–547.

Hudson, P.J. and C. Souriau (2003), 'Engineered antibodies', *Nature Medicine*, Vol. 9, Nature Publishing Group, USA, pp. 129–134.

Kabat, E.A. (1978), 'The structural basis of antibody complementarity', *Advances in Protein Chemistry*, Vol. 32, Elsevier Science, Netherlands, pp. 1–75.

Presta, L.G. (2008), Molecular engineering and design of therapeutic antibodies', *Current Opinion in Immunology*, Vol. 20, No. 4, Elsevier Science, Netherlands, pp. 460–470.

Spiegelberg, H.L. (1974), 'Biological activities of immunoglobulins of different classes and subclasses', *Advances in Immunology*, Vol. 19, Elsevier Science, Netherlands, pp. 259–294.

Chapter 5

Ackerman, A.L. and P. Cresswell (2004), 'Cellular mechanisms governing cross-presentation of exogenous antigens', *Nature Immunology*, Vol. 5, Nature Publishing Group, USA, pp. 678–684.

Brigl, M. and M.B. Brenner (2004), 'CD1: Antigen presentation and T cell function', *Annual Review of Immunology*, Vol. 22, Annual Reviews, California, USA, pp. 817–890.

Germain, R.N. and D.H. Margulies (1993), 'The biochemistry and cell biology of antigen processing and presentation', *Annual Review of Immunology*, Vol. 11, Annual Reviews, California, USA, pp. 403–450.

Jensen, P.E.(2007), 'Recent advances in antigen processing and presentation', *Nature Immunology*, Vol. 8, Nature Publishing Group, USA, pp. 1041–1048.

Nepom, G.T. (1995), 'Class II antigens and disease susceptibility', *Annual Review of Medicine*, Vol. 46, Annual Reviews, California, USA, pp. 17–25.

Sugita, M., M. Cernadas, and M.B. Brenner (2004), 'New insights into pathways for CD1-mediated antigen presentation', *Current Opinion in Immunology*, Vol. 16, Elsevier Science, Netherlands, pp. 90–95.

Chapter 6

Dreyer, W.J. and J.C. Bennett (1965), 'The molecular basis of antibody formation: A paradox', *Proceedings of the National Academy of Sciences*, Vol. 54, National Academy of Sciences, USA, pp. 864–869.

Gellert, M. (2002), 'V(D)J recombination: RAG proteins, repair factors, and regulation', *Annual Review of Biochemistry*, Vol. 71, Annual Reviews, California, USA, pp. 101–132.

Matsuda, F. and T. Honjo (1996), 'Organization of the human immunoglobulin heavy-chain locus', *Advances in Immunology*, Vol. 62, Elsevier Science, Netherlands, pp. 1–29.

Tonegawa, S. (1983), 'Somatic generation of antibody diversity', *Nature*, Vol. 302, Nature Publishing Group, UK, pp. 575–581.

Chapter 7

Arai, K., F. Lee, A. Miyajima, S. Miyatake, N. Arai, and T. Yokota (1990), 'Cytokines: Coordinators of immune and inflammatory responses', *Annual Review of Biochemistry*, Vol. 59, Annual Reviews, California, USA, pp. 783–836.

Borish, L.C. and J.W. Steinke (2003), 'Cytokines and chemokines', *Journal of Allergy and Clinical Immunology*, Vol. 111, Elsevier Science, Netherlands, pp. S460–S475.

Fischer, A., S. Hacein-Bey, and M. Cavazzana-Calvo (2002), 'Gene therapy of severe combined immunodeficiencies', *Nature Reviews Immunology*, Vol. 2, Nature Publishing Group, USA, pp. 615–621.

Leon, L.R. (2002), 'Cytokine regulation of fever: Studies using gene knockout mice', *Journal of Applied Physiology*, Vol. 92, The American Physiological Society, USA, pp. 2648–2655.

Chapter 8

Blackman, M., J. Kappler, and P. Marrack, (1990), 'The role of the T cell receptor in positive and negative selection of developing T cells', *Science*, Vol. 248, American Association for the Advancement of Science (AAAS), USA, pp. 1335–1341.

Davis, D.M. and M.L. Dustin, (2004), 'What is the importance of the immunological synapse?' *Trends in Immunology*, Vol. 25, Elsevier Science, Netherlands, pp. 323–327.

Herman, A.J., J.W. Kappler, P. Marrack, and A.M. Pullen (1991), 'Superantigens: Mechanism of T-cell stimulation and role in immune responses', *Annual Review of Immunology*, Vol. 9, Annual Reviews, California, USA, pp. 745–772.

Krogsgaard, M. and M.M. Davis (2005), 'How T cells "see" antigen', *Nature Immunology*, Vol. 6, Nature Publishing Group, USA, pp. 239–245.

Smith-Garvin, J.E., G. A. Koretzky, and M.S. Jordan (2009), 'T cell activation', *Annual Review of Immunology*, Vol. 27, Annual Reviews, California, USA, pp. 591–619.

Starr, T.K., S.C. Jameson, and K.A. Hogquist (2003), 'Positive and negative selection of T cells', *Annual Review of Immunology*, Vol. 21, Annual Reviews, California, USA, pp. 139–176.

Chapter 9

Celada, A. and C. Nathan (1994), 'Macrophage activation revisited', *Immunology Today*, Vol. 15, Elsevier Science, Netherlands, pp. 100–102.

Murphy, K.M. and S.L. Reiner (2002), 'The lineage decisions of helper T cells', *Nature Reviews Immunology*, Vol. 2, Nature Publishing Group, USA, pp. 933–944.

Russell, J.H. and T.J. Ley (2002), 'Lymphocyte-mediated cytotoxicity', *Annual Review of Immunology*, Vol. 20, Annual Reviews, California, USA, pp. 323–370.

von Andrian, U.H. and C.R. Mackay (2000), 'T-cell function and migration', *The New England Journal of Medicine*, Vol. 343, Massachusetts Medical Society, USA, pp. 1020–1034.

Yokoyama, W.M., S. Kim, and A.R. French (2004), 'The dynamic life of natural killer cells', *Annual Review of Immunology*, Vol. 22, Annual Reviews, California, USA, pp. 405–429.

Chapter 10

Mond, J.J., A. Lees, and C.M. Snapper (1995), 'T cell-independent antigens type 2', *Annual Review of Immunology*, Vol. 13, Annual Reviews, California, USA, pp. 655–692.

DeFranco, A.L. (2000), 'B cell activation', *Immunological Reviews*, Vol. 176, Wiley InterScience, USA, pp. 5–9.

Fearon, D.T. and M.C. Carroll (2000), 'Regulation of B lymphocyte responses to foreign and self-antigens by the CD19/CD21 complex', *Annual Review of Immunology*, Vol. 18, Annual Reviews, California, USA, pp. 393–422.

LeBien, T.W. and T.F. Tedder (2008), 'B lymphocytes: How they develop and function', *Blood*, Vol. 112, American Society of Hematology, USA, pp. 1570–1580.

MacLennan, I.C.M. (1994), 'Germinal centers', *Annual Review of Immunology*, Vol. 12, Annual Reviews, California, USA, pp. 117 139.

Chapter 11

Burton, D.R. and J.M. Woof (1992), 'Human antibody effector function', *Advances in Immunology*, Vol. 51, Elsevier Science, Netherlands, pp. 1–84.

Carroll, M.C. (1998), 'The role of complement and complement receptors in induction and regulation of immunity', *Annual Review of Immunology*, Vol. 16, Annual Reviews, California, USA, pp. 545–568.

Carroll, M.C. (2004), 'The complement system in regulation of adaptive immunity', *Nature Immunology*, Vol. 5, Nature Publishing Group, USA, pp. 981–986.

Ravetch, J.V. and S. Bolland (2001), 'IgG Fc receptors', *Annual Review of Immunology*, Vol. 19, Annual Reviews, California, USA, pp. 275–290.

Tolnay, M. and G.C. Tsokos (1998), 'Complement receptor 2 in the regulation of the immune response', *Clinical Immunology and Immunopathology*, Vol. 88, Academic Press, USA, pp. 123–132.

Chapter 12

Casares, S. and T.L. Richie (2009), 'Immune evasion by malaria parasites: A challenge for vaccine development', *Current Opinion in Immunology*, Elsevier Science, Netherlands, Vol. 21, No. 3, pp. 321–330.

Flynn, J.L. and J. Chan (2001), 'Immunology of tuberculosis', *Annual Review of Immunology*, Vol. 19, Annual Reviews, California, USA, pp. 93–129.

Grau, G.E. and R.L. Modlin (1991), 'Immune mechanisms in bacterial and parasitic diseases: Protective immunity versus pathology', *Current Opinion in Immunology*, Vol. 3, Elsevier Science, Netherlands, pp. 480–485.

Moorthy, V.S., M.F. Good, and A.V.S. Hill (2004), 'Malaria vaccine developments', *The Lancet*, Vol. 363, Elsevier Science, Netherlands, pp. 150–156.

Portnoy, D.A. (2005), 'Manipulation of innate immunity by bacterial pathogens', *Current Opinion in Immunology*, Vol. 17, Elsevier Science, Netherlands, pp. 25–28.

Schofield, L. and G.E. Grau (2005), 'Immunological processes in malaria pathogenesis', *Nature Reviews Immunology*, Vol. 5, Nature Publishing Group, USA, pp. 722–735.

Chapter 13

Ada, G. (2001), 'Vaccines and vaccination', *The New England Journal of Medicine*, Vol. 345, Massachusetts Medical Society, USA, pp. 1042–1053.

Casadevall, A. (2002), 'Passive antibody administration (immediate immunity) as a specific defense against biological weapons', *Emerging Infectious Diseases*, Vol. 8, Centers for Disease Control and Prevention, USA, pp. 833–841.

Casadevall, A., E. Dadachova, and L.A. Pirofski (2004), 'Passive antibody therapy for infectious diseases', *Nature Reviews Microbiology*, Vol. 2, Nature Publishing Group, USA, pp. 695–703.

Donnelly, J.J., B. Wahren, and M.A. Liu (2005), 'DNA vaccines: Progress and challenges', *Journal of Immunology*, Vol. 175, American Association of Immunologists, Maryland, USA, pp. 633–639.

Law, M. and L. Hangartner (2008), 'Antibodies against viruses: Passive and active immunization', *Current Opinion in Immunology*, Vol. 20, No. 4, Elsevier Science, Netherlands, pp. 486–492.

Poland, G. and A. Barrett (2009), 'The old and the new: Successful vaccines of the 20th century and approaches to making vaccines for the important diseases of the 21st century', *Current Opinion in Immunology*, Vol. 21, No. 3, Elsevier Science, Netherlands, pp. 305–307.

Zinkernagel, R.M. (2003), 'On natural and artificial vaccinations', *Annual Review of Immunology*, Vol. 21, Annual Reviews, California, USA, pp. 515–546.

Chapter 14

Busse, W.W. and R.F. Lemanske (2000), 'Asthma', *The New England Journal of Medicine*, Vol. 344, Massachusetts Medical Society, USA, pp. 350–362.

Cohn, L., J.A. Elias, and G.I. Chupp (2004), 'Asthma: Mechanisms of disease persistence and progression', *Annual Review of Immunology*, Vol. 22, Annual Reviews, California, USA, pp. 789–815.

Kay, A.B. (2000), 'Overview of "Allergy and allergic diseases: With a view to the future"', *British Medical Bulletin*, Vol. 56, Oxford University Press, UK, pp. 843–864.

Naparstek, Y. and P.H. Piotz (1993), 'The role of autoantibodies in autoimmune disease', *Annual Review of Immunology*, Vol. 11, Annual Reviews, California, USA, pp. 79–104.

Ravetch, J.V. and S. Bolland (2001), 'IgG Fc receptors', *Annual Review of Immunology*, Vol. 19, Annual Reviews, California, USA, pp. 275–290.

Takeda, K. and E.W. Gelfand (2009), 'Mouse models of allergic diseases', *Current Opinion in Immunology*, Vol. 21, No. 6, Elsevier Science, Netherlands, pp. 660–665.

Theofilopoulos, A.N. and F.J. Dixon (1979), 'The biology and detection of immune complexes', *Advances in Immunology*, Vol. 28, Elsevier Science, Netherlands, pp. 89–220.

Chapter 15

Bluestone, J.A. and V. Kuchroo (2009), 'Autoimmunity', *Current Opinion in Immunology*, Vol. 21, No. 6, Elsevier Science, Netherlands, pp. 579–581.

Feldmann, M. and L. Steinman (2005), 'Design of effective immunotherapy for human autoimmunity', *Nature*, Vol. 435, Nature Publishing Group, UK, pp. 612–619.

Feldmann, M. (2009), 'Translating molecular insights in autoimmunity into effective therapy', *Annual Review of Immunology*, Vol. 27, Annual Reviews, California, USA, pp.1–27.

Kamradt, T. and N.A. Mitchison (2001), 'Tolerance and autoimmunity', *The New England Journal of Medicine*, Vol. 344, Massachusetts Medical Society, USA, pp. 655–664.

Kyewski, B. and L. Klein (2006), 'A central role for central tolerance', *Annual Review of Immunology*, Vol. 24, Annual Reviews, California, USA, pp. 571–606.

Mills, K.H.G. (2004), 'Regulatory T-cells: Friend or foe in immunity to infection?' *Nature Reviews Immunology*, Vol. 4, Nature Publishing Group, USA, pp. 841–855.

Randolph, D.A. and C.G. Fathman (2006), 'CD4$^+$ CD25$^+$ regulatory T cells and their therapeutic potential', *Annual Review of Medicine*, Vol. 57, Annual Reviews, California, USA, pp. 381–402.

Sakaguchi, S. (2004), 'Naturally arising CD4$^+$ regulatory T cells for immunologic self-tolerance and negative control of immune responses', *Annual Review of Immunology*, Vol. 22, Annual Reviews, California, USA, pp. 531–562.

Wucherpfennig, K.W. (2001), 'Mechanisms for the induction of autoimmunity by infectious agents', *Journal of Clinical Investigation*, Vol. 108, American Society for Clinical Investigation, USA, pp. 1097–1104.

Chapter 16

Bonilla, F.A. and R.S. Geha (2006), 'Update on primary immunodeficiency diseases', *Journal of Allergy and Clinical Immunology*, Vol. 117, Elsevier Science, Netherlands, pp. S435–S441.

Buckley, R.H. (2000), 'Primary immunodeficiency diseases due to defects in lymphocytes', *The New England Journal of Medicine*, Vol. 343, Massachusetts Medical Society, USA, pp. 1313–1324.

Douek, D.C., M . Roederer, and R.A. Koup (2009), 'Emerging concepts in the immunopathogenesis of AIDS', *Annual Review of Medicine*, Vol. 60, Annual Reviews, California, USA, pp.471–484.

Duffalo, M.L. and W.J. Christopher (2003), 'Enfuvirtide: A novel agent for the treatment of HIV-1 infection', *The Annals of Pharmacotherapy*, Vol. 37, Harvey Whitney Books Company, USA, pp. 1448–1456.

Letvin, N.L. (2005), 'Progress toward an HIV vaccine', *Annual Review of Medicine*, Vol. 56, Annual Reviews, California, USA, pp. 213–223.

Letvin, N.L. (2006), 'Progress and obstacles in the development of an AIDS vaccine', *Nature Reviews Immunology*, Vol. 6, Nature Publishing Group, USA, pp. 930–939.

Stevenson, M. (2003), 'HIV-1 pathogenesis', *Nature Medicine*, Vol. 9, Nature Publishing Group, USA, pp. 853–860.

Chapter 17

Halloran, P.F. (2004), 'Immunosuppressive drugs for kidney transplantation', *The New England Journal of Medicine*, Vol. 351, Massachusetts Medical Society, USA, pp. 2715–2729.

Kaufman, C.L., B.A. Gaines, and S.T. Iidstad (1995), 'Xenotransplantation', *Annual Review of Immunology*, Vol. 13, Annual Reviews, California, USA, pp. 339–367.

Ricordi, C. and T.B. Strom (2004), 'Clinical islet transplantation: Advances and immunological challenges', *Nature Reviews Immunology*, Vol. 4, Nature Publishing Group, USA, pp. 259–268.

Trowsdale, J. and A.G. Betz (2006), 'Mother's little helpers: Mechanisms of maternal-fetal tolerance', *Nature Immunology*, Vol. 7, Nature Publishing Group, USA, pp. 241–246.

Waldmann, H. and S. Cobbold (2004), 'Exploiting tolerance processes in transplantation', *Science*, Vol. 305, American Association for the Advancement of Science (AAAS), USA, pp. 209–212.

Walsh, P.T., D.K. Taylor, and I.A. Turka (2004), 'Tregs and transplantation tolerance', *Journal of Clinical Investigation*, Vol. 114, American Society for Clinical Investigation, USA, pp. 1398–1403.

Chapter 18

Allison, J.P., A.A. Hurwitz, and D.R. Leach (1995), 'Manipulation of costimulatory signals to enhance antitumor T-cell responses', *Current Opinion in Immunology*, Vol. 7, Elsevier Science, Netherlands, pp. 682–686.

Banchereau, J. and A.K. Palucka (2005), 'Dendritic cells as therapeutic vaccines against cancer', *Nature Reviews Immunology*, Vol. 5, Nature Publishing Group, USA, pp. 296–306.

Dougan, M. and G. Dranoff (2009), 'Immune therapy for cancer', *Annual Review of Immunology*, Vol. 27, Annual Reviews, California, USA, pp. 83–117.

Jansen, K.U. and A.R. Shaw (2004), 'Human papilloma virus vaccines and prevention of cervical cancer', *Annual Review of Medicine*, Vol. 55, Annual Reviews, California, USA, pp. 319–331.

Rabinovich, G.A., D. Gabrilovich, and E.M. Sotomayor (2007), 'Immunosuppressive strategies that are mediated by tumor cells', *Annual Review of Immunology*, Vol. 25, Annual Reviews, California, USA, pp. 267–296.

Rosenberg, S.A. (2001), 'Progress in human tumor immunology and immunotherapy', *Nature*, Vol. 411, Nature Publishing Group, UK, pp. 380–384.

Rosenberg, S.A. and M.E. Dudley (2009), 'Adoptive cell therapy for the treatment of patients with metastatic melanoma', *Current Opinion in Immunology*, Vol. 21, No. 2, Elsevier Science, Netherlands, pp. 233–240.

Srivastava, P.K. (2000), 'Immunotherapy of human cancer: Lessons from mice', *Nature Immunology*, Vol. 1, Nature Publishing Group, USA, pp. 363–366.

von Mehren, M., G.P. Adams, and L.M. Weiner (2003), Monoclonal antibody therapy for cancer', *Annual Review of Medicine*, Vol. 54, Annual Reviews, California, USA, pp. 343–369.

Index

anergy due to lack of 164, 278
by B7 molecules 161
Costimulatory B7 molecules 68, 70,
    161, 196, 278, 295, 344, 349
  B7-1 (CD80) 161, 162
  B7-2 (CD86) 161, 162
  blocking of 169, 332
  in T cell activation 161
  response to 163
CR1 41, 209, 217
  on red blood cells 209
Cross-match test 327, 328
Cross-presentation 164, 342, 343
Cross-reactivity 80, 81, 287, 292
CSFs 12, 149
CTL-precursors, CTL-P 64, 182
CTLA-4-Ig 332
  in donor-specific graft tolerance
    332, 333
CXCR4 147, 311
  as co-receptor for HIV 147, 311
Cyclosporin 166, 294, 321, 331
Cytokine antagonists 149
  Anti-cytokine antibodies 150
  IL-1Ra 149
  soluble TNF receptors 149
Cytokine network 139
Cytokine receptors 146
  signal transduction of 147
Cytokines 20, 136, 349
  and hormones 139
  antagonism in 138
  anti-cytokine antibodies 150
  autocrine action of 138
  cascade induction of 138
  endocrine action of 138
  features of 138
  in therapy 148, 149, 295, 305,
    307, 347, 348, 349
  major families 137
  major roles of 140
  of adaptive immunity 143
  of innate immunity 141
  overproduction of 148
  paracrine action of 138
  pleiotropy in 138
  redundancy of 138, 147
  sources of 137
  synergism of 138

Cytotoxic (type II) hypersensitivity
  267
  haemolytic disease of the newborn
    268
  mismatched blood transfusion
    269
Cytotoxic T cells 64. *See also*
  Cytotoxic T lymphocytes
Cytotoxic T lymphocyte antigen-4
  (CTLA-4) 169, 184, 278, 279,
  281, 286, 332
  in T cell anergy 278, 286
Cytotoxic T lymphocytes 18, 19,
  105, 175, 284, 325, 340, 349
  activation of 164
  antiviral effects 225
  apoptosis by 175, 183, 184
  class I MHC restriction of 105,
    160
  effector functions of 181
  in anti-tumour immunity 175
  in graft rejection 325
  steps in killing by 182

Daudi tumour cells 105
Decay accelerating factor
  (DAF) 217
Defensins 30, 49
Degranulation 13, 36, 264, 267
Delayed-type IV hypersensitivity
  50, 174, 179, 272, 289, 325
  chronic inflammation in 274
  control of 180
  damage in 179, 185
  stages in 272
  stimuli for 272
  TH1 cells in 272
Dendritic cells 14, 38, 68, 69, 111,
  166, 176, 324, 342, 343, 349
  as vaccines 343
  cross-presentation 111, 164
  IDCs 69
  TH1 cell activation by 176
Density gradient centrifugation 378
  separation of mononuclear cells
    by 378
Desensitization 267
Diapedesis 47
DiGeorge syndrome (DGS) 57,
  299, 302

Direct allorecognition 324
Donor-specific tolerance 332, 333
Double electroimmunodiffusion
  370
Double immunodiffusion 368
Double-positive thymocytes 157,
  159
DTH response 289, 325

Enfuvirtide 317
Enzyme-linked immunosorbent assay
  (ELISA) 96, 150, 291, 356, 358
  advantages of 360
  applications 362
  competitive assay 359
  enzymes in 358
  indirect assay 359
  sandwich assay 358
Eosinophil cationic protein (ECP)
  235
Eosinophil chemotactic factor-A
  (ECF-A) 235
Eosinophils 13, 36, 181, 209, 235,
  265, 266
  ADCC by 181
  FcεRI on 209
  interleukin-5 activation of 181
  in degree against helminths 209,
    235
Epitopes 20, 74, 78, 79, 80
  B cell epitopes 78
  immunodominant epitopes 80
  T cell epitopes 79
Epstein–Barr virus (EBV) 223, 227,
  241
  immunosuppression by 227, 241
Experimental autoimmune
  encephalomyelitis 283, 290
  model for 290, 296
Extravasation 46

Fab region 20, 82, 205
  mediated functions 205, 206
Factor B 217
Factor H 217
Factor I 217
Farmer's lung 271
Fas 38, 183, 280
Fas/Fas L pathway 169, 183
Fas ligand (Fas L) 182, 183, 280